Aebi et al. (Eds.) **The Aging Spine**

AF691388

M. Aebi · R. Gunzburg · M. Szpalski
(Editors)

The Aging Spine

With 53 Figures and 40 Tables

Springer

Prof. Dr. Max Aebi
Institute
for Evaluative Research
in Orthopaedic Surgery
University of Bern
Stauffacherstr. 78
3014 Bern
Switzerland

Dr. Robert Gunzburg
Centenary Clinic
Harmoniestraat 68
2018 Antwerp
Belgium

Prof. Dr. Marek Szpalski
Iris South
Teaching Hospitals
142 Rue Marconi
1190 Brussels
Belgium

ISBN 3-540-24408-5 Springer Berlin Heidelberg New York

Also published as Volume 12, Supplement 2, October 2003
of the European Spine Journal
ISSN 0940-6719

Library of Congress Control Number: 2005920460

This work is subject to copyright. All rights are reserved, whether the whole or part of the material is concerned, specifically the rights of translation, reprinting, reuse of illustrations, recitation, broadcasting, reproduction on microfilms or in any other way, and storage in data banks. Duplication of this publication or parts thereof is permitted only under the provisions of the German Copyright Law of September 9, 1965, in its current version, and permission for use must always be obtained from Springer-Verlag. Violations are liable for prosecution under the German Copyright Law.

Springer is a part of Springer Science+Business Media

springeronline.com

© Springer-Verlag Berlin Heidelberg 2005
Printed in Germany

The use of general descriptive names, registered names, trademarks, etc. in this publications does not imply, even in the absence of a specific statement, that such names are exempt from the relevant protective laws and regulations and therefore free for general use. Product liability: The publishers cannot guarantee the accuracy of any information about the application of operative techniques and medications contained in this book. In every individual case the user must check such information by consulting the relevant literature.

Cover design: e STUDIO CALAMAR, Pau/Girona
Typesetting: ROTABENE, Rothenburg o. d. T.
Printing and bookbinding: Mercedes-Druck, Berlin

Printed on acid-free paper 24/3150/PF 5 4 3 2 1 0

Dieter Grob

Foreword

D. Grob (✉)
Spine Unit, Schulthess Clinic,
Lengghalde 2, 8008 Zurich, Switzerland
Tel.: +41-1-3857436,
Fax: +41-1-3857576,
e-mail: Grob@schulthess-clinic.ch

It is the merit of the "Bone and Joint Decade" to draw our attention with increased intensity to the problem of the changes related to aging of our musculoskeletal system and the associated socioeconomic implications. In view of the increasing age of the worldwide population the impact seems to be tremendous. I congratulate the editors of the present supplement of the *European Spine Journal* in picking up this interesting topic and engaging opinion leaders to contribute their knowledge in this supplement. The various contributions cover some of the important problems, which are included in the vast specter of aging spine: osteoporosis, spinal stenosis, and tumors of the spine.

As an introduction Benoist presents an overview of the important issue of the natural history of the aging spine, pointing out that this process is a progressive change ending up in a collapse of the system, a fact that has implications for treatment strategy and disease management.

Some of the authors (Bono et al., Gunzburg et al., Ferguson et al.) emphasize with their contributions the basic changes and problems that develop during a lifetime in our spine. These statements illustrate the complexity of the construction and the variety of responses that the spine is able to provide.

The medical treatment of the aging spine deserves special attention in view of the generally reduced health situation of the involved patients. The important role of the biphosphonates in the treatment, and perhaps even more so in the prevention, of osteoporosis is emphasized by Fleisch.

Any successful surgical treatment starts with accurate diagnostic procedures. The profound knowledge and sophisticated diagnostic techniques of the complex pathoanatomical changes in the spine including the involvement of the neural structures (contribution by Dvorak) often go beyond the capacity of a spine surgeon. Teamwork and adequate communication is mandatory.

The variety of different surgical approaches and options demonstrates the difficulty of the surgery in the aging spine. Reduced general health status, life expectancy with or without cancer that occurs more frequently in elderly persons, and expectations of the patient and social environment are nonsurgical factors to be considered before embarking upon surgery. The extent of intervention and the clinical significance of chronic deformities are questions to be answered at the stage of planning surgery, and finally fragile soft tissue, osteoporosis, and reduced stability are problems to overcome during surgery.

Although the important question of economy is addressed in the contribution by Johnell, we are all aware that the topic of treating elderly patients with all the modern facilities carries the ultimate risk of financial collapse of most health care systems in developed countries. If not at present, we as treating physicians will be confronted in the near future with unpleasant questions. Where does the money come from to treat this increasing section of population? Do we have to decide for selection of our patients due to shortage of money? If yes, for which criteria? Fortunately in most countries these items have not yet become reality, but in a future supplement with the same topic, these questions will be of importance. It remains to be decided who should give the answers. Healthy persons will not put enough energy into the effort due to the lack of actuality for themselves and the involved patient will hardly be in the position to contribute in an objective way. Physicians who stand in front of their patients cannot take over the role of judges in mandating a "yes" or "no" to treatment. Therefore, who else remains than politicians? As opinion leaders of our society it will be their rote to establish rules fair enough to guarantee basic medical treatment. However, these rules must be based on facts and figures for decision making. It is here that the medical professional world must come into action. We must put all our efforts to establish data for the rationale of our activities. The literature search by Lippuner demonstrates the relatively high standard of evaluation of conservative treatment of the osteoporotic spine. Albeit not numerous, there *are* prospective and comparative studies on the efficacy of different treatment modalities. Due to the different nature of medical treatment, this kind of research is found less frequently in the surgical field. For example, vertebroplasty and kyphoplasty as relatively new and apparently successful procedures in the context of the aging spine is explained and described in the contributions by Boszezyk et al. and Mehbod et al. However, a literature research on these techniques does not reveal a single comparative study until today. A serious lack of background knowledge for decision making in view of the giant number of osteoporotic fractures that occur every day worldwide. An important task is waiting for all of us in evaluating carefully existing and new treatment modalities to provide a reasonable base for decision making.

The aging spine will be an ever-present issue in the life of a physician taking care of the different pathologies of the spine. The present supplement of the *European Spine Journal* will help to better understand the nature of the different changes in the spine of the elderly. It contributes to enabling us to diagnose and to treat this complex problem in an appropriate way.

Contents

Marek Szpalski
Robert Gunzburg
Christian Mélot
Max Aebi

The aging of the population: a growing concern for spine care in the twenty-first century

M. Szpalski (✉)
Dept. of Orthopaedics, HIS/C.H.
Molière Longchamp, Brussels, Belgium
e-mail: mszp@win.be

R. Gunzburg
Dept. of Orthopaedics, Euwfeestkliniek,
Antwerp, Belgium

C. Mélot
Intensive Care Unit,
Erasme University Hospital,
Brussels, Belgium

M. Aebi
Maurice E. Müller Institute
for Evaluative Research and Documentation
in Orthopaedic Surgery,
Murtenstr. 35, 3008 Bern, Switzerland

The aging of the population in industrialized countries appears to be a non-reversible phenomenon. Increase in life expectancy, due in great part to the improvement of healthcare, combined with a drastic decrease in birth rates has led to this situation. The world demographic situation has shifted from a pattern of high birth rates and high mortality rates to one of low birth rates and delayed mortality [10].

In Europe, the proportion of subjects over 65 was 10.8% in 1950, 14% in 1970, 19.1% in 1995 and is projected by some sources at 30.1% in 2025 and 42.2% in 2050. The proportion of subjects over 75 has grown from 2.7% in 1950 to 5.2% in 1995 and is projected at 9.1% in 2025 and 14.6% in 2050 [8]. These figures take into account the whole of Europe. When only western Europe is considered, the proportion of individuals over 65 should be over 50% in 2050. These numbers are just a little smaller in the USA [15]. However, this trend is not limited to industrialized countries: the developing countries' share of the world's population above 65 is projected to increase from 59% to 71% [10].

The global consequences of this distortion of the age pyramid on healthcare development, access and costs are huge [4]. In the USA approximately 80% of all individuals over 65 have at least one chronic condition and 50% have two [11]. Approximately 59% of US residents over 65 are affected by osteoarthritis, which is the main cause for disability [3].

All this results in a highly differential distribution of healthcare-related costs heavily skewed towards the elderly population. Costs per capita increase gradually up to the 55–64 age group, and then the costs increase very rapidly and explode after over 85 years [7]. Aging alone will generate an increase of more than 30% in real per capita healthcare expenditures by 2030 [7].

Back and neck pain are among the most frequently encountered complaints of older people and the nature of the spine renders those problems highly complex to investigate and to treat.

The spine is a very specific anatomic and functional unit. Whereas degenerative knee or hip changes visible at imaging will not be found in all elderly subjects, nearly all will exhibit spinal degeneration. Furthermore, few patients with severe gonarthrosis or coxarthrosis are symptom free, while many subjects with severe spinal degenerative images will be asymptomatic. This was demonstrated by several high-quality studies [1]. Furthermore, the existence of degenerative images on MRI of symptom-free subjects does not predict in any way subsequent complaints after several years [2]. The relation between the aging and degenerative process and the possible complaints is far from clear. This in itself may begin to explain why the results of spinal surgery are so mitigated when compared to the excellent outcomes of knee or hip arthroplasty.

Degeneration of the spinal structures induces interactive alterations at many levels: bone, disc, facet joints, ligaments. Some of these degenerative lesions can be responsible for damage to the neural elements by leading to disc herniation or spinal stenosis.

The multifactorial nature of spinal degeneration, the complexity and multiplicity of treatment, the rapid evolution of medical technology and the nature of patient's expectations in terms of quality of life have also resulted in an escalation in costs.

The aging of the western population has increased the number of severely osteoporotic subjects, mostly women. Recent studies have shown that osteoporotic vertebral fractures are associated with an increased risk of mortality [9] and a decreased quality of life. The prevalence in those fractures is around 39% in subjects over 65 years [12, 13].

It does not appear that the preventive treatment strategies applied for the past few decades have yielded very spectacular results in the decrease of the frequency of osteoporotic fractures, including vertebral osteoporotic compression fractures. Whereas those lesions were long considered as a burden with which patients should live, there now exist percutaneous treatment modalities which not only deal with the problem of pain but also aim at restoring the compressed vertebral body height, thus trying to avoid possible kyphotic deformities. [14]. However, those treatments are expensive.

New techniques are also being developed to fight the degenerative process itself. Among those is gene therapy, which could provide a long-term delivery of molecules to retard or even revert degenerative processes. It appears to be a very promising path but, once again, a highly expensive one.

With the delayed mortality and better control of life-threatening chronic diseases the new challenge of care in elderly patients will focus on the preservation or restoration of the quality of life. That will be exactly what elderly subjects will demand and they will expect us to use all the available technological armamentum. New instruments measures such as the Disability Adjusted Life Years (DALY) or Quality Adjusted Life Years (QALY) [6,11] are being developed to try to evaluate this growing variable, and future spinal studies should look at the possibility of integrating them in the outcome assessment, even though they are not without shortcomings.

Although in cost-utility studies DALY's and QALY's have proved their usefulness to fill the gap between population health and medical care, inevitable differences will be seen in the outputs of their estimates of disease burden. Any different outputs may imply different priorities. One study that compared DALY's and QALY's as health-related quality of life weights, but keeping life-expectancy calculations identical, found differences in disease-burden estimates as well as changes in rank order of five common medical conditions [5]. These discrepancies remain a problem to be solved in the near future to allow payers a correct evaluation of the risk and the related costs before defining priorities in an era of budget constraints.

Spinal care in the elderly is, in fact, a very active and fascinating field that combines many different disciplines, from biomechanics to cell engineering. However, the major problem is that of resources. As the expenditures of health care continue to escalade worldwide, competition between medical disciplines for a share of the limited resources will also escalate.

Compared to treatment for cardiovascular disorders or diabetes, the treatment of spinal conditions does not appear to be such a priority. This is even more acute if one considers that there is a large consensus in the handling of these systemic chronic disorders based on high-quality scientific studies, whereas that consensus is painfully lacking in spinal disorders, for which high-quality studies are rare. The comparison with the treatment outcomes in hip and knee degeneration casts further doubt on the appropriateness of treatment of degenerative spine conditions.

The payers in the healthcare field such as governments and insurance companies will not follow forever the increase in costs of treatments for which physicians are not able to demonstrate efficacy through undisputable studies. It is we, spine specialists, who must make sure that we will have resources to meet the growing number of patients who will confront us in the coming years. Not only do we have to fulfill the expectations of the patients but also those of the financing parties. The only way to do this will be to demonstrate, much better than at present, that our expensive treatments are truly efficient and notably improve the duration and quality life of our older patients.

References

1. Boden SD, Davis DO, Dina TS, Patronas NJ, Wiesel SW (1990) Abnormal magnetic-resonance scans of the lumbar spine in asymptomatic subjects. A prospective investigation. Bone Joint Surg 72-A:403–408
2. Borenstein DG, O'Mara JW Jr, Boden SD et al (2001) The value of magnetic resonance imaging of the lumbar spine to predict low-back pain in asymptomatic subjects: a seven-year follow-up study. J Bone Joint Surg Am 83-A: 1306–11
3. CDC (2002) Prevalence of self reported arthritis or chronic joint symptoms among adults – US 2002. MMWR 51:948–950
4. CDC (2003) Public health and aging: trends in aging US and worldwide. MMWR 52:101–106

5. Gold MR, Muennig P (2002) Measure-dependent variation in burden of disease estimates: implication for policy. Med Care 40:260–266
6. Gold MR, Stevenson D, Fryback DG (2002) HALYS and QUALYS and DALYS, oh my: similarities and differences in summary measures of population health. Annu Rev Public Health 23:115–134
7. Hogan S, Hogan S (2002) How will the ageing of the population affect health care needs and costs in the foreseeable future? Commission on the Future of Health Care in Canada. Discussion Paper No. 25, October 2002
8. IIASA/ERD Database (2002) International Institute for Applied Systems Analysis, Laxenburg, Austria. www.iiasa.ac.at/Research/ERD/. Cited 27 April 2003
9. Kado DM, Browner WS, Palermo L et al (1999) Vertebral fractures and mortality in older women: a prospective study. Study of Osteporotic Fractures Research Group. Arch Int Med 159: 1215–1220
10. Kinsella K, Velkoff V (2001) US Census Bureau. An aging world. Washington DC. US Govt Printing Office, series P95/01–1
11. Mullahy J (2001) Live long, live well: quantifying the health of heterogeneous populations. Health Econ 10: 429–440
12. National Center for Chronic Disease Prevention and Health Promotion, CDC (1999) Chronic diseases notes and reports: special focus. Healthy Aging 12:3
13. Pluijm SM, Tromp AM, Smit JH, Deeg DJ, Lips P (2000) Consequences of vertebral deformities in older men and women. J Bone Miner Res 15:1564–1572
14. Szpalski M, Gunzburg R (eds) (2003) Vertebral osteoporotic compression fractures. Lippincott Williams & Wilkins, Philadelphia
15. United States Census 2000 (2000) US Census bureau, US Department of Commerce. www.census.gov. Cited 27 April 2003

Michel Benoist

Natural history of the aging spine

Abstract The unrelenting changes associated with aging progressively affects all structures of the spinal units. The degenerative process starts early during the first decade of life at the disc level. Discal degeneration is associated with biochemical changes followed by macroscopic alterations including tears and fissures, which may lead to discal herniation, the main cause of radiculopathy in the young adult. Moreover, nociceptive nerve fibers have been demonstrated in degenerated discs. They may be a source of nociception and of pure low-back pain. Facet joint changes are usually secondary to discal degeneration. They include subluxation, cartilage alteration and osteophytosis. Facet hypertrophy and laxity, associated with discal degeneration, and enlargement of the ligamentum flavum progressively create narrowing of the spinal canal as well as degenerative instabilities such as spondylolisthesis and scoliosis, which are the main causes of neurogenic claudication and radiculopathy in old persons. Vertebral bodies are the static elements of the spinal unit. With advancing age, osteoporosis weakens the bony structures and facilitates bone remodeling and rotatory deformities. Finally, aging of bone, discs, facets, ligaments, and muscles may ultimately lead to rotatory scoliosis, destabilization, and rupture of equilibrium.

Keywords Lumbar disc degeneration · Age-related intervertebral changes · Disc herniation · Stenosis · Low-back pain

M. Benoist (✉)
Orthopaedic Surgery Unit,
Department of Rheumatology,
Hôpital Beaujon, 100 Bd du Gal Leclerc,
92110 Clichy, France
Tel.: +33-1-45533712,
Fax: +33-1-40871713,
e-mail: deuxmice@aol.com

Introduction

The spine is a flexible, multisegmented column. Its functional role is to maintain stability and an upright position as well as providing mobility at the segmental level. The spine comprises a static, changeless element – the vertebral bodies – and an elastic mobile component – the three-joint complex, consisting of the intervertebral disc and the two posterior facet joints. Spine motion, stability, equilibrium and control of position are assumed by the antagonist action of the powerful flexor and extensor muscle groups.

Changes with age and pathology may modify these structures. Because most of the research work has been devoted to the lumbar spine, the present paper will focus more on this anatomic section of the spine. Aging is a normal process to all structures. As emphasized by Garfin and Herkowitz [9], aging is difficult to distinguish from degenerative changes.

As for every human tissue, aging of the structural components of the spine may be related to a predetermined genetic cell viability and/or to exposure of the tissues to heavy mechanical forces throughout life. Whatever the mechanism, aging will lead to degenerative changes starting with subtle biochemical alterations followed by micro-structural and finally gross structural changes of the spinal unit. The degenerative cycle with its biomechanical consequences will progressively modify the functional anatomy and generate various pain syndromes, rupture of equilibrium and destabilization. Aging affects all the structures of the spine. This review paper will summarize the age-related changes of the various components of the spinal unit in turn.

Aging of the disc

Historically, primary degeneration of the disc has been considered as the initiating event resulting in secondary deterioration of the facets, ligaments, and muscles. The physiology of the intervertebral disc has been recently reviewed [22]. Disc degeneration depends on the failure of cellular activity in charge of producing a normal extracellular matrix. In a normal disc, an equilibrium exists between synthesis and degradation of the matrix elements. Loss of agrecan and water, and a decrease in collagen organization and of disc height are the early modifications of aging. Simultaneously, the level of the proteases responsible for the enzymatic degradation process increases [2, 3, 19]. Rupture of metabolic equilibrium observed with aging is multifactorial, including a predisposed genetic condition [22].

Decrease of nutrient supply of the cells is an important factor in degeneration. The main nutritional pathway of the disc is through the adjacent vertebral end plate [11]. This source of nutrition is at great risk in the aging disc, as the permeability of the end plate diminishes with advancing age. Detrimental effect of a decreased blood supply from the end plate results in tissue breakdown, starting in the nucleus. A recent study has shown that this process may begin early in the second decade of life [3]. The cells of the disc are also sensitive to mechanical signals. They can be negatively affected by mechanical stresses and stimulation undergone throughout life, leading to qualitative and quantitative modulation of the matrix proteinases [17].

The biochemical modifications of the disc are further accompanied by gross anatomic and macroscopic changes. As aging progresses, the boundary between nucleus and annulus becomes less distinct, with an increase of collagen in the nucleus. Concentric fissuring and radial tears may appear during the third and fourth decade of life, with substantial individual differences: elderly persons may have a "young disc" and vice versa. Significant temporospatial variations of histologic and macroscopic changes are also observed across levels and regions [23]. The degenerative changes can be assessed by magnetic resonance imaging, exhibiting variations of signal intensity, with the ultimate loss of disc height and dark signal. Loss of disc height and turgor, secondary to the biochemical events summarized above, have serious biomechanical consequences. Loss of proteoglycans and fluid, lowering of osmotic pressure in the nucleus, as well as alterations of the collagen network, affect the normal absorption and dissipation of the movement forces applied to the normal viscoelastic hydrostatic nature of the disc. Mechanical changes with age and degeneration have been recently reviewed [15]. Loss of mechanical competence and flattening of the disc may generate diffuse bulging, which should be differentiated from focal bulges or true herniations, characterized macroscopically by nuclear migration though radial fissures of the disc. Disc herniation requires pre-existing age-related degenerative changes.

Aging and degeneration are also associated with dramatic changes in vascularization and innervation of the disc. A normal healthy adult disc is avascular, apart from a sparse vascularization at the outer part of the annulus. Presence of blood vessels has been demonstrated in degenerated disc and in herniated disc tissue [2, 10]. Penetration of blood vessels through the rim lesions is promoted by angiogenesis factors [10]. Inflammatory cells as well as macrophages also invade the degenerated disc. Production of various cytokines and proteases by endogenous cells and by the vascular cells of the invading vessels has been demonstrated [18]. Metallo-proteinase (MMP) expression increases with advancing age, thus enhancing the destruction pathway. Correlation of MMPs expression with formation of tears and clefts in the annulus has also been demonstrated [23]. Presence of nerve fibers relevant to pain sensation is a prerequisite for a tissue to be a source of nociception. Recent studies [2, 8, 10, 20] have shown the presence of nociceptive nerve fibers in the annulus and inner nucleus of the degenerated disc. Most nerve fibers identified by immunochemistry accompany blood vessels, suggesting a role of vaso-regulation. However, another set of neural elements, independent of vessels, expressing substance P and with a morphology of nociceptive nerve terminals, have been found in the nucleus of painful discs assessed by provocative discography of patients undergoing anterior surgery for chronic low-back pain [8]. This important finding strongly suggests the role of the nerve terminals of the degenerated disc in the pathogenesis of low-back pain. An innervated disc may be a source of nociception.

In summary, among the various structures of the spine, the process of aging starts in the disc at the beginning of the second decade of life. Failure of the normal cell activity depends on various factors: genetic, nutritional, and mechanical. The initial event is not yet known, but when the degenerative cycle is started, a complex interplay of biochemical and biomechanical factors create a vicious circle, which progressively enhances the degenerative process.

Aging of the facet joint

The facet joints are the only synovial joints in the spine, with hyaline cartilage overlying subchondral bone. Kirkaldy Willis and associates have described a three-joint complex consisting of the intervertebral disc and the two facet joints [7, 9]. In a normal healthy spinal unit, the disc is the major anterior load-bearing structure. The facet joints provide a posterior load-bearing helper, stabilizing the motion segment in flexion and extension and also protecting the disc from excessive torsion. It is generally accepted that degenerative changes of the facets are secondary to disc degeneration. The mechanical consequences of disc degeneration, including loss of disc height and segmental instability, increase the loads on the facets and generate subluxation of the joints and cartilage alteration. Osteoarthritis of the facets is similar to that of all diarthrodial joints. Cartilage degradation leads to the formation of focal and then diffuse erosions, with sclerosis of the subchondral bone. Facet hypertrophy, apophyseal malalignment and osteophyte formation may narrow the spinal canal and create central and/or lateral stenosis. Destabilization of the three-joint complex may lead to degenerative instabilities including degenerative spondylolisthesis and scoliosis. Nociceptive nerve endings have been identified in the facet joint capsules. They may therefore be a source of back pain. Whether so-called "facet joint syndrome" really exists and, if so, how frequently it occurs, remain matters of controversy.

Aging of ligaments and muscles

The ligaments surrounding the spine contribute to its intrinsic stability. They also restrain extremes of motion in all planes. All spinal ligaments have a high content of collagen. Ligamentum flavum, which connects the adjacent vertebrae, has a high percentage of elastin, allowing contraction during flexion and elongation during extension [7]. As part of the aging process, ligaments undergo chemical and macroscopic changes, including a rise in the concentration of elastin, which decreases tensile properties, resulting in ligamentous weakening affecting the stabilizing function of the longitudinal ligaments [13]. In addition, aging and degeneration of the ligamentum flavum leads to increased thickness and bulging, often disclosed during surgery for spinal stenosis.

The trunk and pelvic muscles have a major role in both motion and stabilization of the spine. Their support stabilizes and modifies the load in static and dynamic situations. The postural dorsal and abdominal muscles are constantly active in a standing position. During motion, equilibrium and control of stability are assumed by the antagonist action of the extensor dorsal muscles and abdominal flexors [21]. Aging may induce a "degenerative myopathy," compromising the spine dynamics, and generating a rupture of equilibrium. Camptocormia is a good example of destabilization caused by muscular insufficiency. In this case, fat tissue invades the erector spinal muscles inducing a kyphotic attitude of the lumbar spine.

Aging of the bone

As mentioned earlier, the bony components constitute the static elements of the spinal unit. However, aging of the bony structures, especially osteoporosis, may induce major changes. They will be discussed extensively in the following papers. They include sclerosis and bone formation of the end plate, lowering of the blood supply of the disc, and formation of osteophytes, which increase the surface area of load bearing [7]. Moreover, repetitive torsional loads may progressively induce bone remodeling and rotatory deformities of the posterior elements. These changes generate stenosis and slipping at the intervertebral level, as described by Farfan [6].

Clinical relevance

The biochemical, macroscopic, and biomechanical changes observed with aging, briefly summarized above, are indistinguishable from those disclosed in degenerated discs of symptomatic subjects. Pain and disability are the clinical expression of the aging spine. The role of the clinician is to relate the degenerative changes identified on the imaging studies to the clinical symptoms, and to differentiate the organic pain syndromes from non-organic spinal pain. It is recognized that a degenerated spinal unit may be totally asymptomatic and remain so.

Discal degeneration is generally considered as the primary source of pure low-back pain. The nociceptive nerve fibers identified in the inner annulus and nucleus can be sensitized by the cytokines and neuropeptides present in the degenerated disc [8, 18, 20]. However, other sources of nociception can be found in the spinal unit, including muscles, ligaments, and facets. Nociception coming from these various tissues is difficult to distinguish from discogenic pain. Moreover, recognition of the "painful disc" in multilevel disc degeneration is not easy. Therefore, the exact source of the pain is difficult to identify and often remains unknown at the individual level [4]. It should be remembered that pain is not only nociception: sensitization of the central nervous system may be responsible for chronic low-back pain [5]. Radicular pain is the other possible expression of the degenerative spine. A direct link between discal degeneration and radiculopathy was established many years ago by Mixter and Barr. The biologic activity of the herniated discal tissue has been identified more recently [12]. Discal herniation is not the only cause of nerve root irritation in the degenerated spinal unit. With advancing age, bony overgrowth in the central canal or the lateral recess can compress the nerve roots. The bony encroachment may or may not produce symptoms. The natural history of lumbar spinal stenosis has been recently reviewed [1]. As already mentioned, diffuse annular bulging, buckling of the ligamentum flavum, hypertrophy, and osteophytes of the facets may create midline compression and central stenosis. Lateral bony compression of the nerve root may result from subarticular entrapment, pedicular kinking or foraminal encroachment. Discal degeneration, osteoarthritis of the facets, and bony remodeling may be responsible for degenerative instabilities such as spondylolisthesis, which aggravates the midline and lateral bony compression. These bony constraints are directly related to the changes of the aging spine. Central stenosis with or without slipping is the major cause of neurogenic claudication [16].

Aging of bone, of the segmental mobile spinal unit (disc, facets), and of the muscles may also lead to degenerative rotatory scoliosis, with the possible evolution towards a progressive disorganization of the spine, destabilization, and rupture of equilibrium [13, 14]. As the population ages, stenosis and deformities are more common. As already mentioned, there are substantial differences between individuals: old persons may have a "young" spine. Many factors of degradation of the spinal unit remain unknown. The role of a genetic predisposition appears crucial, but the physical environment is also an important influential factor. Proper nutrition, adequate physical exercise and avoidance of smoking and of inappropriate physical loads are at the present time the only means of prevention at our disposal.

References

1. Benoist M (2001) The natural history of lumbar degenerative spinal stenosis. Joint Bone Spine 69:450–457
2. Bibby S, Jones DA, Lee RB, Jing YU, Urban J (2001) Biochimie. Biologie et physiologie du disque intervertébral. Rev Rhum 68:903–908
3. Boos B, Weissbach S, Rohrbach, et al (2002) Classification of age related changes in lumbar intervertebral discs. Spine 27:2631–2644
4. Carragee EJ, Tanner CM, Khurana M, et al (2000) The rates of false positive lumbar discography in select patients without low-back symptoms. Spine 25: 1373–1381
5. Deleo JA, Winkelstein BA (2002) Physiology of chronic spinal pain syndromes. Spine 27:2526–2537
6. Farfan HF (1980) The pathological anatomy of degenerative spondylolisthesis. A cadaver study. Spine 5:412–418
7. Fraser RD, Bleael JF, Moskowitz RW (1997) Spinal degeneration. Pathogenesis and medical management. In: Frymoyer JW (ed) The adult spine: principles and practice. Lippincott Raven, Philadelphia, pp 735–758
8. Freemont AJ, Peacock TE, Goupille P, et al (1997) Nerve ingrowth into diseased intervertebral disc in chronic low-back pain. Lancet 350:178–181
9. Garfin Sr, Herkowitz H (1996) Lumbar disc degeneration: normal aging or a disease process? In: Wiesel SW, Weinstein JN, Herkowitz H, Dvorak J, Bell G (eds) The lumbar spine. WB Saunders, Philadelphia, pp 458–473
10. Goupille P, Zerkak D, Lemaire V, et al (2000) Rôle des détériorations discales dans la survenue d'une lombalgie. Rev Rhum 67 [Suppl 4]:253–260
11. Holm SH (1996) Nutritional and pathophysiologic aspects of the lumbar intervertebral disc. In: Wiesel SW, Weinstein JN, Herkowitz H, Dvorak J, Bell J (eds) The lumbar spine. WB Saunders, Philadelphia, pp 285–310
12. Olmarker K, Rydevik B (2001) Disc herniation and sciatica. The basic science platform. In: Gunzburg R, Szpalski M (eds) Lumbar disc herniation. Lippincott Williams and Wilkins, Philadelphia, pp 31–41
13. Panjabi MM, Goel VK, Takata K (1982) Physiologic strains in the lumbar spine ligaments: in vitro biomechanical study. Spine 7:192–203
14. Panjabi M, Abumi K, Duranceau J (1989) Spinal stability and inter-segmental muscles forces. A biochemical model. Spine 14:194–199
15. Pope MH (2001) Disc biomechanics and herniation. In: Gunzburg R, Szpalski M (eds) Lumbar disc herniation. Lippincott Williams and Wilkins, Philadelphia, pp 3–21
16. Porter R (1996) Pathophysiology of neurogenic claudication. In: Wiesel SW, Weinstein JN, Herkowitz H, Dvorak J, Bell G (eds) The lumbar spine. WB Saunders, Philadelphia, pp 717–724
17. Rannou F, Poiraudeau S, Corvol M, Revel M (2000) Contraintes mécaniques et disque intervertébral lombaire. Rev Rhum 4:67 [Suppl]:219–224
18. Rannou F, Corvol M, Revel M, Poiraudeau S (2001) Dégénérescence discale et hernie discale: rôle des métalloprotéases et cytokines. Rev Rhum 68:913–920
19. Robert S, Caterson B, Menage J, et al (2000) Matrix metalloproteinases and agrecanase: their rôle in disorders of the human intervertebral disc. Spine 25:3005–3013
20. Roberts S, Johnson E (2000) Innervation du disque intervertebral et lombalgie discale. Rev Rhum 67 [Suppl 4]: 225–232
21. Saillant G, Lemoine J. Instabilité vertébrale et vieillissement du rachis. In: Deburge A, Benoist M, Morvan G, Guigui P (eds) Dégénérescence du rachis lombaire et lombalgies. Sauramps Médical, pp 67–81
22. Urban J (2001) The physiology of the intervertebral disc. In: Gunzburg R, Szpalski M (eds) Lumbar disc herniation. Lippincott Williams and Wilkins, Philadelphia, pp 22–31
23. Weiler C, Nerlich AG, Zipperer Y, et al (2002) Expression of major matrix metallo proteinases is associated with disc degradation and resorption. Eur Spine J 11:308–320

Christopher M. Bono
Thomas A. Einhorn

Overview of osteoporosis: pathophysiology and determinants of bone strength

C. M. Bono (✉)
Department of Orthopaedic Surgery,
Boston University Medical Center,
850 Harrison Avenue, Dowling 2 North,
Boston, MA 02118, USA
Tel.: +1-617-4146281,
Fax: +1-617-4146292,
e-mail: bonocm@prodigy.net

T. A. Einhorn
Department of Orthopaedic Surgery,
Boston University Medical Center,
720 Harrison Avenue,
Doctors Office Building Suite 808,
Boston, MA 02118, USA

Abstract Recent advances in both the pharmacological and surgical treatment of osteoporosis and vertebral compression fractures offer exciting new options for elderly patients. However, these treatments should be considered only with an indepth knowledge of osteoporosis as a metabolic disorder with complex effects on bone, its homeostatic regulation, and vertebral strength. Bone homeostasis is under the influence of both endogenous hormonal changes and external mechanical loads resulting from physical activity. These impart their effects through regulation of the relative activities of bone cells, in particular osteoblasts and osteoclasts, which control bone deposition and resorption, respectively. The strength of a vertebra is directly influenced by the amount and relative proportions of its components, with bone mineral density a useful measure of fracture risk. The purpose of this article is to discuss these issues, among others, in order to offer the reader a better understanding of the pathophysiology of osteoporosis and the determinants of bone strength as they relate to the aging skeleton.

Keywords Osteoporosis · Aging · Mechanical effects · Pathophysiology

Introduction

Decreases in bone mass are inevitable with age. The condition when bone mass drops to a critical level below which fracture risk is substantially higher is termed osteoporosis [17]. Most simply, osteoporosis arises from an imbalance of bone formation and bone resorption. However, understanding the unique characteristics of osteoporosis compared to other metabolic bone disorders requires more indepth knowledge of bone biology and specific pathophysiological mechanisms.

Bone homeostasis is under the influence of both endogenous hormonal changes and external mechanical loads resulting from physical activity [6, 12]. These impart their effects through regulation of the relative activities of bone cells, in particular osteoblasts and osteoclasts. These cells control bone deposition and resorption, respectively. The strength of bone is directly influenced by the amount and relative proportions of its components, with bone mineral density a useful measure of fracture risk [2]. This article will discuss these issues in order to offer the reader a better understanding of the pathophysiology of osteoporosis as well as the determinants of bone strength as they relate to the aging skeleton.

Architectural composition: cortical versus cancellous bone

To understand a pathological process, one must first comprehend relevant normal physiology and microanatomy. There are two contrasting types of bone in the adult human skeleton. Cortical bone is compact and dense. It is found encasing all parts of the skeleton but is most prominent in the diaphyses of long bones such as the femur. The femoral cortex is thick, forming an elliptical tube that surrounds a medullary canal containing sparse trabecular bone. In this example, the mechanical function of cortical

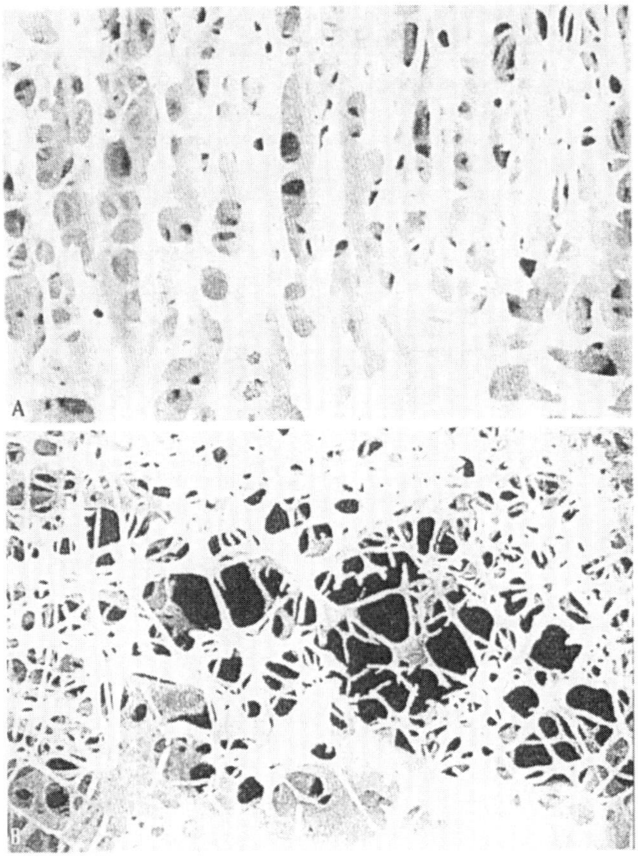

Fig. 1a, b Comparing close-up of views of normal and osteoporotic bone demonstrates a key pathological feature. Note the greater quantity of normal bone (**a**), as well as its greater interconnectivity, compared to osteoporotic bone (**b**)

bone can be best understood. The femur, a major weight-bearing bone, sustains large bending and torsional forces arising during movement. Imagine the forces while ascending a staircase. With extension of the hip and femur, vector forces in opposite directions place huge bending moments along the longitudinal axis of the femoral shaft.

The other type of bone, more abundant in the spine, is trabecular bone. Also known as cancellous bone, it can be considered as a porous interlocking scaffold of vertical and horizontal columns of bone (Fig. 1). Thus, trabecular bone is best at resisting compressive loads. The vertebral body is made up of mostly trabecular bone. In terms of the biomechanics of the spine, this is well suited to the demands of the anterior spinal column. The vertebral body and intervertebral disc sustain approximately 80% of the load during axial compression, with the remaining 20% sustained by the facet joints [21].

The structural differences between cancellous and cortical bone also have metabolic significance. In the densely packed cortical bone, nutrition is supplied by low-pressure vessels within the haversian canalicular system. Considering the amount of bone in relation to the amount of vascularity, the ratio is relatively low. In contrast, cancellous bone is much more richly vascularized by osseous vascular complexes that pass between the less densely packed trabeculae. This arrangement produces a much higher surface-to-volume ratio of bone to extracellular fluids. Therefore, cancellous bone responds more quickly to metabolic alterations and, for this reason, the vertebral bodies are more susceptible to processes that increase bone resorption, such as osteoporosis [9].

Molecular composition: mineralized versus nonmineralized components

While cortical and cancellous bone are architecturally different, they are similar at the molecular and biochemical level. Bone is composed of cells and extracellular matrix (ECM). The cells produce and control the production and removal of bone. The mechanical properties of bone are derived from the composition of the ECM as well as the geometric and architectural characteristics resulting from the way this tissue is distributed in space.

The ECM has mineralized and nonmineralized components. The nonmineralized component is known as osteoid. It is produced and secreted by osteoblasts. The mineralized component is made up of a crystalline material known as calcium hydroxyapatite. The important elements of this material are calcium and phosphate ions. The serum levels of these ions are tightly controlled by various mechanisms that influence bone metabolism and, in turn, bone mass.

Osteoid is made up of both collagenous and noncollagenous proteins. The predominant protein is type I collagen. In general, the collagenous portion of bone is responsible for its tensile strength. The greater the collagen concentration, the higher tensile and shear strength will be. Other noncollagenous proteins include osteonectin, osteopontin, and other various compounds. These noncollagenous proteins affect many of the cellular activities in bone such as the ability of bone cells to attach to the ECM.

The mineralized portion of bone determines its compressive strength. With greater concentrations of calcium, compressive strength increases. Processes that diminish the levels of either bone mineral or collagen substantially decrease the ability of bone to withstand respective loads.

Bones fail and fractures occur when ultimate stress levels are exceeded. Stress is a property defined as an internal resistance to an externally applied load. Tensile and compressive stresses are the result of loads/forces acting along the same line (Fig. 2). Tensile forces act away from each other, while compressive forces act towards each other. Shear forces act towards each other in different, but parallel, planes. Bone can fail under tension, compression, or shear. The relative amounts of mineralized and nonmineralized bone influence its behavior under various loading patterns. Bone fails more easily under shear and ten-

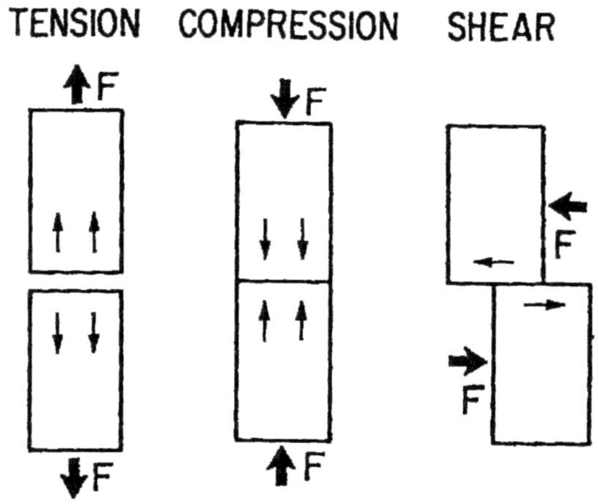

Fig. 2 The three basic types of stress that bone must endure are tension, compression, and shear. *Tension* is produced by forces acting in the same plane but away from each other. *Compression* is produced by forces acting in the same plane but towards each other. *Shear* is produced by two forces acting towards each other but in two different planes

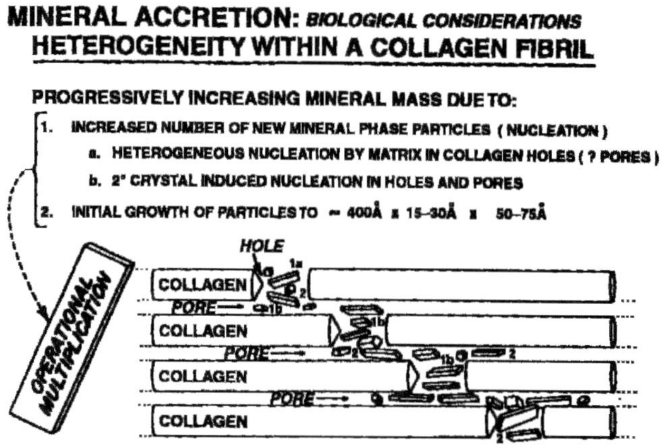

Fig. 3 Bone mineralization is initiated at sites known as *holes* and *pores*. Holes are located between the ends of juxtaposed collagen molecules. Pores are formed longitudinally between collagen molecules

sile forces, while it is strongest in compression. This is true for both cortical and trabecular bone.

These concepts can be illustrated with a simple analogy. Take, for example, a column of bricks stacked one on top of each other, but each connected to its neighbor by a strong rubber band. If one picks up the top brick, while the bottom brick is held fixed to the ground, the bricks will begin to separate, but only as far as the elasticity of the rubber bands will allow it. The rubber bands act like the long fibrils of collagen in bone. Eventually, if the column of bricks is stretched long enough, one of the rubber bands will break. It can be imagined, however, that this would not take an excessive amount of force. Now, consider placing a load on top of the column of bricks. As bricks are used in a similar manner to build a house, they can sustain great loads. One could stand on the column of bricks without fear of the bricks crushing or crumbling. The bricks act like the calcium/mineral component of bone. With this example, it can be understood that (1) the mineral component is responsible for compressive strength, (2) the collagen is responsible for tensile strength, and (3) much greater compressive loads can be endured than tensile loads before failure.

Using the same analogy, shear strength can be illustrated as well. If one were to push the top brick to the right and the bottom brick to the left, the resistance to failure would be from two sources. One would be the elastic tethering effect of the rubber bands. The other would be the friction between the two bricks. Thus shear force would be influenced by both the collagenous and mineral components of bone. In this way, one might also understand why shear strength is dramatically less than compressive strength.

Cellular control of bone mass: osteoblasts and osteoclasts

Osteoblasts are bone-forming cells. They both secrete osteoid and conduct its mineralization. The collagen fibrils within the osteoid are arranged into linear columns, forming pores and holes (Fig. 3). It is at these sites that mineralization is initiated. Osteoblasts have receptors for several factors that are known to control bone metabolism, most notably parathyroid hormone (PTH) and 1,25-dihydroxyvitamin D. Osteoblasts appear to influence the activity of osteoclasts, which suggests that the former may ultimately be in control of both bone formation and resorption.

Recent data have increased the available knowledge of how osteoblasts regulate bone remodeling and resorption. Lacey et al. [13] found that exposing bone marrow cells and osteoblasts to substances like PTH, prostaglandin E_2, and 1,25-dihydroxyvitamin D_3 stimulated osteoclast differentiation and osteoclast activity. This former is effected by expression of an osteoclast differentiation factor known as RANK ligand (receptor activator of NF-κB ligand). RANK ligand binds to a receptor located on the surface of osteoclast precursors. When macrophage colony stimulating factor, a cytokine also produced by bone marrow stromal cells and osteoblasts, binds to its receptor, known as c-fms, the precursor cell then matures into a functioning preosteoclast. This causes an increase in the number of osteoclasts and thus, more bone resorption. To further activate bone resorption, RANK ligand can bind RANK on mature, differentiated osteoclasts. Osteoprotegerin, which is the product of a distinct gene from RANK, inhibits differentiation of osteoclasts by binding RANK as a so-called decoy receptor and preventing its interaction with its ligand [13].

Osteoclasts are bone-resorbing cells. They have several features that make them an ideal vehicle for this function. They have a ruffled border with extensive membrane folding that increases their metabolically active surface area. The cells effect bone resorption by the release of protons (H^+) via a carbonic anhydrase-dependent proton pump. This lowers the pH of (i.e., acidifies) the region surrounding the cell, which in turn activates specific acid proteases. These proteases then break down the bone within the extracellular matrix. The multinucleated osteoclasts reside within bone resorption cavities or pits known as Howship's lacunae, which can be recognized on microscopic examination. Osteoclasts *do not* have receptors for PTH or 1,25-dihydroxyvitamin D. Therefore, these factors appear to influence osteoclastic activity through mechanisms mediated via the osteoblast binding.

Osteocytes are osteoblasts that have terminally divided. Histologically, they are surrounded by, or trapped within, mineralized bone. Metabolically, they are relatively inactive, with a high nucleus-to-cytoplasm ratio. In view of their radiating processes that extend from the cell border to infiltrate the surrounding canaliculi, it is postulated that osteocytes may transmit signals between the bone cells [9, 19]. However, their role still remains unclear.

Circulating factors that influence bone cell function

A number of circulating substances influence the activity of bone cells. As alluded to above, these are mostly directed towards osteoblasts. PTH is secreted by the parathyroid glands and has direct effects on osteoblasts, as these cells have receptors for this hormone. However, PTH also acts to increase bone resorption in response to low serum levels of calcium. It does this by inducing a rounding of the osteoblast, so that it has less surface area contact with the surrounding bone and allows osteoclasts to have more access to the bony surfaces. In addition, it has recently been shown that PTH binding to osteoblasts induces a secondary messenger system involving RANK and RANK ligand, which activates osteoclast activity as described above.

Vitamin D has known effects on bone metabolism. In its initial form (either ingested or produced with exposure to sun), vitamin D is converted to $25(OH)D_3$ in the liver. It is hydroxylated again to its active form, 1,25-dihydroxyvitamin D, in the kidney. 1,25-Dihydroxyvitamin D stimulates intestinal absorption of calcium [15]. Although the exact mechanism is still not known, it also enhances osteoclastic activity. However, as for PTH, osteoclasts do not have receptors for 1,25-dihydroxyvitamin D, so that these effects are most likely mediated by a secondary messenger mechanism with binding of the vitamin D metabolite to an osteoblast receptor.

Osteoclasts have receptors for calcitonin. Calcitonin is produced in the parafollicular cells of the thyroid gland in response to elevated blood levels of calcium. As calcitonin acts to lower serum calcium, binding of this factor to its receptor has an inhibitory effect on the cell's function. Because of this ability, calcitonin administration has been developed as a potential pharmacological treatment for osteoporosis [10].

More recently, a mechanism of hypothalamic control of bone metabolism has been demonstrated. In contrast to the metabolic pathways of PTH and vitamin D, factors are secreted by bone cells and then themselves in turn affect overall bone metabolism through a centrally mediated mechanism. Leptin, a small polypeptide hormone, is secreted by osteoblasts. Its direct effects are thought to be through control of body weight, while its indirect effects may be through modification of gonadal function via interactions within the hypothalamus [1]. In animal studies, mice with leptin deficiency demonstrated obesity, hypogonadism, and increased bone formation and bone mass. This newly discovered interrelationship between the central nervous system and bone metabolism offers an exciting new frontier in the understanding and possible treatment of metabolic bone disorders such as osteoporosis.

Age-related bone loss and osteoporosis

Primary osteoporosis related to aging has been classified as type II, or senile, osteoporosis. The type I disorder is related to the onset of menopause, and is thus termed postmenopausal osteoporosis. Other causes of osteoporosis can be secondary, such as that caused by long-term corticosteroid use or endocrinopathy.

Peak bone mass is achieved between the ages of 16 to 25 years in most people. After this age, bone mass slowly, but continuously, decreases. The greater the amount of bone achieved during the peak period, the lower the chance that a person will develop osteoporosis later in life. Normal rates of bone loss are different in men and women. In men, bone mass is lost at a rate of 0.3% per year, while for women this rate is 0.5%. In contrast, bone loss after menopause, in particular the first 5 years after its onset, can be as high as 5–6% per year [17]. Because women live longer than men, it is believed that increased longevity places women at higher risk of senile osteoporosis.

Besides the difference in age at onset, types I and II osteoporosis have somewhat different effects on the kinds of bone lost. Type I appears to affect mostly trabecular bone, while type II affects both cortical and trabecular bone [16]. While both types substantially increase the risk of fracture in cancellous bone, such as osteoporotic vertebral compression, distal radius, or intertrochanteric hip fractures, patients with type II disease may be at greater risk of fractures through cortical bone, such as the femoral neck, pelvis, proximal humerus, and proximal tibia.

The cellular mechanism of type II osteoporosis is multifactorial. A major factor is probably progressive dietary calcium deficiency [3]. As patients age, appetite can become suppressed, leading to lower intake of foods rich in calcium. Financial constraints, as endured by many elderly individuals with low fixed incomes, can be a disincentive to purchasing foods that support a well-balanced diet. This factor, by itself, has been known to contribute to states of malnutrition in elderly people. Moreover, the presence of osteoporotic vertebral compression fractures and the resultant alterations in the dimensions of the trunk can lead to early satiety in affected individuals [14]. This would have a self-perpetuating effect on osteoporosis, as this can lead to further calcium deficiency and more profound loss in bone density.

Another contributing mechanism is progressive inactivity. Bone mass is positively affected by mechanical loads (i.e., exercise and activity). With age, most people become less active, which can potentiate progressive bone loss. While osteoporosis itself is painless, profound inactivity from the pain of an osteoporotic compression fracture can lead to a vicious cycle of further bone loss, more fractures, and more pain and inactivity.

While not the primary mechanism as in type I osteoporosis, decreases in estrogen levels have been demonstrated in both elderly men and women and this is thought to be an important cause of senile osteoporosis as well.

The cumulative effect of normal aging, dietary calcium deficiency, and lower activity is the upregulation of bone resorption and downregulation of bone formation. While it is commonly held that these effects are mediated by stimulation of osteoclasts and inhibition of osteoblasts, the exact mechanisms by which they lead to age-related bone loss is still not well understood.

Geometry: effects of osteoporosis on cancellous bone

Normal cancellous bone, such as that in the vertebral body, is composed of both horizontal and vertical trabeculae. These trabecular struts are interconnected, much like the scaffolding used to surround buildings during construction. While the individual vertical and horizontal members, are, by themselves, important in resisting loads in particular directions (i.e., anisotropic properties), it is their interaction that gives cancellous bone its great compressive strength.

Osteoporosis is a disorder in which total bone mass is reduced yet the quality of the bone is normal. If a microsection of bone were to be biochemically analyzed, it would demonstrate a normal ratio of osteoid to mineral. Though total bone mass is affected, there is a predisposition to loss of the horizontal trabeculae [4]. This leads to decreased interconnectivity of the internal scaffolding of the vertebral body (Fig. 1b). Without the support of crossing horizontal members, unsupported vertical beams of bone easily succumb to minor, normally subcatastrophic, loads. Clinically, this leads to crush of the cancellous bone within the vertebral body, recognizable as an osteoporotic compression fracture, which may occur with low-energy maneuvers such as picking up a bag of groceries.

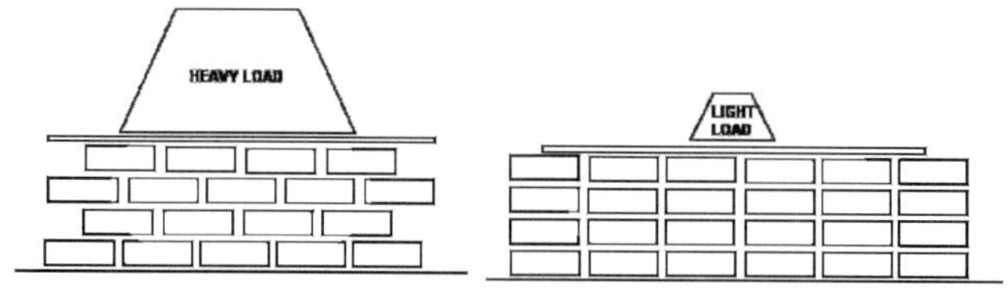

Fig. 4 The importance of interconnectivity of bone is shown by the analogy to a brick wall. Normal bone has interconnectivity, like the overlapping of the brick wall on the *left*. It can sustain heavy loads. Osteoporotic bone has lost its interconnectivity, like the brick wall on the *right*. Its walls can sustain only light loads, as they will collapse and buckle under heavier loads

Using the analogy of the column of bricks detailed above, imagine two different brick buildings. The first is built in the usual manner: the bricks are overlapped with each other in a staggered pattern, representing interconnectivity of the trabeculae. The second building is built with columns of bricks stacked on top of each other with no overlapping, representing loss of interconnectivity (Fig. 4). While both houses might support some weight of objects placed on the roof, the first house would be able to support much greater loads. The walls of the second house would only be able to support much lighter loads. With heavier loads, the walls of the second house will have a tendency to buckle and topple, like an osteoporotic vertebral fracture. Taking the example one step further, consider the first house to be built with bricks made of granite and the second house made of bricks of porous sandstone. The sandstone bricks would have a greater tendency to crumble with loads, as would the osteoporotic vertebral body.

Geometry: effects of osteoporosis on cortical bone

Decreases in bone mass occur throughout the skeleton. As the dense cortices of long bones are designed to withstand bending and torsional loads, decreases in bone mass would potentially diminish loads to failure. Fortunately, long bones exhibit a compensatory mechanism to counteract the mechanical effects of decreased bone mass. In aging individuals, increased endosteal bone resorption and periosteal bone deposition leads to an overall increased diameter of bone. This relationship can be expressed as a formula for the moment of inertia resulting from the loading [4]. Long bones resist failure in bending by their areal moment of inertia and in torsion by their polar moment of inertia properties.

This phenomenon helps explain why mid-shaft long bone fractures do not occur in a proportionately higher frequency in older than younger individuals. Unfortunately, this same adaptive mechanism does not appear to have a role in the vertebral column, as the cortical shell of the vertebral body contributes only about 10% of its overall strength [18].

Geometry: effects on vertebral body strength

The major mechanical role of the vertebral body is to withstand compressive loads. Its broad transverse surface area and primarily trabecular composition are ideal to fulfill these demands. Both bone density and its geometry determine a vertebral body's strength.

The surface area of the vertebral endplates determines the compressive stress concentration imparted to the underlying cancellous bone. In the best case scenario, surface area would be maximized and the compression would be uniform along the entire endplate [20].

In some groups of people, the vertebrae are proportionately smaller. Asians, for example, have a higher rate of vertebral compression fractures than Caucasians. This is thought to be related to the smaller cross-sectional dimensions of the Asian vertebral body. Interestingly, a somewhat opposite relationship is true for osteoporotic hip fractures. Greater hip axis length in Caucasians corresponds to a higher incidence of fracture than the shorter lengths in Asians. This most likely is a result of differences in cantilever bending forces, which would be higher with longer hip axis lengths, as well as with the greater body weights notable in the generally larger Caucasian.

The pattern of loading is another important influence on the amount of weight that can be sustained by the vertebral body. Normal spinal balance dictates that a weight-bearing plumb line dropped from the base of the occiput should fall through the C7 vertebral body, T12–L1 junction, and caudally within or just anterior to the sacral (S2) promontory. This facilitates even distribution of compressive loads to each of the vertebrae in the spinal column. Forward bending of the spine, either fixed or dynamic, leads to a greater percentage of compressive forces along the anterior aspect of the endplates, and thus of the vertebral bodies. Combined with the presence of decreased bone mineral density, this anterior concentration of force can lead to catastrophic failure of the underlying bone. This mode of failure is most common in the thoracic spine, which has a physiologic degree of pre-existing kyphosis [11]. Decreases in cortical bone density with aging within the anterior vertebral body may also predispose to such fracture patterns [7].

The lumbar spine is normally lordotic. Although anterior wedge compression fractures can occur in this region, more commonly fractures demonstrate uniform compression or central (biconcave) types [11]. This may be related to the pattern of loading. One might infer that loads are concentrated within the center of the lumbar endplate if lordosis is maintained at the time of fracture. Ultimately, the pattern of failure, and thus the type of fracture, is most likely influenced by the position of the spine at the time of injury.

Conclusion

As advances in medicine continue to prolong life, an understanding of disorders related to aging becomes increasingly important. Osteoporosis and its complications have important detrimental effects on the quality of life of affected individuals. As with any disorder, a sound understanding of the pathophysiology of the underlying disease process is crucial to effective decision making regarding treatment. Recent advances in both the pharmacological and surgical treatment of osteoporosis and vertebral compression fractures offer exciting new options for elderly patients [5, 8]. However, these treatments should be considered within the context of an indepth knowledge of osteoporosis as a metabolic disorder with complex effects on bone, its homeostatic regulation, and vertebral strength.

References

1. Amling M, Schilling AF, Haberland M, Rueger JM (2001) Leptin: factor in the central nervous system regulation of bone mass. Development of a new understanding of bone remodeling, skeletal reconstruction, skeletal preservation and skeletal repair. Orthopade 30:418–424
2. deLaet CE, vanderKlift M, Pols HA (2002) Osteoporosis in men and women: a story about bone mineral density thresholds and hip fracture risk. J Bone Miner Res 17:2231–2236
3. Eastell R, Lambert H (2002) Strategies for skeletal health in the elderly. Proc Nutr Soc 61:173–180
4. Einhorn TA (1992) Bone strength: the bottom line. Calcif Tissue Int 51:333–339
5. Einhorn TA (2000) Vertebroplasty: an opportunity to do something really good for patients. Spine 25:1051–1052
6. Feskanich D, Willett W, Colditz G (2002) Walking and leisure-time activity and risk of hip fracture in postmenopausal women. JAMA 288: 2300–2306
7. Flynn MJ, Cody DD (1993) The assessment of vertebral bone macroarchitecture with X-ray computed tomography. Calcif Tissue Int 53:S170–S175
8. Garfin SR, Yuan HA, Reiley MA (2001) New technologies in spine: kyphoplasty and vertebroplasty for the treatment of painful ostoeporotic compression fractures. Spine 26:1511–1515
9. Gill SS, Einhorn TA (1998) Bone metabolism and metabolic bone disease. In: JH Beaty (eds) Orthopaedic knowledge update 6. American Academy of Orthopaedic Surgeons, Rosemont, pp 149–165
10. Gur A, Denli A, Nas K, Cevik R, Karakoc M, Sarac AJ, Erdogan F (2002) Possible pathogenetic role of new cytokines in postmenopausal osteoporosis and changes during calcitonin plus calcium therapy. Rheumatol Int 22:194–198

11. Ismail AA, Cooper C, Felsenberg D, Varlow J, Kanis JA, Silman AJ, O'Neill TW (1999) Number and type of vertebral deformities: epidemiological characteristics and relation to back pain and height loss. European Vertebral Osteoporosis Study Group. Osteoporosis Int 9:206–213
12. Kerstetter JE, O'Brien KO, Insogna KL (2003) Low protein intake: the impact on calcium and bone homeostasis in humans. J Nutr 133:855S–861S
13. Lacey DL, Timms E, Tan HL, Kelley MJ, Dunstan CR, Burgess T, Elliott R, Colombero A, Elliott G, Scully S, Hsu H, Sullivan J, Hawkins N, Davy E, Capparell iC, Eli A, Qian YX, Kaufman S, Sarosi I, Shalhoub V, Senaldi G, Guo J, Delaney J, Boyle WJ (1998) Osteoprotegerin ligand is a cytokine that regulates osteoclast differentiation and activation. Cell 93:165–176
14. Leidig-Bruckner G, Minne HW, Schlaich C, Wagner G, Scheidt-Nave C, Bruckner T, Gebest HJ, Ziegler R (1997) Clinical grading of spinal osteoporosis: quality of life components and spinal deformity in women with chronic low back pain and women with vertebral osteoporosis. J Bone Miner Res 12:663–675
15. Norman AW, Roth J, Orci L (1982) The vitamin D endocrine system: steroid metabolism, hormone receptors and biological response. Endocr Rev 3: 331–366
16. Riggs BL, Melton LJ (1983) Evidence for two distinct syndrome of involutional osteoporosis. Am J Med 309: 899–901
17. Riggs BL, Melton LJ (1992) The prevention and treatment of osteoporosis. N Engl J Med 327:620–627
18. Silva MJ, Keaveny TM, Hayes WC (1997) Load sharing between the shell and centrum in the lumbar vertebral body. Spine 22:140–150
19. Silver JJ, Majeska RJ, Einhorn TA (1994) An update on bone cell biology. Curr Opin Orthop 5:50–59
20. Vega E, Ghiringhelli G, Mautalen C, ReyValzacchi G, Scaglia H, Zylberstein C (1998) Bone mineral density and bone size in men with primary osteoporosis and vertebral fractures. Calcif Tissue Int 62:465–469
21. White A, Panjabi M (1990) Clinical biomechanics of the Spine. Lippincott, Philadelphia

Stephen J. Ferguson
Thomas Steffen

Biomechanics of the aging spine

Abstract The human spine is composed of highly specific tissues and structures, which together provide the extensive range of motion and considerable load carrying capacity required for the physical activities of daily life. Alterations to the form and composition of the individual structures of the spine with increasing age can increase the risk of injury and can have a profound influence on the quality of life. Cancellous bone forms the structural framework of the vertebral body. Individual trabeculae are oriented along the paths of principal forces and play a crucial role in the transfer of the predominantly compressive forces along the spine. Age-related changes to the cancellous core of the vertebra includes a loss of bone mineral density, as well as morphological changes including trabecular thinning, increased intratrabecular spacing, and loss of connectivity between trabeculae. Material and morphological changes may lead to an increased risk of vertebral fracture. The vertebral endplate serves the dual role of containing the adjacent disc and evenly distributing applied loads to the underlying cancellous bone and the cortex of the vertebra. With aging, thinning of the endplate, and loss of bone mineral density increases the risk of endplate fracture. Ossification of the endplate may have consequences for the nutritional supply and hydration of the intervertebral disc. The healthy intervertebral disc provides mobility to the spine and transfers load via hydrostatic pressurization of the hydrated nucleus pulposus. Changes to the tissue properties of the disc, including dehydration and reorganization of the nucleus and stiffening of the annulus fibrosus, markedly alter the mechanics of load transfer in the spine. There is no direct correlation between degenerative changes to the disc and to the adjacent vertebral bodies. Furthermore, advancing age is not the sole factor in the degeneration of the spine. Further study is crucial for understanding the unique biomechanical function of the aging spine.

Keywords Aging spine · Biomechanics · Osteoporosis · Vertebral endplate · Disc degeneration

S. J. Ferguson (✉)
M.E. Müller Research Center
for Orthopaedic Surgery,
Institute for Surgical Technology
and Biomechanics, University of Berne,
Murtenstrasse 35, Postbox 8354,
3001 Berne, Switzerland
Tel.: +41-31-6328718,
Fax: +41-31-6324951,
e-mail:
Stephen.Ferguson@MEMcenter.unibe.ch

T. Steffen
Orthopaedic Research Laboratory,
McGill University, Montreal, Canada

Introduction

The vertebral column is built from alternating bony vertebrae, interconnected with fibrocartilagenous discs and diarthrodial facet joints. In total 33 vertebrae (7 cervical, 12 thoracic, 5 lumbar, 5 sacral and 4 coccygeal) all conform to a basic plan. With the exception of the atlas and axis, all vertebra are made of an anterior approximately cylindrical vertebral body and an arch composed of paired pedicles and laminae, the latter joined posteriorly forming the spinous process. The arch on either side also features a transverse process, as well as superior and inferior articular processes forming corresponding synovial joints (called facets) between adjacent vertebrae. The spinous and transverse processes serve as lever arms for many muscles running over single or multiple spinal levels. Only limited movements are possible between adjacent vertebrae, but the sum of these movements amounts to considerable spinal mobility in all major planes. Differences in mobility between regions (cervical, thoracic, lumbar) are due to the splinting effect of the rib cage, differences in shape and size of the articular, and spinous processes.

At birth the spine is generally dorsal convex (kyphotic), but during the first year with the assumption of an upright posture (lifting head, sitting up) the cervical and lumbar regions develop a lordotic shape. The bipedal human erect posture necessitates a tilt of the sacrum between the pelvic bones, increased lumbosacral angulation, and adjustments in size of individual vertebrae and discs. The increasing size of the vertebral bodies from cranial to caudal corresponds to the increasing weights and stresses imposed by successive segments. The sacral (and coccygeal) vertebrae are fused, forming a solid, wedge shaped base, transmitting the axial load of the spinal column over the paired pelvic bones and hip joints into the lower extremities.

The erect posture greatly increases the load carried by the lower spinal joints, and despite millions of years of evolutionary adaptations imperfections seemingly continue to exist, predisposing this region to strains and lower back pain. About three-quarters of axial spinal load is carried by the anterior column. Vertebral bodies, endplates, and intervertebral discs are the principal structures of the anterior column. We describe its elements more in detail below.

The vertebral body

The architecture of a vertebral body is comprised of highly porous trabecular bone, but also of a fairly dense and solid shell. The shell is very thin throughout, on average only 0.4 mm [34]. It is virtually indistinguishable from the trabecular core but rather is a denser arrangement of trabecular elements forming solid and compact bone (histologically different from cortical bone). Finite element analysis estimates the contribution of the shell to the overall load carrying capacity to be less than 15% [23, 35].

Regional variation in bone architecture also exist within any given vertebral body. The regions adjacent to the endplate feature more dense, rodlike trabecular structures. The regions far from the endplate, on the other hand, are less dense, with platelike shaped trabeculae. Mechanical properties tested in normal vertebrae for distinct regions of trabecular bone samples attribute higher strength, stiffness and bone mineral density (BMD) to central trabecular regions [18, 19, 20]. Variability in mechanical properties can be interpreted as adaptive to the environment, in this case to higher vertical stresses transmitted by the central region adjacent to the nucleus pulposus, as opposed to the peripheral region adjacent to the annulus fibrosus. Keller et al. [20] have demonstrated for degenerated intervertebral discs a change in adjacent trabecular mechanical properties, suggesting a more uniform load distribution across the endplate in degenerated spines.

The apparent bone density varies widely (0.05 g/cm^3 to 0.30 g/cm^3) between individuals, between levels, but also as a function of age. Starting in the fourth decade of life, elderly men can easily lose up to 30% and elderly women up to 50% of bone density [22]. Routine estimates of the apparent bone density are obtained using dual energy X-ray absorptiometry (DEXA). Although BMD or bone mineral content (BMC) are not volumetric parameters for bone, they still have proven to be useful predictors for ultimate vertebral strength, since the ultimate vertebral strength is dependent on both the vertebral geometry and the trabecular failure strength. To compare failure strength for vertebral samples from different spinal regions or from different individuals it is best to express the failure strength as a material property, normalized for the endplate's cross-sectional area [4], or expressed as compressive failure stress. The stress at failure for a lumbar vertrebral body is found to range from 1.0 to 5.0 MPa. This measure, however, does not differentiate between trabecular and compact elements of the vertebral body.

Keller [17] established from in vitro testing of isolated trabecular bone samples a relationship between apparent bone density and compressive failure strength. The exponential function [compressive strength=$(97.8\times$apparent bone density$)^{2.30}$] identifies trabecular bone with low apparent density (<0.10 g/cm^3) to feature an ultimate compressive strength of less than 0.2 MPa, which puts this bone at risk to fracture already at axial loads seen in routine and low level daily activity. Resch et al. [30] have shown using quantitative computer tomography that men with 0.11 g/cm^3 apparent bone density have a 25% vertebral fracture risk, whereas individuals with 0.05 g/cm^3 bone density have a 99% vertebral fracture risk.

Osteoporosis is a disease that weakens the structural strength of bone to an extent that normal daily activity can exceed the vertebra's ability for carrying this load, resulting in vertebral fractures. The incidence of fragility fractures doubled within the last decade. It is predominant in women, with an osteoporotic fracture prevalence at age 50 years and above of over 40% ("Bone and joint decade," WHO 2003: http://www.boneandjointdecade.org/background/default.html). Clinically osteoporosis is characterized using DEXA measurements (BMD or BMC) of the lumbar spine that are 2.5 SD or more below the average value for a 30-year-old gender-matched individual [24]. In women the risk for vertebral fractures rises 2.2-fold for every 1 SD loss in BMD or BMC [5].

Decreased structural strength is not only the result of reduced apparent bone density, but also of profound changes in the architecture and the bone remodeling and/or repair rate, resulting in faster damage accumulation for continuous cyclic loading. The increase in bone fragility

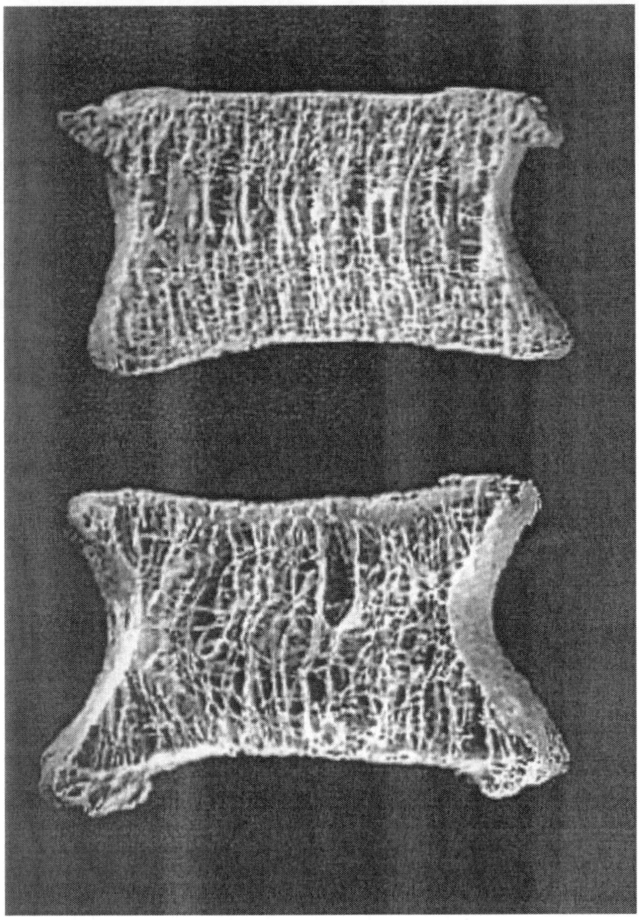

Fig. 1 Normal (*top*) and osteoporotic (*bottom*) vertebral bodies. Decreased structural strength is not only the result of reduced apparent bone density but also changes in the architecture of the trabecular bone. The increase in bone fragility is due to replacement of platelike close trabecular structures with more open, rodlike structures. The more porous cancellous bone appearance is the result of reduced horizontal cross-linking struts

is due to replacement of platelike close trabecular structures with more open, rodlike structures. The more porous cancellous bone appearance is the result of reduced horizontal cross-linking struts, further reducing the buckling strength of vertically oriented trabeculae (Fig. 1).

The typical osteoprotic vertebral fracture leads to a height reduction of the anterior vertebral body, often leaving the posterior vertebral wall intact. This wedge-shaped deformity usually leads to a local increase in kyphosis, and with multiple adjacent vertebral fractures to a progressive kyphotic deformity with postural disfigurement. Multiple vertebral fractures are very common, since the fracture risk of neighboring levels have shown to have a fivefold increased fracture risk compared to normal vertebrae [16].

The vertebral endplate

The vertebral endplate forms a structural boundary between the intervertebral disc and the cancellous core of the vertebral body. Comprised of a thin layer of semiporous subchondral bone, approximately 0.5 mm thick, with an overlying cartilage layer of similar thickness, the principal functions of the endplate are to prevent extrusion of the disc into the porous vertebral body, and to evenly distribute load to the vertebral body. With its dense cartilage layer, the endplate also serves as a semipermeable interface, which allows the transfer of water and solutes but prevents the loss of large proteoglycan molecules from the disc. Finally, the dense subchondral bone of the endplate provides secure anchorage for the collagen network of the intervertebral disc.

The thickness of the endplate varies, with thicker bone found under the annulus than adjacent to the nucleus. The superior endplate is generally thinner than the inferior endplate. A positive correlation between the thickness of the endplate and the proteoglycan content of the disc has been shown, especially for the central endplate under the nucleus. This may be the result of a remodeling process whereby the endplate responds to a greater hydrostatic pressure in discs with higher proteoglycan content [32]. Therefore it is possible that the changes associated with aging and disc degeneration could result in a weakening of the adjacent endplate.

The local material properties of the endplate demonstrate a significant spatial dependence. Grant et al. [9] have shown that the strength and stiffness of the endplate are highest posterolaterally and lowest in the center of the endplate (Fig. 2). Sacral and inferior lumbar endplates are

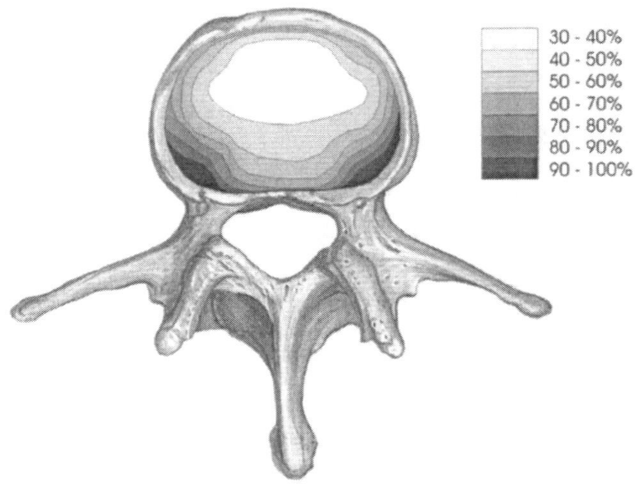

Fig. 2 Spatial distribution of endplate material properties, normalized to maximum values measured. Endplate strength is greatest towards the posterolateral and lowest at the center of the endplate. Regional variation in endplate properties is more pronounced with decreasing bone mineral density. (Adapted from [9])

stronger than superior lumbar endplates, which may indicate an increased fracture risk in the aging spine for the superior endplate. The importance of the endplate for load transfer and the overall structural integrity of the vertebra has been highlighted in laboratory experiments which have shown a significant reduction in the local structural properties of the vertebral body following partial endplate removal [27]. Similar experiments have provided support for the hypothesis that the strength of the central endplate region decreases with increasing disc degeneration due to remodeling, and that logically the overall strength of the endplate decreases with decreasing BMD [10]. With decreasing BMD, the regional variation in material properties becomes more pronounced, which likely plays a significant role in the initiation of the endplate fractures which are a characteristic of the aging spine.

Of particular relevance for the aging spine, the morphology of fatigue fractures of lumbar motion segments has been investigated in laboratory experiments [11, 12]. Under repetitive cyclic loading designed to simulate vigorous physical activity, the weakest part of the vertebral body was shown to be the endplate; failure often occurred after only several hundred cycles. Two main types of fatigue failure occurred, both involving the endplate and the adjacent subchondral cancellous bone of the vertebral body. Fracture morphology was weakly correlated with disc degeneration grade. The development of Schmorl's nodes – the local extrusion of disc material through the endplate – was most often seen with normal intervertebral discs. Central endplate fractures were associated with moderately degenerated discs. In some cases crush or burst fractures were observed. These occurred always on the first loading cycle and were seen in specimens with low BMD.

Deformity of the vertebral body with aging is closely related to BMD loss, i.e., osteoporosis. With aging, increased concavity of the vertebral endplate is seen together with a loss of BMD [36]. The typical loss of stature, often attributed to disc thinning, is more likely a consequence of a fairly normal disc migrating into this concavity. Endplate fracture is significant in the initiation of vertebral body collapse, but is difficult to diagnose from conventional morphometric assessment of spinal osteoporosis; up to 80% of all endplate fractures are missed by conventional diagnostic radiography [21]. However, Schmorl's nodes, which generally evolve from significant traumatic events, are easily recognized on magnetic resonance imaging (MRI) as either a characteristic extrusion of disc material, or as a localized edema in the vertebral body adjacent to the fracture [39].

In contrast to the thinning of the endplate and increased fracture risk often observed with aging, endplate sclerosis with aging has also been reported and can be so substantial as to bias normal measurements of vertebral body bone density [29]. Ossification of the overlying cartilaginous layer has been observed with aging [31]. Localized calcification directly influences the permeability of the endplate, and it has been shown that this may lead to a potential reduction in the volume of fluid exchanged to the disc during daily activity, resulting in a disruption of the nutritional supply to the disc and possible dehydration of the disc [3, 8]. Degenerative changes to the disc are extremely important factors determining the function of the elderly spine, as is outlined below.

The intervertebral disc

The intervertebral disc provides mobility to the spine. Positioned between the bony vertebrae, the disc allows complex motion without the mechanical disadvantages of the opposing articular surfaces of a diarthrodial joint. The disc derives its function from its unique structure, whereby the amorphous, gel-like nucleus pulposus is surrounded by the highly oriented annulus fibrosus. In the healthy disc, a hydrostatic pressure is developed within the nucleus, which is contained by the strong lamellae of the annulus, and loads are thereby evenly distributed across the underlying vertebrae.

The degenerative changes to the vertebral disc which are often observed with aging have been well described in the review by Vernon-Roberts [38]. Macroscopic changes to the disc include the appearance of horizontal splits and clefts midway between the center of the disc and the cartilage endplates, which extend posteriorly and posterolaterally and can eventually lead to fissures through the annulus. Microscopic fragmentation of annulus fibers has been observed, leading to a degeneration of individual fibers. Vertebral rim lesions, annular tears at the corners of the vertebral body separating the annulus from the bony attachment, are commonly present after the age of 50 years. Concentric cracks and cavities and radiating ruptures of the annulus are often present. At the disc boundaries cartilage endplate fissure formation, horizontal cleft formation, death of chondrocytes, vascular penetration, and Schmorl's nodes are observed. Disc thinning occurs due to loss of water content, conversion of the nucleus tissue to a highly organized collagenous tissue, gradual ossification of the endplate and protrusion of disc tissue. While the cartilage endplate and annulus are normally sufficiently strong to contain the nucleus, even under great stress, degeneration of the disc can lead to potential weak points in the subchondral bone and in the posterior and posterolateral segments of the annulus, which are thinner and less firmly attached to the vertebra.

Age- and degeneration-related changes to disc tissue material properties have been extensively evaluated. Based on measurements of the viscoelastic properties of the human nucleus pulposus, Iatridis et al. [14] concluded that changes to the mechanical properties suggest a shift from a "fluid like" behavior to a more "solid like" behavior with degeneration. Due to its crucial role in the containment of the nucleus, changes to the properties of the annulus fibrosus have also been the subject of several studies. An increase in the elastic modulus with progressive degeneration has been shown, likely the results of an increase in tissue density due to water loss. This suggests a shift in the load carriage mechanism of the disc with increasing degeneration from fluid pressurization to elastic deformation of the annulus fibrosus [15]. Although dramatic changes in annulus fibrosus morphology and composition have been documented with aging and degeneration, the tensile mechanical properties of the annulus are not substantially affected by degeneration. A far more important factor for the tensile properties, especially in the radial direction, is the position within the annulus, and this relationship does not change substantially with age or degeneration [1, 7]. Significant changes to the ligamentous structures of the spine with aging have been reported. For example, the elastic modulus of the main substance of the anterior longitudinal ligament increases twofold, while the modulus of the ligament insertion decreases threefold, between 20 and 80 years of age, and the strength of the bone ligament junction decreases twofold with aging [25].

The fluid content of the disc is important for determining its mechanical response. Hydration depends on the proteoglycan content of the disc and also on the balance between external load and the internal swelling pressure of the disc. The influence of age, spinal level, composition and degeneration on disc swelling pressure has been measured for human discs [37]. The natural swelling pressure for human discs was found to be approximately 0.1–0.2 MPa. Proteoglycan content decreased with age, and was lowest at L5–S1, but no substantial change in collagen content was found. Therefore the relationship between equilibrium hydration and swelling pressure could be predicted based on proteoglycan and collagen content, while age and degree of degeneration were not significant factors.

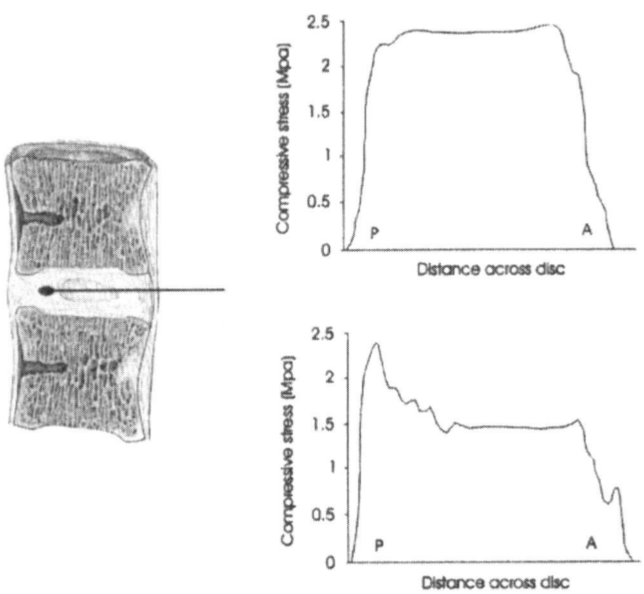

Fig. 3 Typical stress profiles for grade-1 disc (*top*) and for a grade 4 disc (*bottom*). In the healthy disc, a hydrostatic pressure is developed in the nucleus, as indicated by the plateau in the stress plot. For the degenerate disc, nuclear pressure is lower, and stress peaks in the annulus fibrosus are observed. *A* Anterior; *P* posterior. (Adapted from [2])

Aging and disc degeneration have a profound effect on the mechanism of load transfer through the disc. Using the technique of "stress-profilometry," it has been shown that age-related changes to the disc composition result in a shift of load from the nucleus to the annulus [2]. A reduction by approximately 50% of the central hydrostatic region of the disc was observed, and a corresponding 30% reduction in pressure for degenerate discs (Fig. 3). The width of the functional annulus increased by 80% and the height of the compressive stress peak in the annulus by 160% with degeneration. While age and degeneration were closely related, the state of degeneration had the most profound influence on the measured stress distributions. Therefore structural changes in the annulus and endplate with aging may lead to a transfer of load from the nucleus to the posterior annulus, which may cause pain and also lead to annular rupture.

Combined effects of disc degeneration and osteoporosis

The correlation between degenerative changes to the vertebra and the disc remains an open question. Endplate fracture or vertebral body deformity is not necessarily associated with disc degeneration. While disc thinning may be implied from observed stature changes, disc morphometry is altered to accommodate changes to the vertebral body shape by extrusion into the concave endplate, but indicators of degeneration (i.e., MRI signal intensity) are not altered subsequent to throacolumbar spine fractures [26]. Based on MRI imaging and DEXA measurements, a negative correlation between vertebral BMD and intervertebral disc degeneration has been shown [13]. Dai [6] has suggested that, for patients with severe osteoporosis, vertebral bodies adjacent to discs with decreased height or signs of degeneration are less likely to be deformed. In an in vitro study of the influence of disc degeneration on the mechanism of vertebral burst fractures, Shirado et al. [33] demonstrated that disruption of the middle end plate was found only in specimens with normal disc quality. In specimens with severe disc degeneration and osteoporosis, no burst fractures were observed. Further analysis of their test results led to the conclusion that stresses were concentrated towards the center of the vertebral endplate due to hydrostatic pressurization of a normal nucleus pulposus.

The possible mechanical interactions due to disc degeneration and concurrent osteoporotic changes to the vertebrae have been extensively studied using detailed computer simulations of whole spine segments [28]. These analyses have predicted that osteoporosis alone has a substantial influence on the overall stiffness of a spine segment, resulting in a 35–40% reduction in stiffness. Correspondingly, the magnitude of internal vertebral strains for a nominal load level were predicted to increase with the progression of osteoporosis. However, the spatial patterns of strain distribution within the vertebral bodies were similar for the normal and osteoporotic vertebra. Conversely, the simulation of disc degeneration has predicted a substantial load shift from the nucleus towards the annulus, as previously demonstrated in stress-profilometry measurements [2]. While vertebral strain magnitudes for the degenerate disc were similar, there was a marked change in strain distribution, which was an opposite effect to that observed for osteoporosis. Therefore a degenerate disc may moderate the detrimental effects of extreme osteoporosis and it could be hypothesized that the increased fracture risk of an osteoporotic spine segment may be slightly counterbalanced by the material consequences of disc degeneration. This is in agreement with the findings by Shirado et al. [33] and Dai et al. [6], reporting that vertebral bodies next to degenerated discs were less likely to be deformed or fractured for patients with spinal osteoporosis.

Conclusion

The human spine is a highly evolved structure capable of an extensive range of motion and with considerable load carrying capacity. Age-related changes to the form and composition of the individual structures of the spine may increase the risk of injury and limit quality of life for elderly patients. Cancellous bone forms the structural framework of the vertebral body. With aging a loss of BMD, as well as morphological changes including trabecular thinning, increased intratrabecular spacing, and loss of connectivity between trabeculae, may lead to an increased risk of vertebral fracture. The vertebral endplate serves the dual role of containing the adjacent disc and evenly distributing applied loads to the vertebra. Thinning of the endplate and loss of bone density increases the risk of endplate fracture. The intervertebral disc provides mobility to the spine, and transfers load via hydrostatic pressurization of the hydrated nucleus pulposus. Changes to the tissue properties of the disc, including dehydration and reorganization of the nucleus and stiffening of the annulus fibrosus, markedly alter the mechanics of load transfer in the spine. However, advancing age is not the sole factor in the degeneration of the spine and further study is required to understand the mechanisms of degeneration and the unique biomechanical function of the aging spine.

References

1. Acaroglu ER, Iatridis JC, Setton LA, Foster RJ, Mow VC, Weidenbaum M (1995) Degeneration and aging affect the tensile behavior of human lumbar anulus fibrosus. Spine 20:2690–2701
2. Adams MA, McNally DS, Dolan P (1996) 'Stress' distributions inside intervertebral discs. The effects of age and degeneration. J Bone Joint Surg Br 78:965–972
3. Ayotte DC, Ito K, Perren SM, Tepic S (2000) Direction-dependent constriction flow in a poroelastic solid: the intervertebral disc valve. J Biomech Eng 122:587–593
4. Brinckmann P, Biggemann M, Hilweg D (1989) Prediction of the compressive strength of human lumbar vertebrae. Spine 14:606–610
5. Cummings SR, Black D (1995) Bone mass measurements and risk of fracture in Caucasian women: a review of findings from prospective studies. Am J Med 98:24S-28S
6. Dai L (1998) The relationship between vertebral body deformity and disc degeneration in lumbar spine of the senile. Eur Spine J 7:40–44
7. Ebara S, Iatridis JC, Setton LA, Foster RJ, Mow VC, Weidenbaum M (1996) Tensile properties of nondegenerate human lumbar anulus fibrosus. Spine 21:452–461
8. Ferguson SJ, Ito K, Nolte LP (2003) Fluid flow and convective transport of solutes within the intervertebral disc. J Biomech (in press)
9. Grant JP, Oxland TR, Dvorak MF (2001) Mapping the structural properties of the lumbosacral vertebral endplates. Spine 26:889–896
10. Grant JP, Oxland TR, Dvorak MF, Fisher CG (2002) The effects of bone density and disc degeneration on the structural property distributions in the lower lumbar vertebral endplates. J Orthop Res 20:1115–1120
11. Hansson TH, Keller TS, Spengler DM (1987) Mechanical behavior of the human lumbar spine. II. Fatigue strength during dynamic compressive loading. J Orthop Res 5:479–487
12. Hansson T, Keller T, Jonson R (1988) Fatigue fracture morphology in human lumbar motion segments. J Spinal Disord 1:33–38
13. Harada A, Okuizumi H, Miyagi N, Genda E (1998) Correlation between bone mineral density and intervertebral disc degeneration. Spine 23:857–861
14. Iatridis JC, Setton LA, Weidenbaum M, Mow VC (1997) Alterations in the mechanical behavior of the human lumbar nucleus pulposus with degeneration and aging. J Orthop Res 15:318–322
15. Iatridis JC, Setton LA, Foster RJ, Rawlins BA, Weidenbaum M, Mow VC (1998) Degeneration affects the anisotropic and nonlinear behaviors of human anulus fibrosus in compression. J Biomech 31:535–544
16. Jensen ME, Evans AJ, Mathis JM, Kallmes DF, Cloft HJ, Dion JE (1997) Percutaneous polymethylmethacrylate vertebroplasty in the treatment of osteoporotic vertebral body compression fractures: technical aspects. AJNR Am J Neuroradiol 18:1897–1904
17. Keller TS (1994) Predicting the compressive mechanical behavior of bone. J Biomech 27:1159–1168

18. Keller TS, Hansson TH, Abram AC, Spengler DM, Panjabi MM (1989) Regional variations in the compressive properties of lumbar vertebral trabeculae. Effects of disc degeneration. Spine 14:1012–1019
19. Keller TS, Moeljanto E, Main JA, Spengler DM (1992) Distribution and orientation of bone in the human lumbar vertebral centrum. J Spinal Disord 5:60–74
20. Keller TS, Ziv I, Moeljanto E, Spengler DM (1993) Interdependence of lumbar disc and subdiscal bone properties: a report of the normal and degenerated spine. J Spinal Disord 6:106–113
21. Leidig-Bruckner G, Limberg B, Felsenberg D, Bruckner T, Holder S, Kather A, Miksch J, Wuster C, Ziegler R, Scheidt-Nave C (2000) Sex difference in the validity of vertebral deformities as an index of prevalent vertebral osteoporotic fractures: a population survey of older men and women. Osteoporos Int 11:102–119
22. Mazess RB (1982) On aging bone loss. Clin Orthop 239–252
23. McBroom RJ, Hayes WC, Edwards WT, Goldberg RP, White AA III (1985) Prediction of vertebral body compressive fracture using quantitative computed tomography. J Bone Joint Surg Am 67:1206–1214
24. National Institutes of Health (2003) Osteoporosis prevention, diagnosis and therapy. NIH consensus statement 17: 1–36
25. Neumann P, Ekstrom LA, Keller TS, Perry L, Hansson TH (1994) Aging, vertebral density, and disc degeneration alter the tensile stress-strain characteristics of the human anterior longitudinal ligament. J Orthop Res 12:103–112
26. Oner FC, van der Rijt RR, Ramos LM, Dhert WJ, Verbout AJ (1998) Changes in the disc space after fractures of the thoracolumbar spine. J Bone Joint Surg Br 80:833–839
27. Oxland TR, Grant JP, Dvorak MF, Fisher CG (2003) Effects of endplate removal on the structural properties of the lower lumbar vertebral bodies. Spine 28:771–777
28. Polikeit A (2002) Finite element analyses of the lumbar spine: clinical applications. Ph. D. Thesis, University of Berne
29. Recke P von der, Hansen MA, Overgaard K, Christiansen C (1996) The impact of degenerative conditions in the spine on bone mineral density and fracture risk prediction. Osteoporos Int 6:43–49
30. Resch A, Schneider B, Bernecker P, Battmann A, Wergedal J, Willvonseder R, Resch H (1995) Risk of vertebral fractures in men: relationship to mineral density of the vertebral body. AJR Am J Roentgenol 164:1447–1450
31. Roberts S, Urban JP, Evans H, Eisenstein SM (1996) Transport properties of the human cartilage endplate in relation to its composition and calcification. Spine 21:415–420
32. Roberts S, McCall IW, Menage J, Haddaway MJ, Eisenstein SM (1997) Does the thickness of the vertebral subchondral bone reflect the composition of the intervertebral disc? Eur Spine J 6:385–389
33. Shirado O, Kaneda K, Tadano S, Ishikawa H, McAfee PC, Warden KE (1992) Influence of disc degeneration on mechanism of thoracolumbar burst fractures. Spine 17:286–292
34. Silva MJ, Wang C, Keaveny TM, Hayes WC (1994) Direct and computed tomography thickness measurements of the human, lumbar vertebral shell and endplate. Bone 15:409–414
35. Silva MJ, Keaveny TM, Hayes WC (1997) Load sharing between the shell and centrum in the lumbar vertebral body. Spine 22:140–150
36. Twomey LT, Taylor JR (1987) Age changes in lumbar vertebrae and intervertebral discs. Clin Orthop 97–104
37. Urban JP, McMullin JF (1988) Swelling pressure of the lumbar intervertebral discs: influence of age, spinal level, composition, and degeneration. Spine 13:179–187
38. Vernon-Roberts B (1988) Disc pathology and disease states. In: Ghosh P (ed) The biology of the intervertebral disc. CRC, Boca Raton, pp 73–120
39. Wagner AL, Murtagh FR, Arrington JA, Stallworth D (2000) Relationship of Schmorl's nodes to vertebral body endplate fractures and acute endplate disk extrusions. AJNR Am J Neuroradiol 21:276–281

Mikayel Grigoryan
Ali Guermazi
Frank W. Roemer
Pierre D. Delmas
Harry K. Genant

Recognizing and reporting osteoporotic vertebral fractures

Abstract Vertebral fractures are the hallmark of osteoporosis, and occur with a higher incidence earlier in life than any other type of osteoporotic fractures. It has been shown that both symptomatic and asymptomatic vertebral fractures are associated with increased morbidity and mortality. Morbidity associated with these fractures includes decreased physical function and social isolation, which have a significant impact on the patient's overall quality of life. Since the majority of vertebral fractures do not come to clinical attention, radiographic diagnosis is considered to be the best way to identify and confirm the presence of osteoporotic vertebral fractures in clinical practice. Traditionally, conventional lateral radiographs of the thoracolumbar spine have been visually evaluated by radiologists or clinicians to identify vertebral fractures. The two most widely used methods to determine the severity of such fractures in clinical research are the semiquantitative assessment of vertebral deformities, which is based on visual evaluation, and the quantitative approach, which is based on different morphometric criteria. In our practice for osteoporosis evaluation we use the Genant semiquantitative approach: an accurate and reproducible method tested and applied in many clinical studies. The newest generation of fan-beam DXA systems delivering "high-resolution" lateral spine images offers a potential practical alternative to radiographs for clinical vertebral fracture analysis. The advantages of using DXA over conventional radiographic devices are its minimal radiation exposure and high-speed image acquisition. It also allows combined evaluation of vertebral fracture status and bone mass density, which could become a standard for patient evaluation in osteoporosis. The disadvantage of DXA use is that upper thoracic vertebrae cannot be evaluated in a substantial number of patients due to poor imaging quality. We truly believe that the that there is a major role for radiologists and clinicians alike to carefully assess and diagnose vertebral fractures using standardized grading schemes such as the one outlined in this review. Quantitative morphometry is useful in the context of epidemiological studies and clinical drug trials; however, the studies would be flawed if quantitative morphometry were to be performed in isolation without additional adjudication by a trained and highly experienced radiologist or clinician.

Keywords Osteoporosis · Vertebral fractures · Semiquantitative assessment · Bone mineral density · Quantitative morphometry

M. Grigoryan · A. Guermazi
F. W. Roemer · H. K. Genant (✉)
Osteoporosis and
Arthritis Research Group,
Department of Radiology,
University of California San Francisco,
350 Parnassus Avenue,
San Francisco, CA 94117, USA
Tel.: +1-415-4763680,
Fax: +1-415-4768550,
e-mail: Harry.Genant@oarg.ucsf.edu

P. D. Delmas
Hopital Edouard Herriot,
Place d'Arsonval, Pavillion F,
69347 Lyon, Cedex 03, France

Introduction

Osteoporosis is a serious public health problem. The incidence of osteoporotic fractures increases with age. As life expectancy increases for a greater proportion of the world's population, the financial and human costs associated with osteoporotic fractures will multiply exponentially. According to the International Osteoporosis Foundation, more than 40% of middle-aged women in Europe will suffer one or more osteoporotic fracture during their remaining lifetime [23].

Vertebral fractures are the hallmark of osteoporosis and occur with a higher incidence earlier in life than any other type of osteoporotic fractures, including hip fractures [34]. The importance of fragility fractures, of which vertebral fractures are the most common, was acknowledged by the World Health Organization classification criteria for osteoporosis evaluation [51]. The criterion of the World Health Organization defines "severe osteoporosis" as "low bone mass (T score below –2.5) in the presence of one or more fragility fractures."

The definition of osteoporosis is centered on the level of bone mass, which is measured as bone mineral density (BMD). BMD measurements are widely used to estimate the risk of osteoporotic fractures and individuals who are at risk for osteoporotic fractures are usually referred for BMD measurements under the current standard of care. In addition, many other risk factors have been identified, some of which are known to add to the risk independently of BMD measurements. The combination of BMD with such risk factors increases the gradient of risk/standard deviation than that achieved by BMD alone. Several clinical trials have demonstrated that a substantial improvement in the assessment of the risk for future fractures can be accomplished by the assessment of prevalent vertebral fractures in combination with BMD measurements [2, 5, 15, 27, 31, 36, 39, 41]. Nonetheless, it remains a common clinical practice to consider "low" BMD to be a risk factor irrespective of the presence of vertebral fractures.

Clinical identification of vertebral fractures

It has been shown that both symptomatic and asymptomatic vertebral fractures are associated with increased morbidity [9] and mortality [8, 22, 35]. Morbidity associated with these fractures includes decreased physical function and social isolation, which have a significant impact on the patient's overall quality of life [16]. Still, it remains difficult to determine the exact incidence of osteoporotic vertebral fractures that occur annually, as a substantial proportion remains clinically undetected. Large-scale prospective studies demonstrate that only about one of four vertebral fractures becomes clinically recognized [7]. This is due to both the absence of specific symptoms in some and the difficulty in determining the cause of possible physical symptoms such as pain or height loss. Therefore the evaluation of spinal radiographs for prevalent and incident vertebral fractures is important in both clinical and epidemiological evaluation of patients with established osteoporosis and populations at risk for developing it. Fewer than 1% of back pain episodes are related to vertebral fractures [10]. Therefore vertebral fractures are often not suspected in patients reporting back pain, unless associated with trauma. Trauma-related fractures, however, are not considered as classical osteoporotic fractures. Historical height loss is also difficult to assess clinically. Some height loss is expected with aging due to compression of the intervertebral discs and postural changes. However, height loss could also be due to multiple fractures, which represent significant and irreparable damage. Therefore it has been concluded that height loss is an unreliable indicator of fracture status until it exceeds 4 cm [9]. As a result vertebral fractures are often not being considered in clinical patient evaluation, and it is relatively uncommon for patients to be referred for radiographs in the course of osteoporosis testing. Improvements in detecting and reporting vertebral fractures in patients with osteoporosis would increase the potential of therapeutic intervention to prevent subsequent fractures.

Radiographic assessment of vertebral fractures

Radiographic diagnosis is considered to be the best way to identify and confirm the presence of osteoporotic vertebral fractures in clinical practice. Traditionally, conventional lateral radiographs of the thoracolumbar spine have been visually evaluated by radiologists or clinicians to identify vertebral fractures. However, there is still no internationally agreed definition for vertebral fracture. One global prospective study (the IMPACT study [6]) compared the results of local radiographic reports from five continents with that of subsequent central readings in more than 2,000 postmenopausal women with osteoporosis. This study demonstrated that vertebral fractures were frequently underdiagnosed radiologically worldwide, with false-negative rates as high as 30% despite a strict radiographic protocol that provided an unambiguous vertebral fracture definition and minimized the influence of inadequate film quality. It was concluded that the failure was a global problem attributable to either lack of radiographic detection or use of ambiguous terminology in reports. Therefore it is very important to use standardized methods for the visual assessment of vertebral fractures.

Several standardized approaches to describe vertebral fractures have been proposed. They may serve to facilitate the diagnosis of osteoporosis and to assess the severity or progression of the disease as well as to rule out nonfracture deformities or normal variants.

Visual semiquantitative methods of vertebral fracture assessment

The first standardized approach was introduced by Smith et al. [44] in 1960. They introduced a classification of vertebral deformities as diagnosed from lateral thoracolumbar radiographs for the purpose of diagnosing the severity of osteoporosis. This method grades only the most severely deformed vertebra on the radiograph. In 1968 Meunier [33] proposed an approach in which each vertebra is graded according to its shape or deformity. Grade 1 is assigned to a normal vertebra that has no deformity, grade 2 to a biconcave vertebra, and grade 4 to an endplate fracture or a wedged or crushed vertebra. Using this approach vertebral bodies T3 (or T7) to L4 are evaluated. A "radiological vertebral index" can be calculated as the sum of the grades of all vertebrae, or as the quotient of this sum and the number of the vertebrae.

Kleerkoper et al. [26] modified Meunier's radiological vertebral index and introduced the so-called "vertebral deformity score." In the vertebral deformity score each vertebra from T4 to L5 is assigned an individual score from 0 to 3 depending on the type of deformity. This grading scheme is based on the reduction in the anterior, middle, and posterior vertebral heights (h_a, h_m, and h_p, respectively). A vertebral deformity (graded 1–3) is present when h_a, h_m, or h_p is reduced by at least 4 mm or 15%. This score, as with Meunier's radiological vertebral index, still relies very much on the type of deformity, i.e., the vertebral shape, and there would have to be changes in vertebral shape in order to account for incident vertebral fractures on follow-up radiographs. Furthermore, the majority of vertebral fractures consist of a combination of wedge and endplate deformities, and less frequently posterior deformities. Therefore an examiner's distinction among these deformities is often quite subjective.

A vertebral deformity does not always represent a vertebral fracture, but a vertebral fracture is always a vertebral deformity. From a radiological prospective, there are many potential differential diagnoses for vertebral deformities – osteoporotic fracture, posttraumatic deformity, degenerative remodeling, Scheuermann's disease (juvenile kyphosis), congenital anomaly, neoplastic deformity, and Paget's disease – and the correct qualitative classification of vertebral deformities can be accomplished only by visual inspection and expert interpretation of the radiograph. This perspective on vertebral fracture diagnosis is perhaps reflected at its best in the semiquantitative fracture assessment method proposed by Genant et al. [12, 13, 14, 15] This method provides an insight into the severity of a

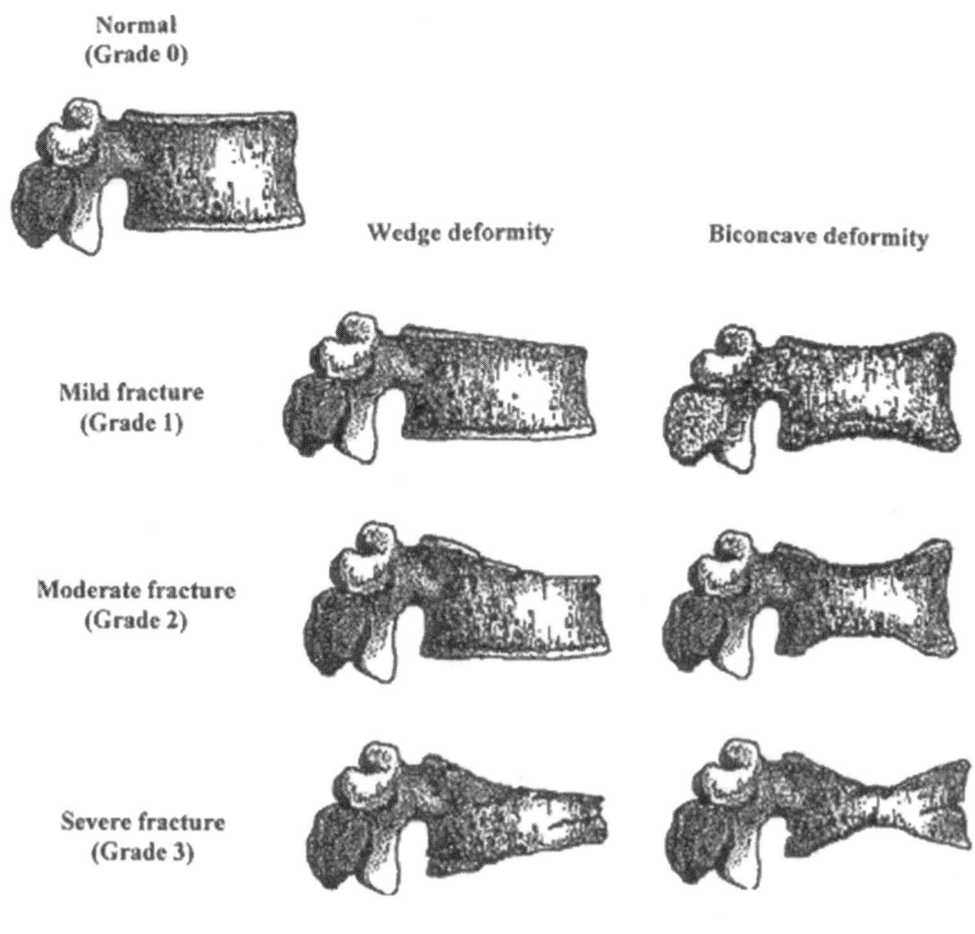

Fig. 1 Schematic diagram of semiquantitative grading scale for vertebral fractures. (From Genant et al. [13])

fracture which is assessed solely by visual estimation of the extent of a vertebral height reduction and morphological change, and vertebral fractures are differentiated from other, nonfracture deformities. In Genant's visual semiquantitative assessment (Fig. 1) each vertebra receives a severity grade based upon the visually apparent degree of vertebral height loss. Unlike the other approaches the type of the deformity (wedge, biconcavity, or compression) is no longer linked to the grading of a fracture in this approach.

Thoracic and lumbar vertebrae from T4 to L4 are graded on visual inspection and without direct vertebral measurement as normal (grade 0), mildly deformed (grade 1: reduction of 20–25% of height and 10–20% of projected vertebral area), moderately deformed (grade 2: reduction of 26–40% of height and 21–40% of projected vertebral area), and severely deformed (grade 3: reduction of >40% of height and projected vertebral area; Fig. 2). A grade 0.5 designates "borderline" vertebrae that show some deformation but cannot be clearly assigned to grade 1 fractures is sometimes also utilized. In addition to height reductions, careful attention is given to alterations in the shape and configuration of the vertebrae relative to adjacent vertebrae and expected normal appearances. These features add a strong qualitative aspect to the interpretation. For example, vertebral deformities due to degenerative changes should be ruled out, whereas an endplate vertebral fracture can be identified without a 20% reduction in the vertebral height. Nevertheless, in experienced, highly trained hands, it makes the approach both sensitive and specific. A "spinal fracture index") can be calculated from this semiquantitative assessment as the sum of all grades assigned to the vertebrae divided by the number of the evaluated vertebrae.

An advantage of this semiquantitative approach over other standardized visual approaches is that the severity of the deformation as the reduction in vertebral height means can be assessed from serial films and is especially useful for the interpretation of incident fractures. It considers the continuous character of vertebral fractures and makes a meaningful interpretation of follow-up radiographs possible. Furthermore, inevitably arbitrary decisions regarding wedge, endplate, or crush deformities, as assessed in some grading schemes, are not necessary since most fractures

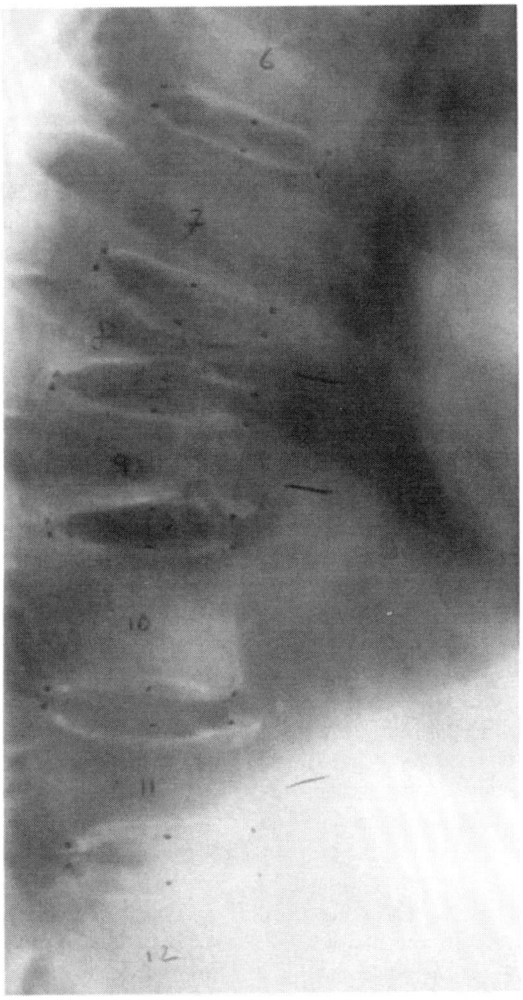

Fig. 2 Lateral thoracic radiograph shows a grade 3 fracture T8 and grade 2 fractures of T9 and T11

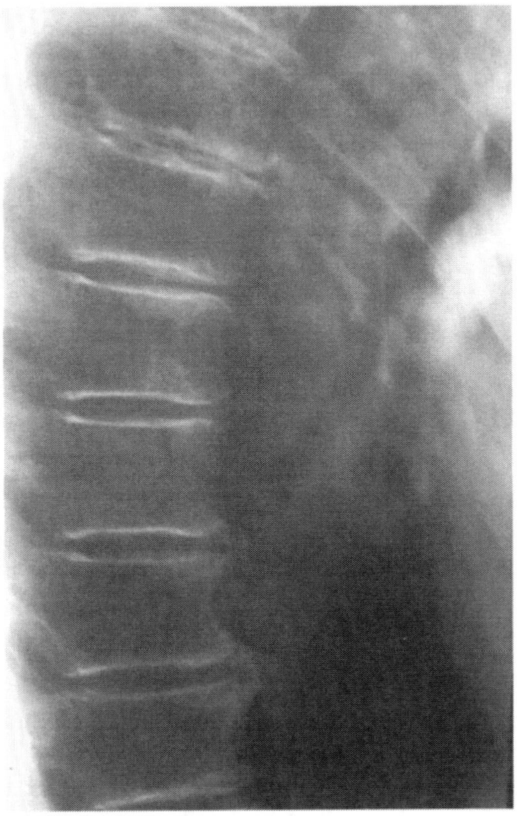

Fig. 3 Degenerative remodeling in middle-thoracic region simulating wedge deformities

contain a combination of these features, influenced by the local biomechanics of the spinal level.

The Genant's semiquantitative method has been tested and applied in a number of clinical drug trials and epidemiological studies [15, 20, 47, 50, 52]. The reproducibility of the method for the diagnosis of prevalent and incident vertebral fractures was found to be high, with intraobserver agreement of 93–99% and interobserver agreement of 90–99%. This indicates that close agreement among readers can be reached using this standardized visual semiquantitative grading method, and that subjectivity in the readings can be reduced. This accounts for experienced and relatively inexperienced readers with reasonable results.

There are limitations of this semiquantitative grading scheme that may also apply to other standardized approaches. For example, from the morphometric data on normal subjects we know that vertebrae in the middle thoracic spine (especially in women) and thoracolumbar junction (especially in men) are slightly more wedged than in other regions (Fig. 3) [3, 30, 32, 40]. As a result these normal variations may be misinterpreted as mild vertebral deformities, thereby falsely increasing prevalence values for vertebral fractures. The same applies to a lesser extent to the middle to lower lumbar spine, where some degree of biconcavity is frequently observed [26, 45]. Accurate diagnosis of prevalent fractures which requires distinguishing between normal variations and the degenerative changes from true fractures still depends on the experience of the observer. It has been argued that the diagnosis of mild vertebral fractures (grade 0.5–1) in particular may be quite subjective, and that these fractures may be unrelated to osteoporosis [45]. However, mild fractures are also associated with a lower bone density and to a certain extend predict future vertebral fractures [1].

Other limitations may apply for the diagnosis of incident fractures. The reader may sometimes feel that even though a further height reduction is seen in a previous vertebral fracture, it may not be justified to assign a higher fracture grade on a serial radiograph, since some degree of settling or remodeling generally occurs. Therefore in general, serial radiographs including the baseline radiograph of a patient should be viewed together so that incident fractures can be readily identified as only those progressive changes that lead to a full increase in deformity grade or from a questionable deformity (grade 0.5) to a definite fracture.

Quantitative morphometry and its comparison with the semiquantitative methods

Quantitative morphometric assessment of vertebral deformity was introduced in order to obtain an objective and reproducible measurement, using rigorously defined point placement and well-defined algorithms for fracture definition [3, 42]. Typically six points are used to derive the anterior height (h_a), the central (middle or middle-vertebral, h_m) height, and the posterior height (h_p; Fig. 4). This exclusively quantitative approach has, however, a number of drawbacks including projectional effects that significantly influence the reliability of these measures performed in isolation.

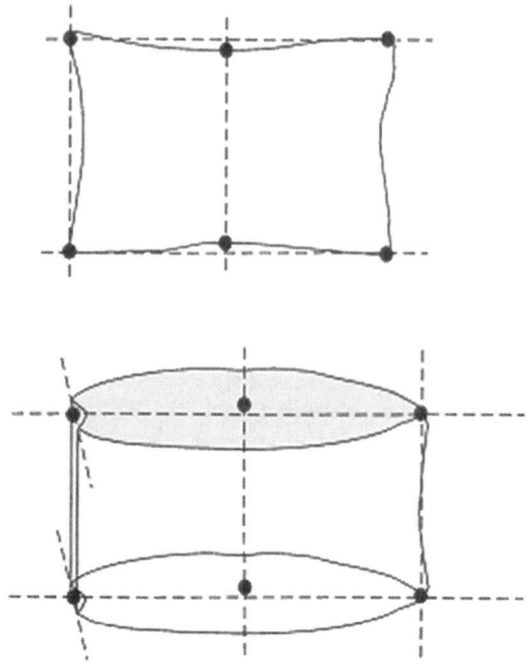

Fig. 4 Example of six-point placement in quantitative vertebral morphometry

In general, a substantial number of mild deformities detected by visual reading are missed by the quantitative technique when applying the common threshold values for reduction in vertebral heights such as 15–20% or 3 SD decrease. Furthermore, a significant number of false positives are found with quantitative techniques. The choice of point placement in the quantitative technique, but especially the choice of the threshold for defining vertebral deformity, gives results that vary in specificity and sensitivity. Most of the moderate to severe deformities are detected by both techniques. However, only expert visual evaluation can detect mild and subtle deformities, as well as appreciate anatomical, pathological and technical issues that bear on the evaluation of fracture detection.

The strength of a semiquantitative approach is that it makes use of the entire spectrum of visible features that are helpful in identifying deformities [15, 49]. The visual interpretation, when performed by the expert eye, also separates true deformities from normal or anomalous vertebrae. In addition to changes in dimension, vertebral deformities are generally detected visually by the presence of endplate deformities, the lack of parallelism of the endplates, and the general altered appearance compared with neighboring vertebrae. Some of these visual characteristics are not captured by the six-digitization points used in quantitative techniques; this can cause some deformities to remain undetected. For example, only an experienced observer can make the subtle distinctions between a fractured endplate and wedge shaped appearance caused by the remodeling of the vertebral bodies in degenerative disc disease (Fig. 3). This is often interpreted as a wedge fracture in quantitative studies.

In the absence of distinct characteristics of a fracture, however, a reader using a visual approach could rather arbitrarily consider a mild wedge deformity normal, anomalous, or fractured; in such a case, a well-defined quantitative criterion could be useful. Even here, however, with borderline wedge deformity, small subjective difference in joint placement could result in considerable variation in fracture/nonfracture discrimination of sequential films or even on the same film.

Most incident fractures, as with prevalent fractures, are easily identifiable visually on sequential radiographs. The unavoidable variation in position and parallax may result in differences in point placement on follow-up radiographs. This can result in the morphometric detection of an incident fracture that would be interpreted visually as simply an alteration in projection. These sources of false-positive or false-negative interpretation are especially common when parallax problems due to radiographic technique or patient positioning are encountered.

Intraobserver variability for a semi-quantitative approach depends on experience and training. The same however, is true for digitizing techniques: an experienced observer is more consistent in the placement of the points for digitization.

A number of comparative studies have evaluated the relative performance of the quantitative morphometric and the semiquantitative methods and moderate correlations were found in most of them [1, 17, 29, 52]. The concordance was high for fractures defined as moderate or severe by semiquantitative reading. There was, however, a significant discordance for fractures defined as mild in the semiquantitative reading. Additionally, the interobserver agreement was demonstrated to be better for the visual semiquantitative approach. The authors of these studies concluded that quantitative morphometry should not be performed in isolation, particularly when applying highly sensitive morphometric criteria at low threshold levels without visual assessment to confirm the detected prevalent or incident vertebral deformities as probable fractures.

Standardization of visual approaches to vertebral fracture assessment

In an effort to develop a standardized consensus protocol for the visual assessment of vertebral fractures, the United States National Osteoporosis Foundation's Working Group on Vertebral Fractures suggested the following procedural requirements for a qualitative (semiquantitative) assessment of vertebral fractures in osteoporosis research [25]:

- Assessments should be performed by a radiologist or trained clinician who has specific expertise in the radiology of osteoporosis.
- Qualitative and semiquantitative assessments should be performed according to a written protocol of fracture definitions, which are sufficiently detailed that the readings can be reproduced by other experts. Reference to an atlas of standard films or illustrations may be helpful. It is recommended that a standardized protocol be developed by a consensus of expert radiologists.
- The definition of fracture should include deformities of the endplates and anterior borders of vertebral bodies, as well as generalized collapse of a vertebral body.
- Grading of the extent of each fracture should employ discrete, mutually exclusive categories. An atlas of standard films and illustrations may again help to assure consistency.

There is some subjectivity in each method, and performing the grading in discrete, exclusive categories may be problematic at times, particularly for prevalent fractures. However, for the assessment of vertebral fractures in the form of a fracture/nonfracture dichotomy, trained readers have achieved excellent results. After all, the fracture/nonfracture distinction may be the most important, and the semiquantitative standardized grading schemes may be the instruments to make this diagnosis reliable and valid.

Ensuring the reliability of the interpretation of incident vertebral fractures on serial radiographs requires close attention to the procedure. Serial radiographs of a patient should always be viewed together in chronological order to accomplish a thorough and reliable analysis of all new fractures. Because a vertebral fracture is a permanent event that is unlikely to vanish on follow-up radiograph, temporal blinding does not appear to be any use: most readers easily identify a temporal sequence of films by new deformities as well as by progressive disc degeneration and osteophyte formation, which are universal among the elderly.

Alternatives to radiographic assessment of vertebral fractures

Because of the difficulty in identifying vertebral fractures clinically, and the practical difficulties preventing routine radiographic assessment at the point of care, vertebral fracture status is frequently unknown at the time of patient evaluation for BMD [18]. Hence the interest in morphometric assessment from dual X-ray absorptiometry (DXA) images was a natural consequence of the need for quantitative fracture evaluation in pharmaceutical trials. The main advantage of the morphometric X-ray absorptiome-

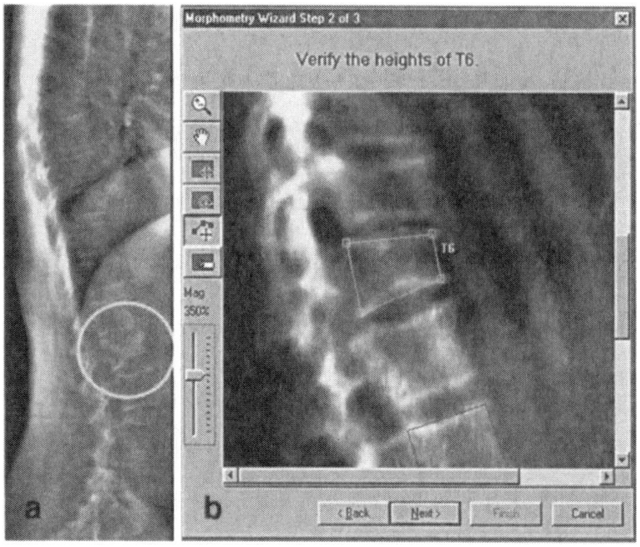

Fig. 5 Rapid (10-s) "high-resolution" fan-beam DXA imaging allows both visual (**a**) and quantitative (**b**) assessment of vertebral fractures

try technique is that the radiation dose to the patient is substantially reduced compared with conventional radiography. The use of "high-resolution" lateral spine images, obtained with fan-beam X-ray bone densitometry systems (Fig. 5), offers a potential practical alternative to radiographs for clinical vertebral fracture analysis. "High-resolution" fan-beam DXA systems, utilizing technology similar to that used by computed tomography (CT) systems, can image the lateral spine in as little as 10 s. In fact CT scout scans, with about the same image resolution as fan-beam DXA scans, have been used for vertebral fracture identification [24, 43, 48].

As with radiographs, however, CT images are expensive and are not available clinically without referral. Consequently CT is not generally an option unless performed in conjunction with quantitative CT for BMD assessment. In contrast, DXA images can be performed at the point of care, in conjunction with standard BMD determination, with a radiation dose as much as 100 times lower than that of conventional radiographs. The most notable strength of radiographs, of course, is image resolution, which is superior to that of DXA images.

DXA images provide several advantages. The digital nature allows for electronic data storage, digital image enhancement and processing, as with magnification and contrast adjustment, which is not possible with conventional radiographic techniques. Cone-beam distortion, inherent in the radiographic technique, is not present when using the scanning fan-beam geometry of DXA devices. Low-dose, single-energy acquisition modes are substantially faster than dual energy scan modes due to substantially lower signal to noise in the images and can be performed during suspended respiration. High-dose, dual-energy acquisitions, while slower, generally provide higher bone contrast images and sometimes reduce artifacts.

The use of fan-beam DXA images for quantitative (morphometric) assessment of spinal fractures has been reported in both research applications and pharmaceutical trials [4, 11, 19, 21, 28, 37, 38, 46]. Clinical studies demonstrated the feasibility of visual evaluation of fan-beam lateral DXA spine images compared to conventional lateral spine radiographs in postmenopausal women, with a strong overall agreement of 96.3% [37, 38]. This agreement was approximately as strong as that found among different morphometric techniques [15, 21]. The images permitted visual assessment of about 90% of all vertebrae. The main shortcoming of the MXA scans in comparison with conventional radiographs is the inferior image quality that limits the evaluation of vertebrae in the upper thoracic spine. This is less of a concern if MXA is used as a screening tool for conventional radiography and this approach may help reduce the radiation dose in the diagnosis and monitoring of osteoporosis.

Conclusion

Vertebral fractures are the most common type of osteoporotic fracture, occurring in a substantial portion of the elderly population. Most new vertebral fractures, even painful ones, remain unrecognized by patients and their physicians. It is established that the presence of a vertebral fracture is a strong risk factor for subsequent osteoporotic fractures, and that those with low bone density and vertebral fractures are at highest risk. Large-scale clinical trials have demonstrated that osteoporosis therapies can reverse bone loss and reduce fracture rates, and that these benefits are most pronounced in patients with low BMD and vertebral fractures. Clinical guidelines promulgated by the National Osteoporosis Foundation, International Osteoporosis Foundation, and others recognize the importance of vertebral fractures, along with BMD, as the key risk factors for use in patient evaluation. However, while BMD is widely used in patient evaluation, radiological assessment of vertebral fractures is commonly not performed, or if performed, is inadequately standardized and interpreted. By understanding the clinical principles of osteoporosis diagnosis and management provided in this document and by adopting the radiological guidelines for assessing vertebral fractures provided herein, clinicians worldwide can contribute substantially to reducing the consequences of this important disease.

References

1. Black D, Palermo L, Nevitt MC, Genant HK, Epstein R, San Valentin R, Cummings SR, and the Study of Osteoporotic Fractures Research Group (1995) Comparison of methods for defining prevalent vertebral deformities: the study of osteoporotic fractures. J Bone Miner Res 10:890–902
2. Black DM, Arden NK, Palermo L, Pearson J, Cummings SR (1999) Prevalent vertebral deformities predict hip fractures and new vertebral deformities but not wrist fractures. Study of Osteoporotic Fractures Research Group. J Bone Miner Res 14:821–828
3. Black DM, Cummings SR, Stone K, Hudes E, Palermo L, Steiger P (1991) A new approach to defining normal vertebral dimensions. J Bone Miner Res 6:883–892
4. Blake GM, Rea JA, Fogelman I (1997) Vertebral morphometry studies using dual-energy X-ray absorptiometry. Semin Nucl Med 27:276–290
5. Davis JW, Grove JS, Wasnich RD, Ross PD (1999) Spatial relationships between prevalent and incident spine fractures. Bone 24:261–264
6. Delmas PD, Watts N, Eastell R, von Ingersleben G, van de Langerijt L, Cahall DL (2001) Underdiagnosis of vertebral fractures is a worldwide problem: The IMPACT Study. J Bone Miner Res 16 Suppl. 1:S139
7. Ensrud KE, Nevitt MC, Palermo L, Cauley JA, Griffith JM, Genant HK, Black DM (1999) What proportion of incident morphometric vertebral fractures are clinically diagnosed and vice versa? J Bone Miner Res 14:S138
8. Ensrud KE, Thompson DE, Cauley JA, Nevitt MC, Kado DM, Hochberg MC, Santora AC 2nd, Black DM (2000) Prevalent vertebral deformities predict mortality and hospitalization in older women with low bone mass. Fracture Intervention Trial Research Group. J Am Geriatr Soc 48:241–249
9. Ettinger B, Black DM, Nevitt MC, Rundle AC, Cauley JA, Cummings SR, Genant HK (1992) Contribution of vertebral deformities to chronic back pain and disability. The Study of Osteoporotic Fractures Research Group. J Bone Miner Res 7:449–456
10. Ettinger B, Cooper C (1995) Clinical assessment of osteoporotic vertebral fractures. In: Genant HK, Jergas M, van Kuijk C (ed) Vertebral fracture in osteoporosis. Radiology Research and Education Foundation, San Francisco, pp 15–20
11. Ferrar L, Jiang G, Eastell R, Peel NF (2003) Visual identification of vertebral fractures in osteoporosis using morphometric X-ray absorptiometry. J Bone Miner Res 18:933–938
12. Genant HK, Jergas M (2003) Assessment of prevalent and incident vertebral fractures in osteoporosis research. Osteoporos Int 14 Suppl 3:S43–S55
13. Genant HK, Jergas M, Palermo L, Nevitt MC, Valentin RS, Black D, Cummings SR (1996) Comparison of semiquantitative visual and quantitative morphometric assessment of prevalent and incident vertebral fractures in osteoporosis. The Study of Osteoporotic Fractures Research Group. J Bone Miner Res 11:984–996
14. Genant HK, van Kuijk C, Jergas M (1995) Vertebral fracture in osteoporosis. Radiology Research and Education Foundation, San Francisco
15. Genant HK, Wu CY, van Kuijk C, Nevitt MC (1993) Vertebral fracture assessment using a semiquantitative technique. J Bone Miner Res 8:1137–1148
16. Gold DT (2001) The nonskeletal consequences of osteoporotic fractures. Psychologic and social outcomes. Rheum Dis Clin North Am 27:255–262
17. Grados F, Roux C, de Vernejoul MC, Utard G, Sebert JL, Fardellone P (2001) Comparison of four morphometric definitions and a semiquantitative consensus reading for assessing prevalent vertebral fractures. Osteoporos Int 12:716–722
18. Guermazi A, Mohr A, Grigorian M, Taouli B, Genant HK (2002) Identification of vertebral fractures in osteoporosis. Semin Musculoskelet Radiol 6:241–252
19. Hans D, Baiada A, Dubouef F, Vignot E, Bochu M, Meunier P. Expert-XL (1996) Clinical evaluation of a new morphometric technique on 21 patients with vertebral fracture. Osteoporos Int 6:79
20. Heuck AF, Block J, Glueer CC, Steiger P, Genant HK (1989) Mild versus definite osteoporosis: comparison of bone densitometry techniques using different statistical models. J Bone Miner Res 4: 891–900
21. Jergas M, Lang TF, Fuerst T (1995) Morphometric X-ray absorptiometry. In: Genant HK, Jergas M, van Kuijk C (ed) Vertebral fracture in osteoporosis. Radiology Research and Education Foundation Publishers, San Francisco, pp 331–348
22. Kado DM, Duong T, Stone KL, Ensrud KE, Nevitt MC, Greendale GA, Cummings SR (2003) Incident vertebral fractures and mortality in older women: a prospective study. Osteoporos Int 14: 589–594
23. Kanis JA, Delmas P, Burckhardt P, Cooper C, Torgerson D (1997) Guidelines for diagnosis and management of osteoporosis. The European Foundation for Osteoporosis and Bone Disease. Osteoporos Int 7:390–406
24. Katragadda CS, Fogel SR, Cohen G, Wagner LK, Morgan C 3rd, Handel SF, Amtey SR, Lester RG (1979) Digital radiography using a computed tomographic instrument. Radiology 133: 83–87
25. Kiel D (1995) Assessing vertebral fractures. National Osteoporosis Foundation Working Group on Vertebral Fractures. J Bone Miner Res 10:518–523
26. Kleerekoper M, Nelson DA (1992) Vertebral fracture or vertebral deformity. Calcif Tissue Int 50:5–6
27. Kotowicz MA, Melton LJ 3rd, Cooper C, Atkinson EJ, O'Fallon WM, Riggs BL (1994) Risk of hip fracture in women with vertebral fracture. J Bone Miner Res 9:599–605
28. Lang T, Takada M, Gee R, Wu C, Li J, Hayashi-Clark C, Schoen S, March V, Genant HK (1997) A preliminary evaluation of the lunar expert-XL for bone densitometry and vertebral morphometry. J Bone Miner Res 12:136–143
29. Leidig-Bruckner G, Genant HK, Minne HW, Storm T, Thamsborg G, Bruckner T, Sauer P, Schilling T, Soerensen OH, Ziegler R (1994) Comparison of a semiquantitative and a quantitative method for assessing vertebral fractures in osteoporosis. Osteoporos Int 4:154–161
30. McCloskey EV, Spector TD, Eyres KS, Fern ED, O'Rourke N, Vasikaran S, Kanis JA (1993) The assessment of vertebral deformity: a method for use in population studies and clinical trials. Osteoporos Int 3:138–147
31. Melton LJ III, Kan SH, Frye MA, Wahner HW, O'Fallon WM, Riggs BL (1989) Epidemiology of vertebral fractures in women. Am J Epidemiol 129: 1000–1011
32. Melton LJ 3rd, Atkinson EJ, Cooper C, O'Fallon WM, Riggs BL (1999) Vertebral fractures predict subsequent fractures. Osteoporos Int 10:214–221
33. Meunier P (1968) La dynamique du remaniement osseux humain, etudiee par lecture quantitative de la biopsie osseuse. Lyon

34. Meunier PJ, Delmas PD, Eastell R, McClung MR, Papapoulos S, Rizzoli R, Seeman E, Wasnich RD (1999) Diagnosis and management of osteoporosis in postmenopausal women: clinical guidelines. International Committee for Osteoporosis Clinical Guidelines. Clin Ther 21:1025–44. Review
35. Nevitt MC, Ettinger B, Black DM, Stone K, Jamal SA, Ensrud K, Segal M, Genant HK, Cummings SR (1998) The association of radiographically detected vertebral fractures with back pain and function: a prospective study Ann Intern Med 128:793–800
36. Nevitt MC, Ross PD, Palermo L, Musliner T, Genant HK, Thompson DE (1999) Association of prevalent vertebral fractures, bone density, and alendronate treatment with incident vertebral fractures: effect of number and spinal location of fractures. The Fracture Intervention Trial Research Group. Bone 25:613–619
37. Rea JA, Li J, Blake GM, Steiger P, Genant HK, Fogelman I (2000) Visual assessment of vertebral deformity by X-ray absorptiometry: a highly predictive method to exclude vertebral deformity. Osteoporos Int 11:660–668
38. Rea JA, Steiger P, Blake GM, Fogelman I (1998) Optimizing data acquisition and analysis of morphometric X-ray absorptiometry. Osteoporos Int 8:177–183
39. Ross PD, Davis JW, Epstein RS, Wasnich RD (1991) Pre-existing fractures and bone mass predict vertebral fracture incidence in women. Ann Intern Med 114:919–923
40. Ross PD, Davis JW, Epstein RS, Wasnich RD (1992) Ability of vertebral dimensions from a single radiograph to identify fractures. Calcif Tissue Int 51: 95–99
41. Ross PD, Genant HK, Davis JW, Miller PD, Wasnich RD (1993) Predicting vertebral fracture incidence from prevalent fractures and bone density among non-black, osteoporotic women. Osteoporos Int 3:120–126
42. Ross PD, Yhee YK, He YF, Davis JW, Kamimoto C, Epstein RS et al (1993) A new method for vertebral fracture diagnosis. J Bone Miner Res 8:167–174
43. Sener RN, Ripeckyj GT, Otto PM, Rauch RA, Jinkins JR (1993) Recognition of abnormalities on computed scout images in CT examinations of the head and spine. Neuroradiology 35: 229–231
44. Smith RW, Eyler WR, Mellinger RC (1960) On the incidence of osteoporosis. Ann Intern Med 52:773–781
45. Spector TD, McCloskey EV, Doyle DV, Kanis JA (1993) Prevalence of vertebral fracture in women and the relationship with bone density and symptoms: the Chingford Study. J Bone Miner Res 8:817–822
46. Steiger P, Cummings SR, Genant HK, Weiss H (1994) Morphometric X-ray absorptiometry of the spine: correlation in vivo with morphometric radiography. Study of Osteoporotic Fractures Research Group. Osteoporos Int 4: 238–244
47. Storm T, Thamsborg G, Steiniche T, Genant HK, Sørenson OH (1990) Effect of intermittent cyclical etidronate therapy on bone mass and fracture rate in women with postmenopausal osteoporosis. N Engl J Med 322:1265–1271
48. Takada M, Wu CY, Lang TF, Genant HK (1998) Vertebral fracture assessment using the lateral scoutview of computed tomography in comparison with radiographs. Osteoporos Int 8: 197–203
49. Van Kuijk C, Genant HK (1995) Radiology in osteoporosis. In: Riggs BL, Melton LJ (eds) Osteoporosis. Raven, New York
50. Watts NB, Harris ST, Genant HK, Wasnich RD, Miller PD, Jackson RD, Licata AA, Ross P, Woodson GCI, Yanover MJ, Mysiw J, Kohse L, Rao MB, Steiger P, Richmond B, Chesnut CHI (1990) Intermittent cyclical etidronate treatment of postmenopausal osteoporosis. N Engl J Med 323:73–79
51. World Health Organization (1994) Assessment of fracture risk and its application to screening for postmenopausal osteoporosis. Report of a WHO study group. WHO technical report series, Geneva, pp 843:1–129
52. Wu CY, Li J, Jergas M, Genant HK (1994) Semiquantitative and quantitative assessment of incident fractures: comparison of methods. J Bone Miner Res 9:S157

REVIEW

Alexander G. Hadjipavlou
Paul G. Katonis
Michael N. Tzermiadianos
George M. Tsoukas
George Sapkas

Principles of management of osteometabolic disorders affecting the aging spine

Abstract Osteoporosis is the most common contributing factor of spinal fractures, which characteristically are not generally known to produce spinal cord compression symptoms. Recently, an increasing number of medical reports have implicated osteoporotic fractures as a cause of serious neurological deficit and painful disabling spinal deformities. This has been corroborated by the present authors as well. These complications are only amenable to surgical management, requiring instrumentation. Instrumenting an osteoporotic spine, although a challenging task, can be accomplished if certain guidelines for surgical techniques are respected. Neurological deficits respond equally well to an anterior or posterior decompression, provided this is coupled with multisegmental fixation of the construct. With the steady increase in the elderly population, it is anticipated that the spine surgeon will face serious complications of osteoporotic spines more frequently. With regard to surgery, however, excellent correction of deformities can be achieved, by combining anterior and posterior approaches. Paget's disease of bone (PD) is a non-hormonal osteometabolic disorder and the spine is the second most commonly affected site. About one-third of patients with spinal involvement exhibit symptoms of clinical stenosis. In only 12–24% of patients with PD of the spine is back pain attributed solely to PD, while in the majority of patients, back pain is either arthritic in nature or a combination of a pagetic process and coexisting arthritis. In this context, one must be certain before attributing low back pain to PD exclusively, and antipagetic medical treatment alone may be ineffective. Neural element dysfunction may be attributed to compressive myelopathy by pagetic bone overgrowth, pagetic intraspinal soft tissue overgrowth, ossification of epidural fat, platybasia, spontaneous bleeding, sarcomatous degeneration and vertebral fracture or subluxation. Neural dysfunction can also result from spinal ischemia when blood is diverted by the so-called "arterial steal syndrome". Because the effectiveness of pharmacologic treatment for pagetic spinal stenosis has been clearly demonstrated, surgical decompression should only be instituted after failure of antipagetic medical treatment. Surgery is indicated as a primary treatment when neural compression is secondary to pathologic fractures, dislocations, spontaneous epidural hematoma, syringomyelia, platybasia, or sarcomatous transformation. Five classes of drugs are available for the treatment of PD. Bisphosphonates are the most popular antipagetic drug and several forms have been investigated.

Keywords Osteoporosis · Fractures · Neurological deficit · Deformity · Paget's disease · Back pain · Spinal stenosis · Myelopathy · Treatment

A. G. Hadjipavlou (✉) · P. G. Katonis
M. N. Tzermiadianos
School of Health Sciences,
University of Crete,
Department of Orthopaedic Surgery
& Traumatology,
University General Hospital,
PO Box 1352,
71110 Heraklion, Crete, Greece
Tel.: +30-2810-3923724,
Fax: +30-2810-392370,
e-mail: ahadjipa@med.uoc.gr

A. G. Hadjipavlou
Division of Spine Surgery,
Department of Orthopaedic Surgery,
University of Texas Medical Branch
at Galveston, Galveston, Texas, USA

G. M. Tsoukas
Department of Endocrinology,
Montreal General Hospital,
McGill University School of Medicine,
Montreal, Quebec, Canada

G. Sapkas
School of Medicine,
National University of Greece,
Athens, Greece

Introduction

Osteoporosis and Paget's disease of bone are two metabolic conditions that usually affect the aging population. The former is a very common skeletal disorder, whereas Paget's disease affects about 3% of the population. This paper looks at both conditions. It first addresses principles of surgical management of complications caused by osteoporosis of the spine (minimally invasive surgery for these complications will be addressed in a separate paper in this issue). Secondly, it describes spinal involvement of Paget's disease in bone and outlines the best treatment options.

Osteoporosis

Surgical treatment of osteoporosis is still not widely accepted by orthopedic surgeons, nor well known among the medical community at large. However, recently, it has been gaining support for two main reasons. The first is that more in-depth studies, which are detailed below, have shown that osteoporosis is not an innocent disease characterized by minor complications and disabilities, but a serious health problem that can create devastating complications with substantial morbidity and mortality. The second reason is the advancement of medical knowledge and technology, which allows the use of more sophisticated instrumentation and makes it possible to operate successfully on high-risk patients of advanced age who no longer accept physical conditions limiting their life enjoyment.

The extent of disability and the socioeconomic consequences associated with osteoporosis are well known through widely cited publications [24, 94, 112]. It is not the scope of this paper to review this aspect of osteoporosis. However, it is worth highlighting some pertinent statistics regarding the magnitude and implications of osteoporotic vertebral compression fractures (OVCF) in order to emphasize the need for a more specific treatment. OVCF is the most common fracture that may occur after minimal trauma (e.g. bending, turning, etc), or even in the absence (silent) of any obvious trauma [25].

The estimated incidence of OVCF in European Union Member States is 438,700 clinically diagnosed vertebral fractures (117 per 100,000 person-years) [25], while the US epidemiological databases give an annual rate of 700,000 cases [111].

The average duration of hospitalization ranges from 8 to 30 days [111].

The reported periods of disability for cases of OVCF required for bed rest are 25.8 days for the lumbar region and 12.6 days for the thoracic region. The periods of disability required for limited activity are 158.5 days and 73.6 days respectively. Whereas the figures for hip fracture are 21.6 days for bed rest and 101.5 days for limited activity [37].

Apart from physical impairment incurred by the OVCF [87, 126], these patients also experience a substantial deterioration in quality of life and a cascading of psychosocial disorders, such as sleep disturbance, increased depression, lower self-esteem, increased anxiety, diminished social poles and increased dependency on others [127].

The overall mortality rate also appears to be equivalent to hip fractures. A prospective study of 9575 women, followed over 8 years, demonstrated that patients with OVCF have a 23–34% increased mortality rate when compared to patients without OVCF [69]. This study echoes the findings of Cooper et al. [25], who demonstrated in a retrospective study that the 5-year survival rate in patients with OVCF is significantly lower than the expected normal survival rate (61 vs 76%), and almost comparable to the 5-years survival rate after hip fracture. However, in hip fractures, the excess mortality rate occurs within 6 months of the fracture event, whereas in OVCF survival declines steadily after the fracture [25]. Most common causes of death in patients with OVCF are pulmonary problems caused by chronic obstructive pulmonary disease (COPD) and pneumonia (hazard ratio 2.1) [69]. Lung function (FVC, FEV1) is significantly decreased in patients with thoracic and lumbar fracture. It has been estimated that one OVCF may result in 9% loss of forced vital capacity (FVC) [82, 121, 122].

Eighty-five percent of cases of radiologically diagnosed OVCF are associated with back pain, which in the majority of patients is expected to subside within 2–3 months [34]. However, it has been postulated that in one-third of patients, this pain remains as chronic pain, with varying degrees of physical disability [29]. Several reports also indicate that patients with OVCF are at increased risk for subsequent fractures [68, 84, 114]. Most cases of OVCF are wedge compression fractures (type A1), creating varying degrees of kyphotic deformity of the spine, usually not associated with neurological deficit. These fractures are manageable either conservatively (braces, corsets, analgesics and antiresorptive osteoporotic drugs such as calcitonin and bisphosphonates, or parathyroid hormone, apparently the most effective antiosteoporotic drug) [22, 70, 88], or surgically by means of minimally invasive surgery (vertebroplasty, balloon kyphoplasty). These procedures have been recently introduced in the treatment armamentarium for OVCF as a more effective treatment [42, 83].

According to a study by Parfitt and Duncan, published in 1982 [101], spontaneous crush fractures in osteoporotic patients do not result in spinal cord compression requiring decompressive surgery. However, several reports have since appeared in the literature highlighting the fact that spontaneous osteoporotic fracture with serious spinal cord compression and variable degrees of neurological deficit do occur [6, 8, 26, 27, 63, 71, 72, 75, 77, 90, 97, 98, 118, 119, 125, 132].

There are five main reasons for operating on osteoporotic spines:

1. Acute or subacute osteoporotic fractures that can be corrected or stabilized by minimally invasive surgery (vertebroplasty or balloon kyphoplasty)

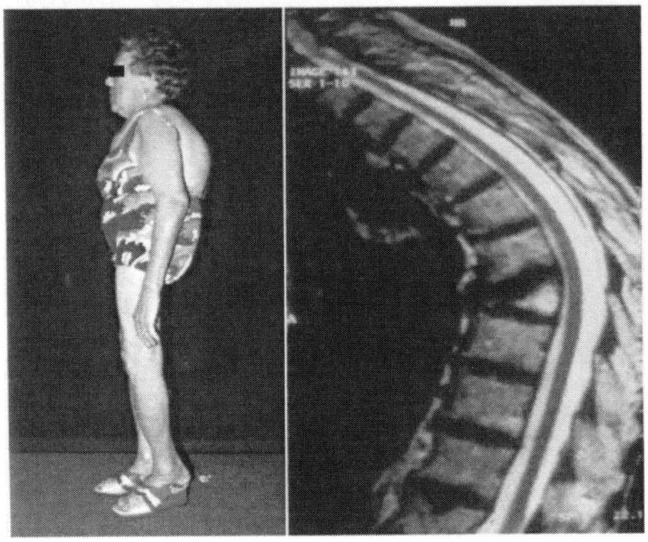

Fig. 1 A patient with painful kyphosis. Could this deformity have been prevented?

2. Conditions requiring spinal instrumentation, such as extensive laminectomy, which may destabilize an osteoporotic spine
3. Prevention of severe kyphotic deformity developing from osteoporotic fractures (Fig. 1)
4. Established painful deformities (kyphosis/scoliosis), and
5. Symptomatic neurocompression caused by osteoporotic fractures

Review of a series of 29 cases

A review recently conducted by the present authors of 29 patients treated for serious musculoskeletal spinal and neurological complications from osteoporosis of the spine shows how serious the condition can be and how important it is to maintain surgery as a treatment option. The patients were managed surgically between January 1994 and January 2001 at the University of Texas Medical Branch at Galveston, at the University of Crete, Heraklion, and at the National University of Greece in Athens.

Fifteen patients were treated for severe neurological compromise, ranging from paraplegia to paraparesis (Frankel A: n=1, Frankel B,C and D: n=14) and 14 for intractable back pain complicating kyphoscoliotic osteoporotic deformities. Acute burst fractures were observed in five patients and were associated with serious neurological complications (Frankel B in four and Frankel A in one). Ten patients suffered from wedge compression fractures, two developed acute onset of symptoms, and in the remaining eight, the neurological deterioration was gradual. (The neurological deficit grading was Frankel B in two, with the rest ranging between C and D.)

Surgical treatment

Anterior decompression was accomplished through an anterior approach in 15 patients (8 for painful deformity and 7 for neurological deficit). Anterior stabilization alone was achieved by means of a Kostuik rod: n=1, a Kaneda device: n=4, or a plate: n=1. Posterior stabilization was performed in three cases, and combination of anterior Kaneda and posterior instrumentation (Varigrip hook) in another six cases. Anterior reconstruction was achieved by means of bone graft in four cases (femoral ring allograft: n=2 and ribs: n=2), and Harms titanium cages filled with bone graft in 11 cases. A posterior approach alone was used in 11 cases, and consisted of either wide laminectomy and stabilization (eight cases), or indirect reduction and stabilization (three cases). More specifically, instrumentation consisted of multisegmental fixation with either transpedicle screws (bone cement augmentation n=2; triangular technique n=2) or laminar claws (Varigrip) or a combination of the two.

Three patients who had serious co-morbid diseases were treated with morphine pump. One had a partial paraparesis and the other two intractable painful deformities.

Outcomes

The patient with complete paraplegia never recovered (Fig. 2), whereas patients with Frankel B, C, or D improved by two grades. All patients with serious neurolog-

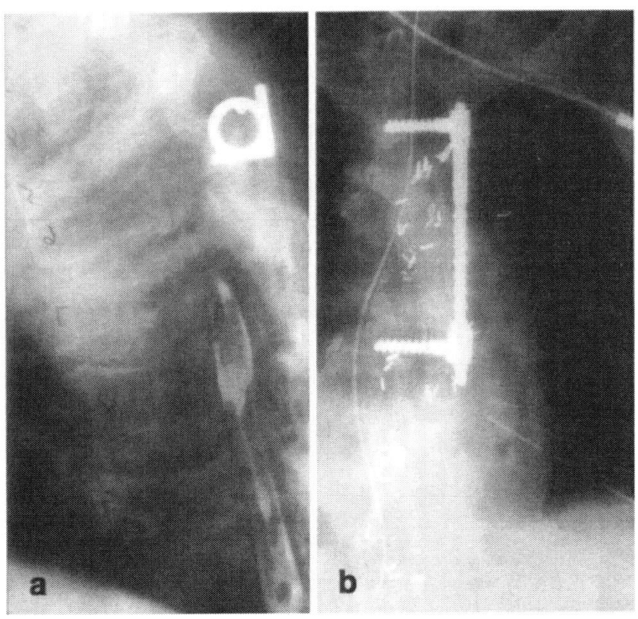

Fig. 2 Osteoporotic pathological fracture of T6, resulting in severe kyphosis and rapid progression of neurological deficit to complete paraplegia (**a**). The patient failed to recover after anterior decompression and stabilization (**b**)

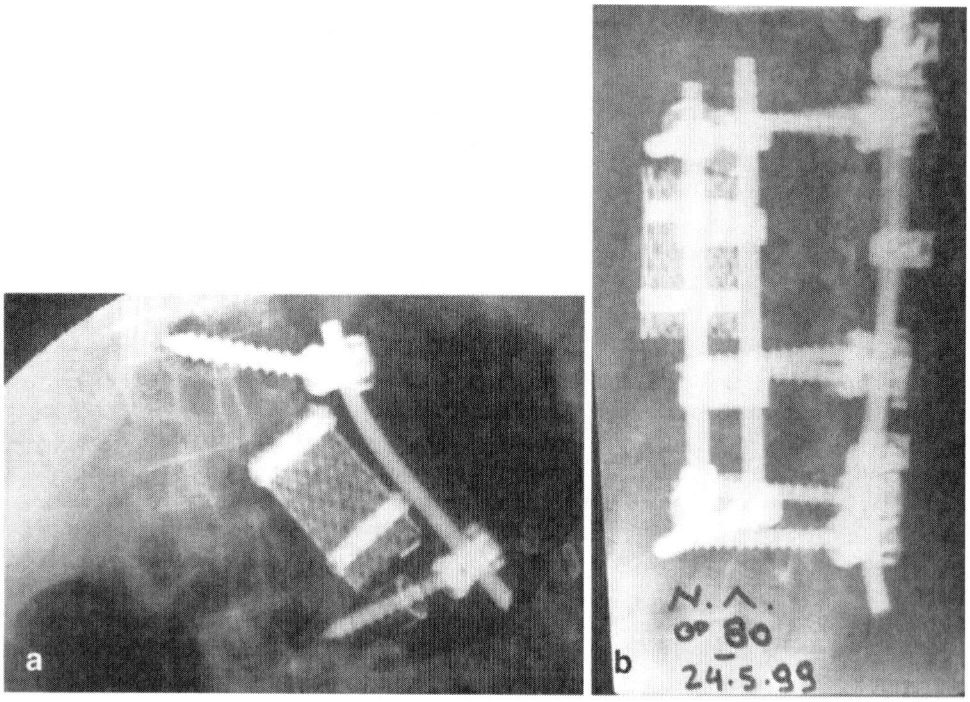

Fig. 3 Dislodgment of anterior instrumentation construct in an osteoporotic L1 fracture (**a**). This resulted from poor application of instrumentation principles in an osteoporotic spine. It was successfully revised using anterior and posterior multisegment fixation constructs (**b**)

Table 1 Outcomes of surgery for spinal cord neurocompression and painful deformities

Procedure	Serious neurological deficit[a]			Painful deformities (kyphosis/scoliosis)			Combined		
	Total	Improvement	Failure	Total	Success	Failure	Total	Success	Failure
Anterior decompression + graft or cages	7	6/7	1/7	8	5/8	3/8	15	11/15	4/15
Anterior stabilization	3	2/3	1/3[b]	3	0	3/3[c]	6	2/6	4/6
Posterior stabilization	–	–	–	3	3/3	0	3	3/3	0
Combined	4	4/4	0	2	2/2	0	6	6/6	0
Posterior decompression, indirect reduction + stabilization	3	3/3	0	–	–	–	3	3/3	0
Posterior decompression + stabilization	4	3/4	1/4	4	2/4	2/4	8	5/8	3/8
Morphine pump	1	0	1/1	2	1/2	1/2	3	1/3	2/3

[a] "Serious neurological deficit" indicates Frankel B–D. "Improvement" denotes patients' neurological status improved by at least two Frankel grades. The patient with morphine pump deteriorated from Frankel D to Frankel B

[b] One patient with complete paraplegia never recovered

[c] Two patients developed junctional kyphosis. One was successfully corrected by supplementing posterior instrumentation. The other healed in a kyphotic deformity with residual pain. Complete dislodgement of instrumentation occurred in the third patient, who was revised successfully through a combined approach.

ical deficit underwent anterior decompression. Pain improved substantially in all patients, as well as in the patients who underwent revision surgery. Two of the patients in the deformity group who underwent anterior decompression and anterior stabilization developed junctional kyphosis, which was corrected by indirect reduction in hyperextension and stabilization with posterior instrumentation. In one patient, complete dislodgement of a cage and an anterior device occurred soon after surgery, and responded well to revision surgery (Fig. 3). In the patient with paraparesis, morphine pump was successful as a pain management modality; however, his neurological status deteriorated and the patient died after a few months.

A morphine pump substantially improved the pain in one patient with painful deformity and failed in the other patient (Table 1).

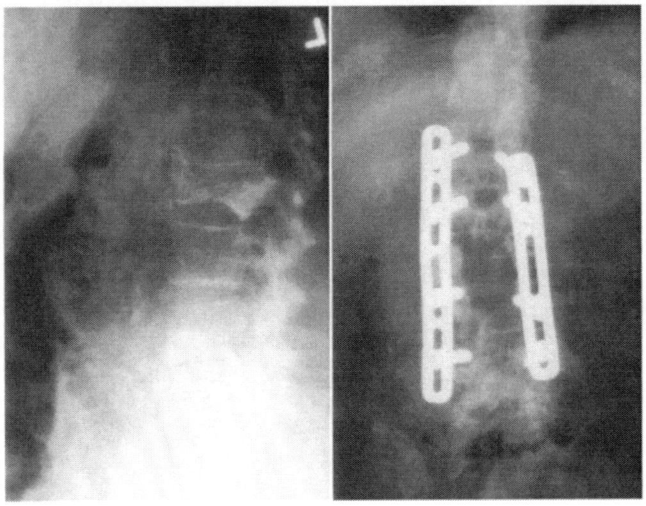

Fig. 4 Acute burst fracture in a patient on chronic use of steroids, who sustained the fracture after a minor trauma (bending over and lifting a heavy object). The onset of severe paraparesis was late, gradual and crippling. Neurological status responded successfully to posterior decompression and stabilization, but the treatment failed to correct the deformity and the patient remained with severe back pain

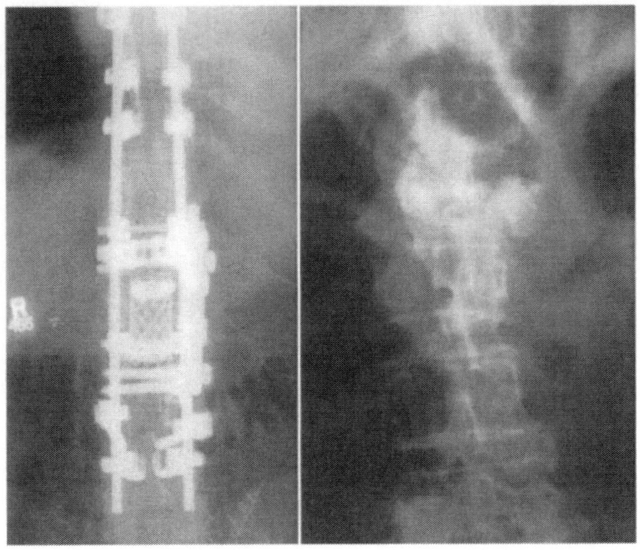

Fig. 5 Correction of a rigid painful post-fracture kyphoscoliotic deformity by means of anterior and posterior instrumentation

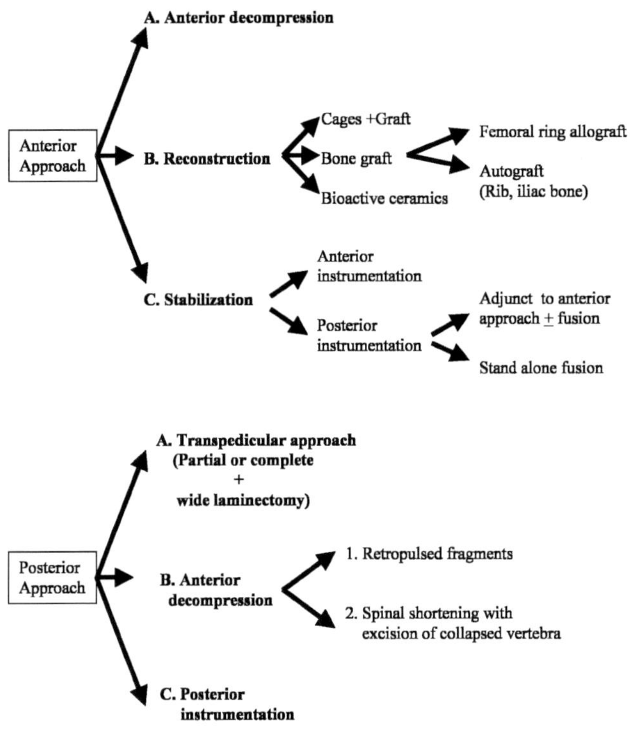

Fig. 6 Principles of surgery of osteoporotic vertebral fracture with neurological deficit or severe painful kyphotic-scoliotic deformity. A,B,C signify sequential steps for each approach

Discussion

With the increasing size of the elderly population (people at risk), it is expected that the rate of osteoporotic vertebral fracture and resulting neurological complications will rise dramatically.

Acute kyphotic deformity as a result of OVCF is not usually associated with neurological deficit, but may continue to remain as a painful crippling condition requiring major surgical intervention (Fig. 1). The type of OVF that can cause neurocompression results from either acute crush fracture [77, 98, 102] (Fig. 4) or delayed collapse of an antecedent wedge fracture that leads to retropulsion of a vertebral body fragment and contribution to progressive kyphotic deformity [71, 75, 97].

The reported time period from the original injury to clinical manifestation of neurocompression varies between 1 and 18 months [8, 71, 75]. The cord is compromised either by the severity of the kyphotic deformity or by retropulsion of a posterior wall fragment [8, 63, 71, 75, 97]. The postulated mechanisms of delayed vertebral collapse are attributed to either bone ischemia and necrosis [13, 18, 71, 75], or pseudarthrosis [60]. Apparently, it is a combination of both these factors [71, 75]. Repeated microtraumas have been postulated as the causative factor for pseudarthrosis [75], which produces an unstable kyphotic spine and severe pain [75].

Neurological deficit can range from acute paraplegia (usually after an acute crush fracture) [98, 102] to delayed onset of insidious paralysis that gradually deteriorates to severe paraplegia [69, 73]. The latter phenomenon is usually associated with delayed vertebral collapse and progressive kyphotic deformity [75]. Within this context, therefore, it is not unreasonable to entertain balloon kyphoplasty, a recently introduced minimally invasive surgery, as a preventative intervention for progressive kyphotic deformity (Fig. 1).

Table 2 Reported cases of severe neurological deficit caused by osteoporotic vertebral fractures

Authors	No. of cases	Neurological status	Type of fracture	Treatment	Results and remarks
Salomon et al. 1988 [119]	1	Spastic paraparesis	Wedge fracture with acute retropulsion	Combined posterior and anterior approach	Complete recovery
Kaplan et al. 1989 [72]	3	Neurological deficit	Burst with retropulsion		Spontaneous Fx, no trauma
Arciero et al. 1989 [6]	2	Paraparesis: acute onset 1, delayed onset 1	Acute burst fracture	Anterior decompression	Nearly complete recovery
Shikata et al. 1990 [125]	7	Delayed paraparesis	5 burst Fx, 5 wedge Fx	Posterior decompression	Substantial improvement
Kaneda et al. 1992 [71]	22	Gradual onset incomplete paralysis	Wedge fracture with delayed bone retropulsion	Anterior decompression	Excellent
Heggeness 1993 [63]	9	Gradual onset of neurological symptoms	Delayed collapse with bone retropulsion		Benign appearing compression Fx may progress to serious situation
Tanaka et al. 1993 [132]	1	Delayed conus medullaris syndrome	L1 burst fracture	Anterior decompression and fusion	Restoration of vesicorectal function
Korovessis et al. 1994 [77]	7	Delayed cord compression; paraplegia 1	Burst fracture with progression	Anterior or posterior or combined approach	6 recovered, 1 (with paraplegia) died
Cortet et al. 1995 [26]	6	Gradual onset: paraplegia 1, paraparesis 3, leg weakness 2, sphincteric dysfunction 2	Vertebral crush Fx	Surgery: 3 Conservative: 3	1 recovered, 1 improved, 1 unchanged 1 improved, 2 unchanged
Baba 1995 [8]	27	Gradual late paralysis	Delayed collapse with bone retropulsion	Anterior or posterior decompression	Recommend transpedicular posterolateral decompression
Hu 1997 [66]	1	Gradual progression of leg weakness	Progressive loss of vertebral height; retropulsion of fragments; progressive kyphosis	Combined anterior and posterior approach	Recovery
Courtois et al. 1998 [27]	1	Cauda equina syndrome	L2 Fx with osteonecrosis		Imaging failed to diagnose oseteonecrosis. Diagnosis made from the biopsy.
Saita et al. 2000 [118]	1	Acute onset with gradual deterioration	Wedge compression	Spondylectomy	Excellent
O'Connor et al. 2002 [98]	1	Acute onset of complete paraplegia	Crush with retropulsion	Conservative	Died
Kim et al. 2003 [75]	14	Gradual onset of severe paraparesis	Wedge fracture with delayed retropulsion	Anterior cord decompression	Excellent
Nguyen et al. 2003 [97]	10	Frankel D: 7, Frankel C: 3; late onset: 9, acute onset: 1	Burst with retropulsion	Surgery	8/10 survived, 6/10 improved, 1/10 deteriorated

Based on our findings and the experience of others, we have shown that posterior instrumentation alone, after wide laminectomy, can improve neurological deficits even in seriously spinal cord-compromised patients in the acute fracture where indirect reduction of kyphotic deformity is feasible. However, for rigid curves (Fig. 5), a combined anterior and posterior approach seems a more appropriate treatment. For an experienced surgeon, anterior decompression and stabilization with or without posterior stabilization can achieve excellent results in terms of neurological decompression and correction of painful deformities [22]. Anterior decompression and stabilization can also be achieved through a posterior or posterolateral translaminar approach.

Fig. 6 outlines the techniques of surgical management of OVF when the spinal cord is compromised, and Table 2

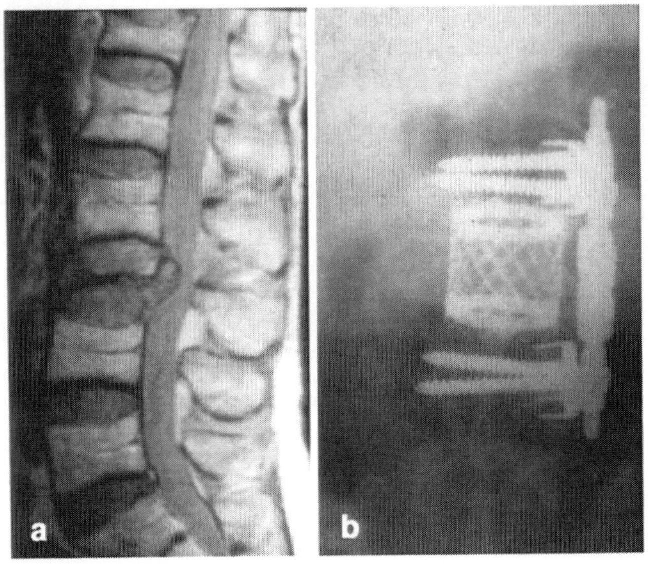

a b

Fig. 7 Paraparesis after spontaneous osteoporotic fracture (**a**), corrected by anterior decompression and reconstruction (**b**)

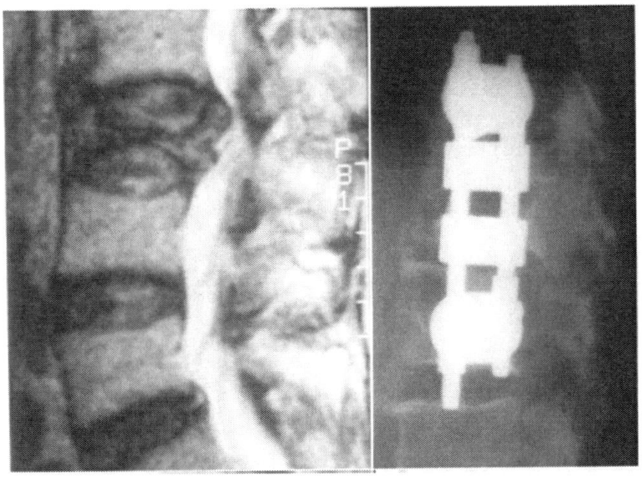

Fig. 8 Pathological osteoporotic fracture with complete restoration of neurological deficit after anterior decompression, iliac bone graft and Kaneda stabilization

summarizes the published reports of serious neurocompression complicating osteoporotic fractures.

Surgical approach

Through an anterior approach, decompression of a retropulsed bone fragment can be easily and safely performed. Reconstruction and fusion can be achieved either by femoral ring bone allograft, rib struts, iliac bone, cages filled with bone chips, or bioactive ceramic [71] (we do not use methylmethacrylate as a reconstruction material advocated by others) [6]. Stabilization can be accomplished using a Kaneda device or similar rigid anterior instrumentation (Fig. 7, Fig. 8). Because screw holding grip is incomplete in osteoporotic bone, we advocate that the screw should stabilize the contralateral vertebral body cortex. Stabilization can also be obtained through a posterior approach (Fig. 9). Alternatively the surgeons could elect first to stabilize the spine posteriorly and, in the same sitting, proceed with an anterior decompression [119].

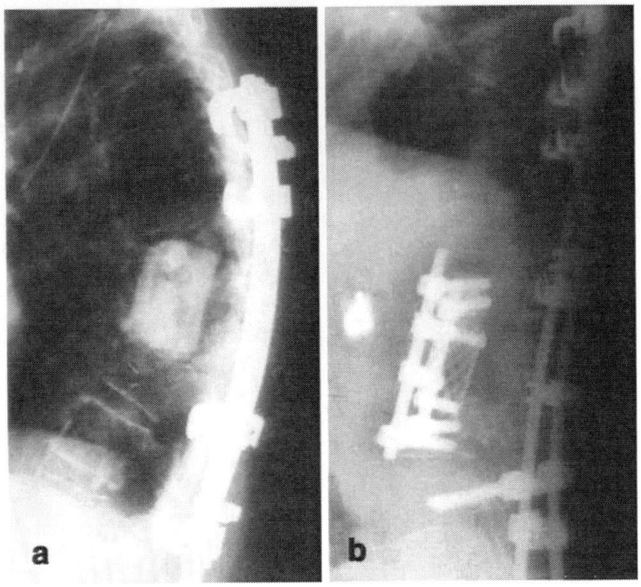

a b

Fig. 9 **a** Anterior decompression and reconstruction with femoral ring bone graft and posterior stabilization. **b** Anterior decompression and reconstruction with titanium mesh cage filled with bone chips; stabilization was obtained though a combined anterior and posterior long multisegmental stabilization construct

Anterior cord decompression can also be performed through a posterior transpedicle or posterolateral approach. In general, many surgeons who are more familiar with the posterior approach prefer this method, which also avoids the need for sectioning the diaphragm – especially advantageous in elderly patients with serious pulmonary problems [75, 125]. Through this approach, cord decompression can be achieved either by:

- Partial posterior vertebrectomy and bone grafting [75]
- Driving forward the retropulsed fragment by gentle direct tapping [125], or
- Performing a vertebrectomy to accomplish shortening and decompression of the spinal cord [118]

The spine is then stabilized through a posterior instrumentation, preferably by using transpedicular screw fixation two to three levels above and below the decompression. The only technical complication reported with this approach is dural tear (14%) [75]. Laminectomy, as a stand-alone procedure, should be rejected, because it does not deal with the anterior cord compression, and further deterioration of neurological deficit from progressive kyphotic deformity has been observed [73].

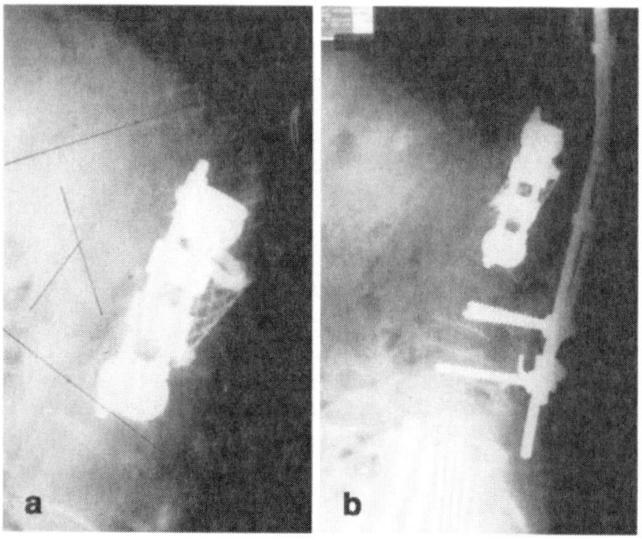

Fig. 10 Junctional kyphosis after anterior instrumentation (**a**), corrected by posterior instrumentation combining screws and hooks (**b**)

Options for instrumentation

Hardware loosening or cut-out with dislodgment of instrumentation construct are the most serious technical complications when operating on osteoporotic spines. To avoid this, the surgeon should be aware of certain well-established surgical principles when instrumenting osteoporotic spines, as suggested by Hu [66]:

1. Try to avoid the use of hooks or screws as the sole fixation device.
2. Avoid ending the instrumentation within kyphotic segments [66] (Fig. 10) to prevent junctional kyphotic complications [66, 86].
3. Use multiple sites of fixation to dissipate stresses and therefore decrease stresses at any site [66] (Fig. 9b, Fig. 5). Similarly, the excessive forces on the instrumentations, can be sufficiently dissipated by combining anterior and posterior surgical approaches and instrumentation [14].
4. Accept a lesser degree of deformity correction (Fig. 11), in order to avoid hardware pull-out from excessive corrective forces [66].

And, finally, one should keep in mind that fixation may not be feasible!

As an ultimate salvage approach one may consider a morphine pump, as the last attempt to control musculoskeletal pain in moribund patients.

In relation to point (1) above, there are a number of considerations to bear in mind. Laminar hooks are considered to be more resistant to posteriorly directed forces, because laminar bone is more cortical than cancellous and will therefore have been affected by osteoporosis [21]. Hooks in a claw configuration spanning two vertebral levels can augment the holding grip of the construct. Experimental work indicates that transpedicular screw axial pull-out is correlated to the vertebral bone mineral density [21, 58, 99, 131]. Triangulation of pedicle screws apparently resists axially directed screw pull-out [54, 55]. Augmentation of transpedicle screw fixation in osteoporotic patients using polymethylmethacrylate has been accepted as a sound technical principle [22, 85, 96, 131]. A combination of pedicle screw and laminar hooks will provide the greatest resistance to pull-out forces [7, 17, 58, 61, 92] (Fig. 11). Hu thinks that sublaminar wire fixation of spinal rods is a sound surgical principle in osteoporotic spine [66]. Although sublaminar wires pose a potential risk for neurological complications, they are ideal because the multiple sites of wire fixation decrease the stresses generated at points of fixation [66].

Osteoporosis: conclusion

In conclusion, several caveats deserve to be highlighted here. Osteoporotic fracture of the spine is not always an innocent occurrence, as most people are led to believe, but

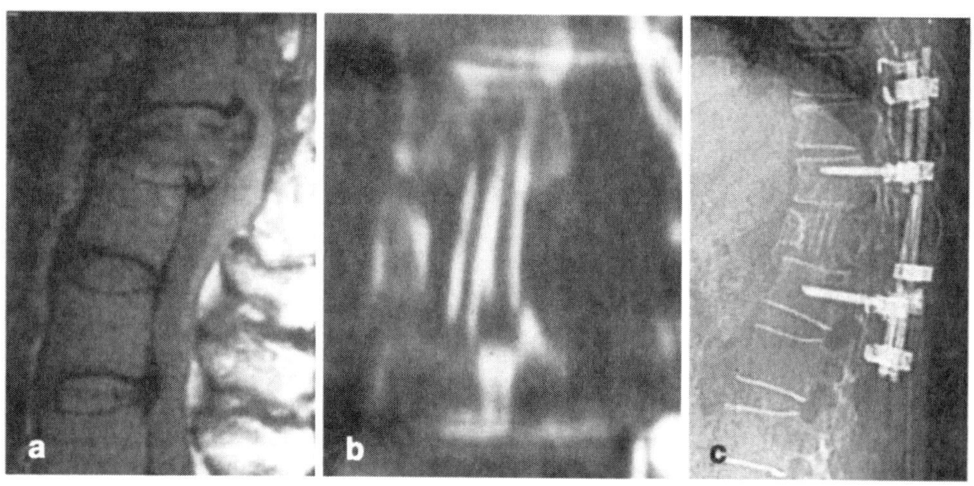

Fig. 11 Pathological fracture with severe delayed neurocompresion (**a**), treated by means of anterior decompression and reconstruction with rib strut graft (**b**). **c** Posterior stabilization with screws and Varigrip claws

can give rise to serious and crippling neurological complications and painful deformities as well. Surgery in these cases is apparently the sole alternative approach, and may turn out to be a formidable task. However, the clinician who is armed with knowledge of the best options in surgical treatment can effectively and safely manage the problem, which is anticipated to be seen more frequently in the near future. The aging population should be rewarded with the enjoyment of life without pain and disabilities.

Paget's disease of the spine

The second part of this paper looks at Paget's disease, another osteometabolic disorder that can affect the aging spine. It describes the spinal involvement of Paget's disease in bone and outlines best treatment options.

Etiology

The original disease was described by Sir John Paget [100] in 1877, and despite recent intensive studies, its etiology remains obscure. Paget's disease of bone (PD), a mono-ostotic or polyostotic non-hormonal osteometabolic disorder, is postulated to be caused by a viral infection [10, 49, 127]. This claim is supported by circumstantial evidence garnered from electron microscopic, immunologic, and epidemiologic studies [56].

PD is found more commonly in populations of Anglo-Saxon origin, and is rarely encountered in Asia, Scandinavia, or the Middle East [9]. A survey of PD in South Africa revealed a prevalence of 1.3% among the black population and 2.4% among the white population [44], suggesting that PD may not be uncommon in Africans, as was previously believed [128]. Autopsy and radiographic studies indicate that the overall prevalence of PD is 3–3.7% [23, 104, 123], with a tendency to increase with age. At the age of 90, the expected prevalence is about 10% [123]. A very recent report on radiographic examination of the pelvis [5] revealed an estimated overall prevalence in the US of 1–2%, with near equal distribution between whites and blacks and between sexes.

Genetic factors also play a role in the pathogenesis of PD [62, 65, 129]. A positive family history in patients of siblings was reported in 12.3% of cases, as compared to 2.1% of controls. In another study, the prevalence of PD was found to be approximately seven times higher in relatives of cases than controls.

Viral infection may also help explain the genetic predisposition, by gene mutation, of PD [93]. Circumstantial evidence thus supports the plausible hypothesis that viral infection may trigger the onset of PD as well stimulate inheritable gene mutation. Future research hopefully will cast light on these issues [56].

Histopathology

The histopathology of PD is characterized by two entities: osseous lesions and bone marrow fibrosis. The former is characterized by its so-called mosaic appearance, which is the hallmark of the pagetic lesion. The pagetic cellularity consists of variable sizes of osteoblasts and large osteoclasts with multiple nuclei (up to 100) [106].

Prevalence of back pain and spinal stenosis

The spine is the second most commonly affected site in PD [2, 30, 95], predisposing patients to low back pain and

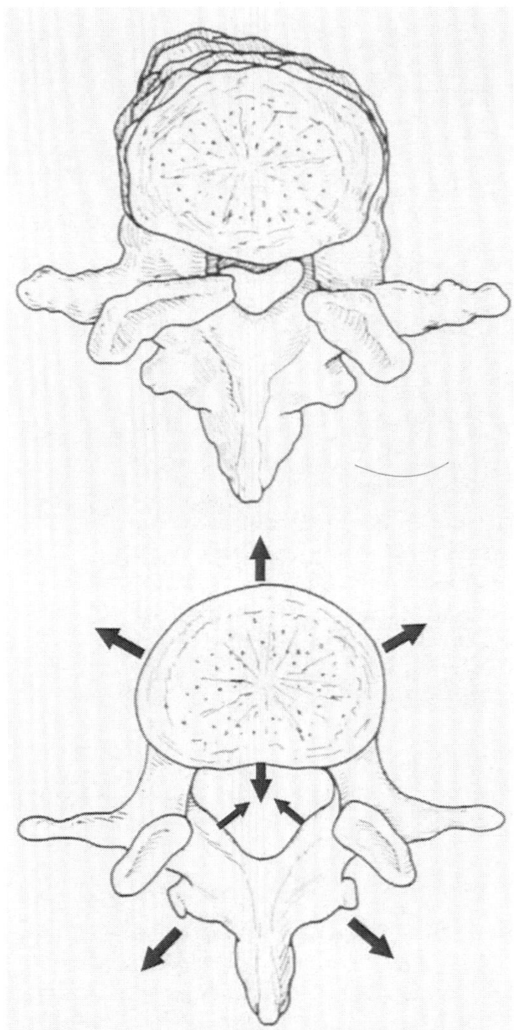

Fig. 12 Bone modeling of vertebra depicted diagrammatically to demonstrate tendency of bone expansion in all directions, leading to hypertrophic facet osteoarthropathy and spinal stenosis. [Reprinted, with permission, from Hadjipavlou A, Lander P (1995) Paget's disease. In: White AH, Schofferman JA (eds) Spinal care. Mosby, St Louis, pp 1720–1737]

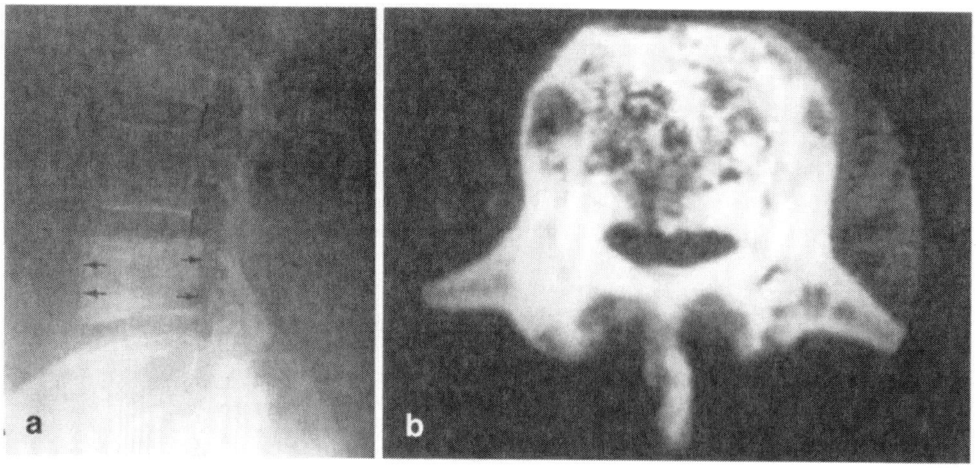

Fig. 13 **a** Plain radiography demonstrating pagetic involvement of L4 vertebra with typical expansion in the mixed-blastic phase. **b** Axial computed tomography scan of the third lumbar vertebra, demonstrating circumferential expansion of a mixed-blastic-phase lesion of Paget's disease (PD) causing severe spinal stenosis. [Reprinted, with permission, from Hadjipavlou A, Gaitanis I, Katonis P, Lander P (2001) Paget's disease of the spine and its management. Eur Spine J 10:370–384]

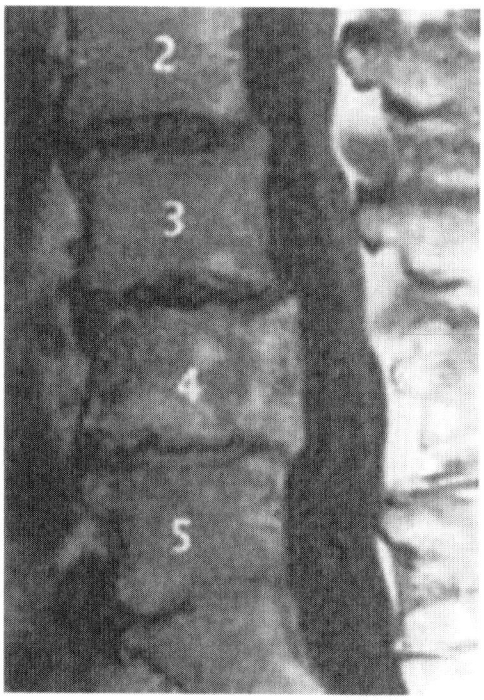

Fig. 14 T1-weighted magnetic resonance image showing posterior expansion of the vertebral body. [Reprinted, with permission, from Hadjipavlou A, Gaitanis I, Katonis P, Lander P (2001) Paget's disease of the spine and its management. Eur Spine J 10:370–384]

spinal stenosis [4, 52, 64, 137]. Hartman and Dohn have shown that 15.2% of patients with PD had involvement of the vertebrae, and 26% of these patients had symptoms of spinal stenosis [59]. The reported incidence of back pain in PD ranges from 11% [40] to 34% [2] and as high as 43% [113]. The causal relationship between vertebral PD and back pain has been disputed [2], with low back pain in PD being attributed to coexisting osteoarthritis of the spine in 88% of patients and to PD alone in only 12%. Others consider PD to cause back pain even more rarely [45]. However, in our population, 33% of patients with PD demonstrated pagetic involvement of the spine; 30% had clinical symptoms of spinal stenosis and 54% of these patients suffered back pain (24% attributed clearly to PD alone, 50% to degenerative changes and 26% to a combination of PD and degenerative changes) [46].

Spinal pain (back pain and neck pain)

PD can be defined as an abnormal disturbance of bone remodeling, giving rise to the four phases of the disease observed radiologically: the osteolytic, mixed, osteoblastic, and osteosclerotic phases [79]. This leads to abnormal modeling, which determines the shape and geometry of the bone [43] (Fig. 12) leading, in turn, to spinal stenosis [79] (Fig. 13, Fig. 14) and facet arthropathy [50, 57].

Pagetic facet arthropathy is a major contributing factor to both back pain and spinal stenosis, and the more advanced the facet joint arthropathy, the greater the likelihood that patients will suffer clinical spinal stenosis and/or back pain [46]. However, this does not necessarily preclude that, though present, severe facet arthropathy may remain asymptomatic [46]. Back pain in PD may also be attributed to blood engorgement of the vertebral body caused by vascular and disorganized, hyperactive remodeling processes.

Other factors implicated in spinal pain may include invasion of the vertebral disc space by the pagetic process (Fig. 15) [80], and spinal stenosis [137]. The authors hypothesize that microfractures of pagetic vertebral bodies, especially in the osteolytic or mixed phase, can also lead to back pain [46].

Spinal stenosis

Involvement of the cervical and thoracic spine tends very often to predispose to clinical spinal stenosis with my-

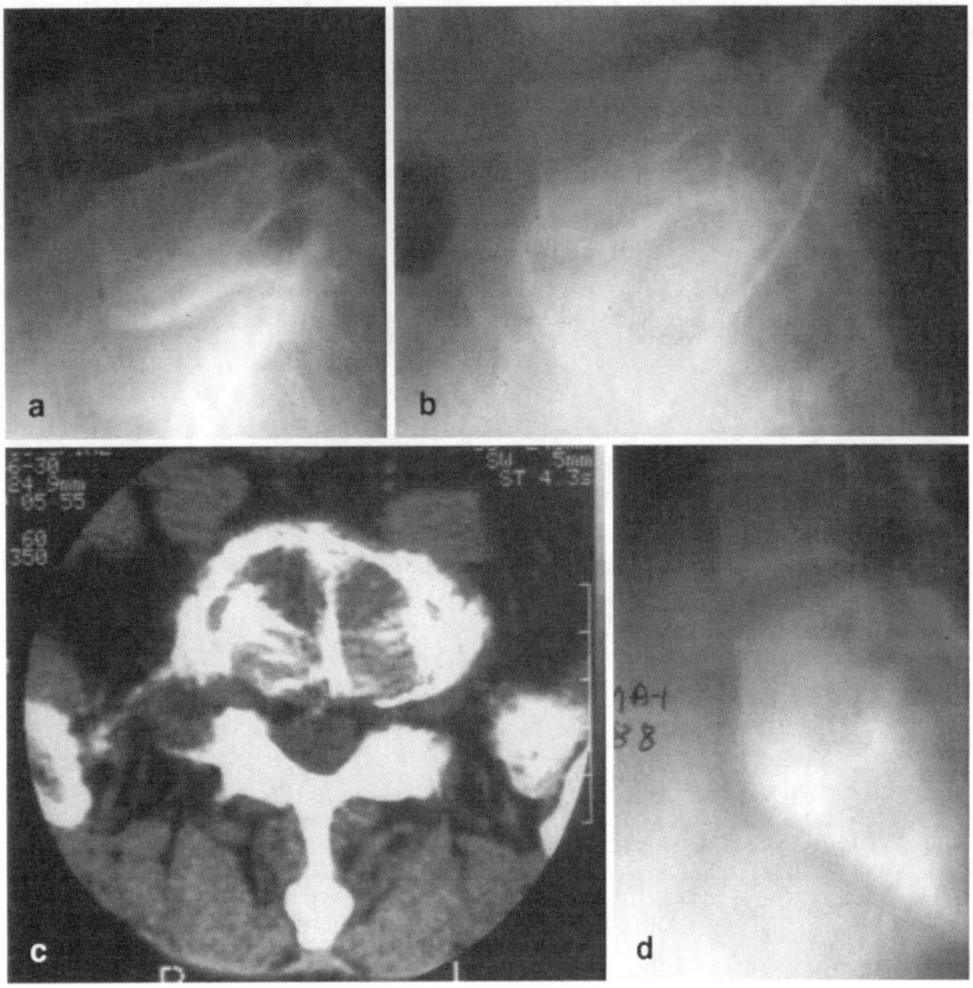

Fig. 15 **a** Lateral radiograph of the lumbosacral junction demonstrating mixed phase Paget's disease of the first sacral segment with moderate narrowing of the L5-S1 disc space. **b** Pagetic bone extension across the disc space with adjacent anterior bridging with sclerotic bone noted 3 years after the initial radiograph. **c** The corresponding axial CT scan of the L5-S1 disc demonstrates pagetic bone within the disc. **d** Lateral tomogram demonstrating the intradiscal bone extension from the adjacent S1 vertebra resulting in complete bony ankylosis 4 years after the initial radiograph. [Reprinted, with permission, from Lander P, Hadjipavlou A (1991) Intradiscal invasion of Paget's disease of the spine. Spine 16: 46–51]

elopathy [46]. Ten distinct mechanisms have been implicated in the development of neural element dysfunction in patients affected by PD:

1. Compression of the neural elements by pagetic bone overgrowth [31, 46, 76]
2. Compression by pagetic intraspinal soft tissue [46, 51] (Fig. 16)
3. Ossification of the epidural fat similar to ankylosing spondylitis [20]
4. Neural ischemia produced by blood diversion, causing the so-called "arterial steal phenomenon" [16, 59, 64, 103] (Fig. 17)
5. Interference with blood supply to the cord due to arterial compression by the expanding pagetic bone [123] or other factors not well defined [91]
6. Vertebral fracture or atlantoaxial subluxation [124, 135]
7. Platybasia with impingement on the medulla [28]
8. Spinal cord compression by epidural hematoma from spontaneous bleeding [81, 110]
9. Formation of syringomyelia as a complication of PD of the spine, especially after cranial settling (basilar invagination) [35, 110], and
10. Rarely, neurocompression can be caused by pagetic sarcomatous degeneration [67].

Bone compression by the expanding pagetic vertebrae is by far the most common cause of neural dysfunction [46]; it was first reported by Wyllie in 1923 [136]. However, severe stenosis, as seen on computed tomographic (CT) scan, may remain asymptomatic, suggesting adaptability of the thecal sac and its neural elements to severe spinal stenosis without significant loss of function [124].

The mechanism of neural ischemia is, however, still hypothetical, and supported only by circumstantial evidence. For example, patients with spinal cord symptomatology respond to calcitonin treatment better than patients with spinal nerve root lesions [28]; some patients experience progressive deterioration of neural function without evidence of myelographic block, which is not easily explained by mechanical effect alone [117]; neurologic signs do not always correlate with the site of skeletal involvement; and rapid clinical improvement occurs in some patients with medical antipagetic treatment alone. These observations suggest that neural dysfunction in PD may also result from mechanisms other than simple bone encroach-

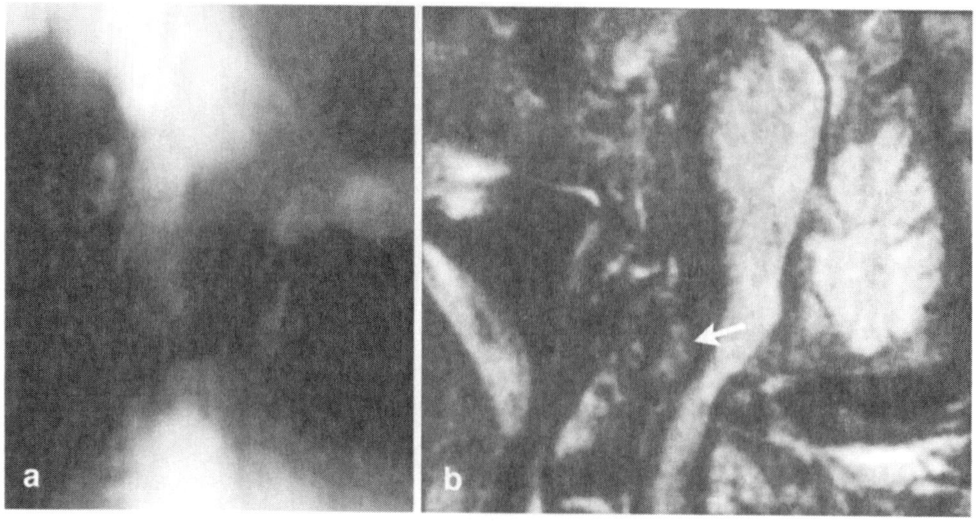

Fig. 16 A 63-year-old male patient with pagetic soft tissue expansion originating from the dens and compressing the medulla as seen on: **a** lateral tomogram of dens (bony element), and **b** MRI scan of soft tissue (*see arrow*). The patient was treated successfully with surgical decompression

ment on the neural element [32, 47, 64, 74, 103, 134, 136], such as deprivation of blood supply to the neural elements by the rapidly remodeling hypervascular pagetic bone, which produces "arterial steal phenomenon".

Other associated conditions

Malignant transformation

Malignant transformation is the most dreaded complication of PD of bone. Fortunately, this complication is relatively rare, occurring in about 0.7% [52] of cases. In our series of PD patients [52, 53] we have not seen any cases with sarcomatous degeneration in the spine. In Schajowicz et al. [120], of 62 patients with sarcomatous transformation, five of the sarcomas occurred in the spine. Surgical decompression offers little, if any, true relief of pain, with the longest survival reported at just over 5 months [67].

One should be aware of the appearance of "pseudosarcoma" or "pumice bone," which is a localized extracortical periosteal pagetic bone expansion or a bulky juxtacortical soft tissue mass, giving the erroneous appearance of sarcomatous transformation [62, 78] (Fig. 18).

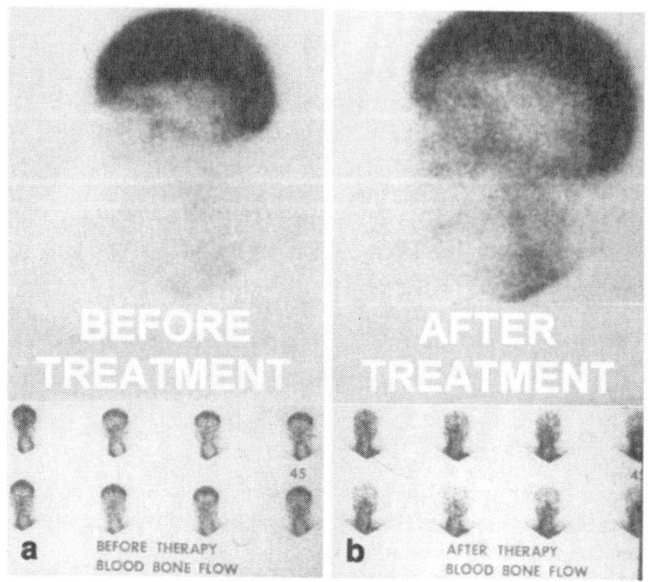

Fig. 17 A 78-year-old male patient presented himself with unsteady gait and confusion. **a** Bone scan (^{99}Tc MDP) revealed increased uptake in the skull, and bone blood flow revealed increased engorgement of the skull. **b** After treatment with i.v. mithramycin, bone scan activity improved somewhat, while bone blood flow was restored to normal. This coincided with improvement of the patients gait and mental status, suggesting that the brain had most likely been deprived of its blood supply (steal syndrome by the skull hypervascularity)

Rheumatic and arthritic conditions

Forestier's disease, or disseminated idiopathic hyperostosis (DISH), can frequently affect patients with PD. However, care should be taken not to confuse DISH with Paget's extraosseous bone formation [15]. The incidence of DISH in PD was reported to range from 14% [48] to 30% [5]. Pagetic tissue may invade the hyperostotic lesions produced by DISH and transform them into pagetic exostosis [46], which may progress to vertebral ankylosis [89].

PD has also been noted to be associated with an increased incidence of gout [40] and pseudogout [105]. These conditions, however, are not clearly implicated in the production of back pain. One has to keep in mind that treatment with sodium etidronate may be responsible for the accumulation of pyrophosphate crystals in the synovial joint, producing pseudogout [41].

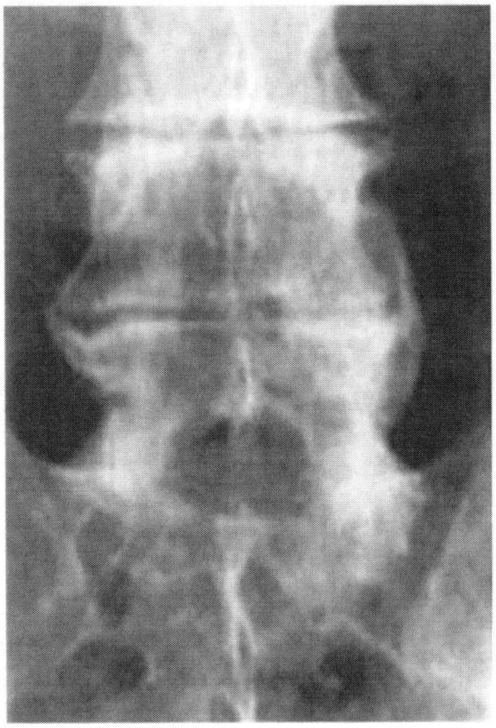

Fig. 18 Anteroposterior radiograph of the lumbar spine showing a localized bulky juxtacortical bone expansion of the lateral aspect of L4-L5 vertebrae resulting in bone union. The appearance of the lesion may be misconstrued as sarcomatous degeneration (pseudosarcoma or pumice bone). The cortical margins are well defined in contrast to the usual appearance of sarcomatous transformation, which remains poorly delineated. [Reprinted, with permission, from Hadjipavlou A, Gaitanis I, Katonis P, Lander P (2001) Paget's disease of the spine and its management. Eur Spine J 10:370–384]

Treatment

Treatment of back pain

One must be certain before attributing back pain to PD, otherwise the results of antipagetic treatment may not be rewarding [3]. For patients with low back pain and PD, suppressive therapy with EHDP (disodium etidronate) was beneficial to 36% of patients in one report [4]. This suggests that unless a well-defined lesion is related to low back pain, antipagetic therapy is not expected to be effective. If antipagetic medical therapy is ineffective within 3 months, a concomitant nonsteroidal anti-inflammatory drug and other treatment methods (physical therapy, corsets, etc) for back pain should be prescribed, especially when the presenting back pain is mechanical or arthritic in nature [50, 130].

Treatment of spinal stenosis

Because antipagetic medical therapy is rewarding in the treatment of pagetic spinal stenosis syndrome, one should start with antipagetic drug treatment. Calcitonin, mithramycin, sodium etidronate, pamidronate disodium, and clodronate have been reported to either improve or to completely reverse the clinical symptoms of spinal stenosis [1, 16, 36, 107]; however, relapse of spinal stenosis symptomatology after medical antipagetic treatment is not uncommon [32, 33]. Therefore, patients should be closely monitored and cyclical therapy should be continued if necessary until biochemical bone indices normalize.

Severe spinal stenosis of lytic type has been shown to respond successfully to antipagetic treatment with clodronate [36]. It has been suggested that, for pagetic spinal stenosis in the lytic phase of the disease, administration of vitamin D and calcium supplements to improve mineralization of lytic pagetic spinal lesion causing canal block can enhance the effectiveness of bisphosphonate therapy [36].

If the symptoms persist, in spite of bone remodeling markers normalization, surgery is an alternative treatment. Decompression of spinal stenosis should be implemented promptly after failure of antipagetic therapy. In these circumstances, delaying decompression may result in irreversible myelopathy or radiculopathy [80]. On the other hand, the results of surgery have shown variable improvement in 85% of patients [117], with frequent relapses or failures, which may improve with subsequent medical antipagetic therapy [1, 16, 107]. In our series, patients who demonstrated either partial or temporary improvement after laminectomy and were treated with further antipagetic medical treatment exhibited marked improvement of their symptomatology with sustained relief [50]. From our experience and from other reports, spinal surgery for pagetic spinal stenosis may fail to reverse the neurological deficit completely [15], and may be associated with serious complications such as a mortality rate of 11% [117] and dangerously profuse, if not torrential, bleeding [116]. To avoid such catastrophes, we recommend the preoperative assessment of bone vascularity by means of radionuclide bone blood flow in the affected spinal region. We have found this test reliable, simple and reproducible [11]. To decrease potential bleeding during surgery, if there is increased vascularity in the affected region, we strongly recommend a course of medical antipagetic treatment until the bone blood flow normalizes [50]. This may take 2–3 months with calcitonin therapy, or 2–3 weeks with mithramycin treatment [56, 57, 114]. The new generation of IV bisphosphonates can also be used effectively in this situation. In emergency situations, embolization of the region may be indicated. Because of the anticipated massive bleeding during laminectomy, the use of a cell saver is strongly recommended [115].

Surgery for spinal stenosis, when indicated, should be tailored to the pathology responsible for neural compression. If neural compression is caused by the posterior expansion of vertebral bodies, an anterior approach with corpectomy and fusion is indicated. If neural compression is caused by posterior vertebral elements, then posterior decompression should be the approach of choice [50]. An acute onset of spinal compression seems to bear a graver prognosis than the more gradual development of symptoms; the former tends to respond better to surgical decompression [126]. Surgery is also indicated as a primary treatment when neural compression is secondary to pathological fracture, dislocation, epidural hematoma, syringomyelia, platybasia, or sarcomatous transformation.

Pharmacologic treatment

A pressing issue regarding treatment is whether physicians should treat asymptomatic patients. The progressive nature of PD, the severity of its associated complications, the potential negative impact on patients' quality of life, and the availability of effective and relatively safe new antipagetic drugs have led many experts to recommend treatment for asymptomatic patients who have active disease [50, 93, 133]. According to Meunier et al., in a long-term follow up study of 41 cases of PD, antipagetic therapy that did not normalize biochemical markers in 71% of patients did not prevent new complications in 62% of patients [95], suggesting that antipagetic therapy should continue until normalization of biochemical markers is achieved. However, there are no conclusive data to support the theory that complications are preventable by controlling bone-remodeling with drug therapy [133]. Patients who are asymptomatic and inactive by biochemical and imaging parameters do not require treatment. However, patients who are clinically asymptomatic but demonstrate increased disease activity as shown by biochemical markers, bone scan uptake activity, or increased engorgement by radionuclide investigation should be treated repeatedly until a normalization of these indices is accomplished [95, 130].

Five classes of drugs are available for the treatment of PD: bisphosphonates, calcitonin, mithramycin (plicamycin), gallium nitrate, and ipriflavone. Bisphosphonates appear more effective than calcitonin in suppressing the histological and biochemical activity of PD. Therefore, calcitonin is no longer considered the treatment of choice for this condition. Some of these drugs are still experimental and can be obtained only through clinical trials. A major advantage of the use of bisphosphonates over calcitonin in PD is that biochemical and histological suppression of disease activity may persist for many years after the cessation of treatment [108].

Bisphosphonates. The mechanism of action of bisphosphonates on bone was originally ascribed to their physicochemical effect on hydroxyapatite crystals [38]. They bind strongly to hydroxyapatite crystals and inhibit both their formation and dissolution in vitro. Although such an effect is characteristic of their overall action, their influence on cells is probably of greater importance. The mechanism of action appears to be complex [39], involving several components:

1. A direct effect on osteoclastic activity
2. A direct effect on osteoclast recruitment
3. An indirect effect on osteoclast recruitment mediated by cells of osteoclastic lineage that are capable of stimulating or inhibiting osteoclastic recruitment (macrophages are osteoclast precursors), and
4. A shorter osteoclast life-span due to apoptosis

Bisphosphonates can be classified into nitrogen and non-nitrogen containing groups; two pharmacologic classes with distinct molecular mechanisms. Several bisphosphonates have been investigated [56, 57], but only the following bisphosphonates have been approved for clinical use: disodium etidronate, clodronate, pamidronate, alendronate, risedronate, neridronate, tiludronate, ibadronate, amino-hydroxybutilene bisphosphonates (ABDP), olpadronate, and zoledronate.

Oral administration of alendronate at a dose of 40 mg per day for 6 months has demonstrated efficacy in normalization of serum alkaline phosphatase [56, 109]. The present authors assessed the effects of an unpublished study of a higher dose (60 mg per day) of oral alendronate (Fosamax, Merck and Co., inc) on PD over a shorter period (3 months) in 28 patients, 18 male and 10 female with a mean age of 68 years. Ten patients had never been treated before, and 18 had previously received drug therapy. The mean period without treatment prior to alendronate was 14 months. Sites of Paget's were visually scored from +1 to +4 for radiological assessment. Quantitative uptake by region of interest (ratio of Paget's to normal bone) was also determined for scintigraphic examination.

As a result of treatment, alkaline phosphatase levels fell from 266.6 to 82.2 IU/l (mean difference 183.8 IU/l, P=0.000). Osteocalcin levels fell from 5.1 to 8.7 pmol/l (mean difference 3.6 pmol/l, P=0.0002). All patients normalized their alkaline phosphatase levels. Follow-up was carried out on all 28 patients 2 years after the 3-month treatment. All but three were in remission, giving a rate of 89.2%. No side effects were noted in any of the patients treated. The response to therapy was similar between patients who had previously received antipagetic therapy and those who had not. Similarly, there was a marked radiological (Fig. 19) and scintigraphic improvement (Fig. 20).

A major advantage of the bisphosphonates over calcitonin is that biochemical and histological suppression of the disease activity may persist for many years after the cessation of treatment [108].

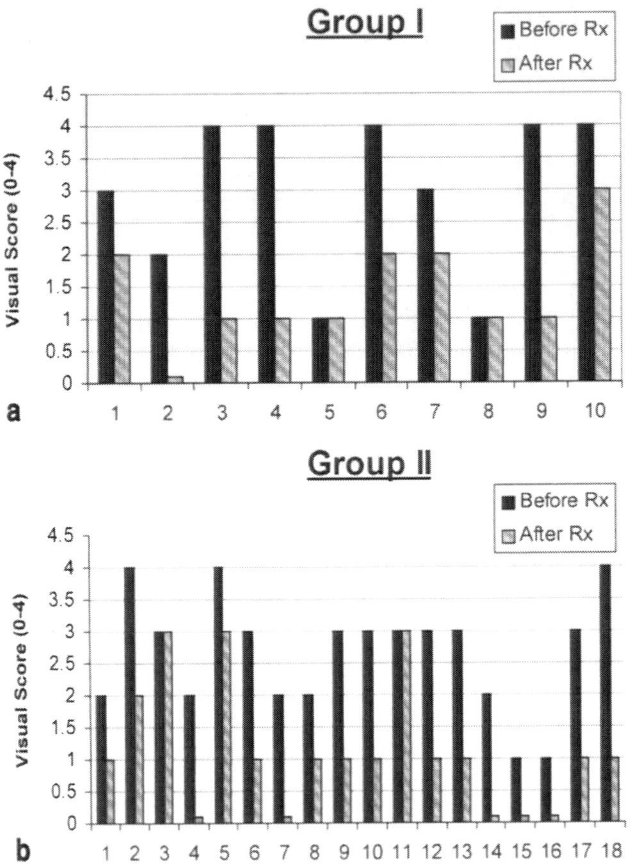

Fig. 19 Radiographic effects of alendronate treatment. Patients in group I had never been treated before alendronate treatment. Group II patients had previously received drug therapy

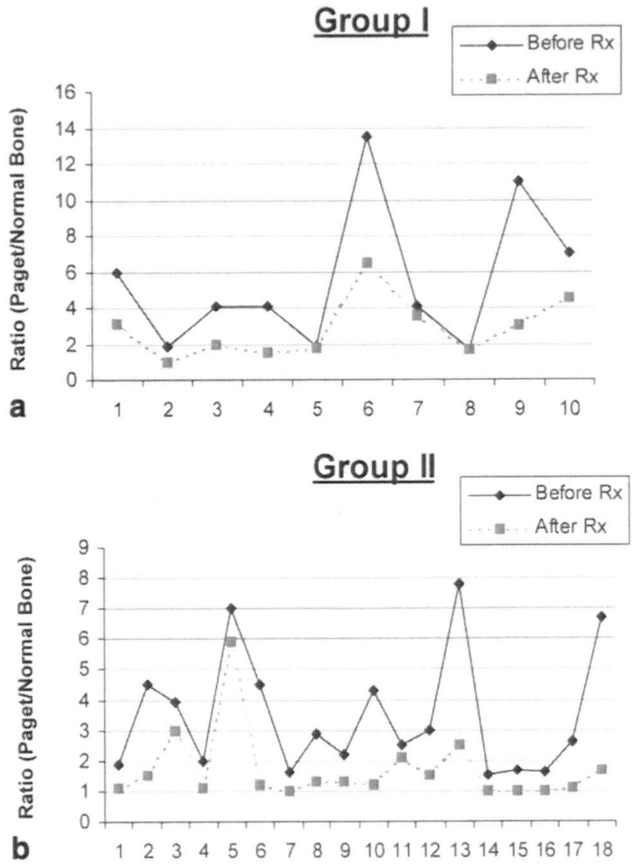

Fig. 20 Scintigraphic evaluation of alendronate treatment. Patients in group I had never been treated before alendronate treatment. Group II patients had previously received drug therapy

Laboratory methods for clinical assessment and monitoring antipagetic drug treatment

Imaging resources

The effects of treatment are monitored by the patient's clinical response, imaging modalities, and bone remodeling markers [56, 57].

Radionuclide bone blood flow can be used to monitor vascularity. Therefore, it can be used:

1. To assess a relevant pagetic region for potential profuse bleeding before proceeding with surgery, and
2. To monitor the effectiveness of an emergency intravenous administration of antipagetic agents

Conventional bone scan is recommended before and 6 months after treatment, and 12 months thereafter depending on the behavior of the pagetic lesion. Twenty-four hour retention scan, a more quantitative radionuclide assessment, can be used as an adjunct to bone scan [11]. Quantitative bone scan scintigraphy allows early and objective assessment of PD when evaluating the effects of therapy. Radiographic images should be obtained before treatment and every 1 to 2 years thereafter, to monitor the modeling (bone expansion) and remodeling changes (phase of the disease activity). Although PD can be diagnosed cost effectively with conventional radiography, magnetic resonance (MR) imaging is well suited for demonstrating specific characteristics of certain complications, including basilar invaginations, spinal stenosis, and secondary neoplasm [12].

Biomechanical bone markers

Recently, the assessment and effectiveness of treatment of patients with Paget's disease have been improved by new emerging biochemical markers for bone remodeling, promptly applied.

Common bone markers used for the evaluation of bone turnover in PD are:

- In serum: total alkaline phosphatase (tAP) and bone alkaline phosphatase (βAP), procollagen type 1 N-terminal polypeptide (PINP), beta-carboxyterminal telopeptide of type 1 collagen (SCTx); osteocalcin and serum bone sialoprotein
- In urine: hydroxyproline (Hyp), amino (NTX) and beta-carboxyterminal (CTX) telopeptides of collagen type I, total pyridinoline (PYD) and deoxypyridinoline (DPD)

Markers of bone resorption representing degradation of type I collagen are: N-telopeptides, C-telopeptides, hydroxyproline and collagen crosslinks-pyridinoline and dexopyridinoline, and urinary calcium.

Serum tartrated-resistant acid phosphatase is a marker for osteoclastic activity. Bone formation markers include bone-specific alkaline phosphatase and N terminal and C terminal extension peptides of procollagen and osteocalcin.

Resorption markers respond approximately 1–3 months after treatment intervention, whereas markers of formation respond much later, usually after 6–9 months [19].

The serum markers of bone turnover show lower biological variability than urinary markers, and are therefore more sensitive indices of disease activity.

Paget's Disease: conclusions

The natural history of PD affecting the spine is therefore progressive, characterized by bone proliferation, vertebral expansion, and structural changes, leading to spinal stenosis and facet arthropathy, clinical entities that are not always symptomatic. Pagetic facet arthropathy is a major contributing factor to both back pain and spinal stenosis, and the more advanced the facet joint arthropathy, the greater the likelihood that patients will suffer clinical spinal stenosis and/or back pain. In the majority of cases the clinical picture of pagetic spinal stenosis and facet osteoarthropathy is not expected to differ from that of degenerative spondylosis. A minority of patients (13%), however, exhibits constant spinal pain attributed to the pagetic pathologic remodeling process. Treatment of pagetic spinal stenosis symptoms should start with medical antipagetic therapy, with surgery being the alternative choice only if the symptoms persist in spite of normalization of bone remodeling markers.

References

1. Alexandre C, Trillet M, Meunier P, et al (1979) Traitement des paraplegics pagetiques par les disphosphonates. Ren Neurol (Paris) 135:625–632
2. Altman RD (1980) Musculoskeletal manifestation of Paget's disease of bone. Arthritis Rheum 23:1121–1127
3. Altman RD (1999) Paget's disease of bone: rheumatologic complications. Bone 24 [5 Suppl]:47–48
4. Altman RD, Brown M, Gargano F (1987) Low back pain in Paget's disease of bone. Clin Orthop 217:152–161
5. Altman RD, Bloch DA, Hochberg MC, Murphy WA (2000) Prevalence of pelvic Paget's disease of bone in the United States. J Bone Miner Res 15:461–465
6. Arciero RA, Leung KY, Pierce JH (1989) Spontaneous unstable burst fracture of the thoracolumbar spine in osteoporosis. Spine 14:114–117
7. Argenson C, Lovet J, De Peretti F, et al (1990) The treatment of spinal fractures with Cotrel-Dubousset instrumentation: results of the first 85 cases. Orthop Trans 14:776–777
8. Baba H, Maezawa Y, Kamitani K, Furusawa N, Imura S, Tomita K (1995) Osteoporotic vertebral collapse with late neurological complications. Paraplegia 33:281–289
9. Barry HC (1969) Paget's disease of bone. Churchill Livingstone, Edinburgh
10. Basle MF, Rebel A, Fournier JG, et al (1987) On the trail of paramyxoviruses in Paget's disease of bone. Clin Orthop 217:9–15
11. Boudreau RJ, Lisbona R, Hadjipavlou A (1983) Observation on serial radionuclide blood flow studies in Paget's disease. J Nucl Med 24:880–885
12. Boutin RD, Spitz DJ, Newman JS, et al (1998) Complications in Paget disease at MR imaging. Radiology 209: 641–651
13. Brower AC, Downey EF (1981) Kummel disease: report of a case with serial radiographs. Radiology 1341: 363–364
14. Byrd JA, Scoles PV, Winter RB, Bradford DS, Lonstein JE, Moe JH (1987) Adult idiopathic scoliosis treated by anterior and posterior spinal fusion. J Bone Joint Surg Am 69:843–850
15. Cartlidge N, McCollum JPK, Ayyar RDA (1972) Spinal cord compression in Paget's disease. J Neurol Neurosurg Psychiatry 35:825–828
16. Chen JR, Richard SCR, Wallach S, et al (1979) Neurologic disturbances in Paget's disease of bone: response to calcitonin. Neurology 29:448–457
17. Chiba M, McLain RF, Yerby SA, et al (1996) Short-segment pedicle screw fixation: biomechanical analysis of supplemental hook fixation. Spine 21:288–294
18. Chou LH, Knight RQ (1997) Idiopathic avascular necrosis of a vertebral body. Spine 22:1928–1932
19. Christenson RH (1997) Biochemical markers of bone metabolism: an overview. Clin Biochem 30:573–593
20. Clarke PR, Williams HI (1975) Ossification in extradural fat in Paget's disease of the spine. Br J Surg 62: 571–572
21. Coe JD, Warden KE, Herzig MA, McAfee PC (1990) Influence of bone mineral density on the fixation of thoracolumbar implants: a comparative study of transpedicular screws, laminar hooks, and spinous process wires. Spine 15:902–907
22. Cohen LD (1990) Fractures of the osteoporotic spine. Orthop Clin North Am 21:143–150
23. Collins DH (1956) Paget's disease of bone: incidence and subclinical forms. Lancet 2:51–56
24. Consensus Conference (1984) Osteoporosis. JAMA 252:799–802
25. Cooper C, Atkinson EJ, O'Fallon WM, Melton LJ 3rd (1992) Incidence of clinically diagnosed vertebral fractures: a population-based study on Rochester, Minnesota, 1985–1989. J Bone Mineral Res 7:221–227
26. Cortet B, Solau-Gervais E, Labbe P, et al (1995) Tassements vertébraux ostéoporotiques avec complications neurologiques sévères. A propos de six observations. Rev Med Interne 16:891–896

27. Courtois I, Lauwers A, Prades B, Alexandre C (1998) Can an osteoporotic vertebral fracture cause compression of the spinal cord or cauda equina. Rev Rhum Engl Ed 65:207–211
28. Curran JE (1975) Neurological sequelae of Paget's disease of the vertebral column and skull bone. Austral Radiol 19:15–19
29. Cyteval C, Sarrabere MP, Roux JO, Thomas E, Jorgensen C, Blotman F, Sany J, Taourel P (1999). Acute osteoporotic vertebral collapse: open study on percutaneous injection of acrylic surgical cement in 20 patients. AJR 173:1685–1690
30. Danais S, Hadjipavlou A (1977) Etude scintigraphique comparative des lésions osseuses et de la moelle osseuse dans la maladie de Paget. Union Med Can 106:1100–1109
31. Direkze M, Milnes JN (1970) Spinal cord compression in Paget's disease. Br J Surg 57:239–240
32. Douglas DL, Duckworth T, Kanis JA, et al (1980) Biochemical and clinical responses to dichloromethylene disphosphonate (CI 2MDP) in Paget's disease of bone. Arthritis Rheum 23:1185–1192
33. Douglas DL, Duckworth T, Kanis JA, et al (1981) Spinal cord dysfuction in Paget's disease of bone: has medical treatment a vascular basis? J Bone Joint Surg Br 63:495–503
34. Eck JC, Hodges SD, Humphreys SC (2002) Vertebroplasty: a new treatment strategy for osteoporotic compression fractures. Am J Orthop 31: 123–128
35. Elisevich K, Fontaine S, Bertrand C (1987) Syringomyelia as a complication of Paget's disease. J Neurosurg 67:611–613
36. Eulry F, Poirier JM, Perard D, et al (1997) Cauda equina syndrome with pagetic vertebral fusion. Clinical recovery under calcium-vitamin D supplementation plus clodronate after apparent failure of pamidronate and acquired resistance to etidronate. Rev Rhum Engl Ed 64:495–499
37. Fink HA, Ensrud KE, Nelson DB, et al (2003) Disability after clinical fracture in postmenopausal women with low bone density: the fracture intervention trial (FIT). Osteoporos Int. Jan;14(1):69-76
38. Fleisch H (1987) Experimental basis for the use of bisphosphonates in Paget's disease of bone. Clin Orthop 217:72–78
39. Fleisch H (1997) Mechanisms of action of the bisphosphonates. Medicina (B Aires) 57 [Suppl 1]:65–75
40. Franck WA, Bress NM, Singer FR, et al (1974) Rheumatic manifestations of Paget's disease of bone. Am J Med 56:592–603
41. Gallagher SJ, Boyle IT, Capell HA (1991) Pseudogout associated with the use of cyclical etidronate therapy. Scott Med J 36:49–54
42. Garfin (2001) New technologies in spine: kyphoplasty and vertebroplasty for the treatment of painful osteoporotic compression fractures. Spine 26:1511–1515
43. Gray RE (1988) Paget's disease of bone: comments by eight specialists. Excerpta Medica, Princeton
44. Guyer PB, Chamberlain AT (1988) Paget's disease of bone in South Africa. Clin Radiol 39:51–52
45. Guyer PB, Shepherd DFC (1980) Paget's disease of lumbar spine. Br J Radiol 53:286–288
46. Hadjipavlou A, Lander P (1991) Paget's disease of the spine. J Bone Joint Surg Am 73:1376–1381
47. Hadjipavlou A, Tsoukas G, Siller T, et al (1977) Combination drug therapy in treatment of Paget's disease of bone: clinical and metabolic response. J Bone Joint Surg Am 59:1045–1051
48. Hadjipavlou A, Lander P, Srolovitz H (1986) Pagetic arthritis: pathophysiology and management. Clin Orthop 208:15–19
49. Hadjipavlou A, Begin LR, Abitbol JJ (1986) Observations morphologiques, histochimiques et ultrastructurales de culture cellulaires in vitro d'os pagetique et normal. Union Med Can 115: 746–750
50. Hadjipavlou AG, Lander PH, Enker P (1986) Paget's disease of bone: orthopedic management. In: Arthritis pathology and management. Current Concepts of Bone Fragility Uttof Springer, Berlin Heidelberg New York
51. Hadjipavlou A, Shaffer N, Lander P, Srolovitz H (1988) Pagetic spinal stenosis with extradural pagetoid ossification: a case report. Spine 13:128–130
52. Hadjipavlou A, Lander P, Srulovitz H, Enker P (1992) Malignant transformation in Paget's disease of bone. Cancer 70:1802–1808
53. Hadjipavlou AG, Lander PH (1995) Paget's disease. In: White AH, Schofferman JA (eds) Spinal care. Mosby, St Louis, pp 1720–1737
54. Hadjipavlou A, Enker P, Dupuis O, Katzman S, Silver J (1996) The causes of failure of lumbar transpedicular spinal instrumentation and fusion: a prospective study. Int Orthop 20: 35–42
55. Hadjipavlou AG, Nicodemus C, Al-Hamden FA, Simmons JW, Pope MH (1997) Correlation of bone equivalent mineral density to pull out resistance of triangulated pedical screw construct. J Spinal Disord 10:12–19
56. Hadjipavlou A, Gaitanis I, Katonis P, Lander P (2001) Paget's disease of the spine and its management. Eur Spine J 10:370–384
57. Hadjipavlou A, Gaitanis I, Kontakis G (2002) Paget disease of the bone and its management. J Bone Joint Surg Br 84:160–169
58. Halvorson TL, Kelley LA, Thomas KA, Whitecloud TS, Cook SD (1994) Effects of bone mineral density on pedicle screw fixation. Spine 19:2415–2420
59. Hartman JT, Dohn DF (1966) Paget's disease of the spine with cord or nerve root compression. J Bone Joint Surg Am 48:1079–1084
60. Hasegawa K, Homma T, Uchiyama S, et al (1988) Vertebral pseudarthrosis in the osteoporotic spine. Spine 23: 2201–2206
61. Hasegawa K, Takahashi HE, Uchiyama S, et al (1997) An experimental study of a combination of methods using a pedicle screw and laminar hook for the osteoporotic spine. Spine 22:958–963
62. Haslam SI, Van Hul W, Morales-Piga A, et al (1998) Paget's disease of bone: evidence for a susceptibility locus on chromosome 18q and for genetic heterogeneity. J Bone Miner Res 13:911–917
63. Heggeness MH (1993) Spine fracture with neurological deficit in osteoporosis. Osteoporos Int 3:215–221
64. Herzberg L, Bayllis E (1980) Spinal cord syndrome due to compressive Paget's disease of bone: a spinal artery steal phenomena reversible with calcitonin. Lancet 2:13–15
65. Hocking L, Slee F, Haslam SI, et al (2000) Familial Paget's disease of bone: patterns of inheritance and frequency of linkage to chromosome 18q. Bone 26:577–580
66. Hu SS (1997) Internal fixation in the osteoporotic spine. Spine 22 [24 Suppl]: 43–44
67. Huang TL, Cohen NJ, Sahgal SA, et al (1979) Osteosarcoma complicating in Paget's disease of the spine with neurologic complication. Clin Orthop 14:260–265
68. Hyde C, et al (2002) Secondary osteoporotic compressive vertebral fracture after kyphoplasty. Eur Spine J [Suppl 1]:34–35

69. Kado DM, Browner W, Palermo L, Nevitt MC, Genant HK, Cumming S (1999) Vertebral body fractures and mortality in older women: a prospective study. Study of osteoporotic fracture research group. Arch Intern Med 159:1215–1220
70. Kane WJ (1988) Spinal osteoporosis. Spinal deformity: what's the latest and what's the best? Presented at the AAOS Meeting, Baltimore, 29 September
71. Kaneda K, Asano S, Hashimoto T, Satoh S, Fujiya M (1992) The treatment of osteoporotic-posttraumatic vertebral collapse using the Kaneda device and a bioactive ceramic vertebral prosthesis. Spine 17 [8 Suppl]: 295–303
72. Kaplan PA, Orton DF, Asleson RJ (1987) Osteoporosis with vertebral compression fractures, retropulsed fragments, and neurologic compromise. Radiology 165:533–535
73. Kempinsky WH (1958) Osteoporotic kyphosis with paraplegia. Neurology 8:181–186
74. Kennedy BJ (1970) Metabolic and toxic effects of mithromycin during tumor therapy. Am J Med 48:494–503
75. Kim K, Suk K, Kim J, Lee S (2003) Delayed vertebral collapse with neurological deficits secondary to osteoporosis. Intern Orthop 27:65–69
76. Klenerman L (1966) Cauda equina and spinal cord compression in Paget's disease. J Bone Joint Surg Br 48:365–370
77. Korovessis P, Maraziotis T, Piperos G, Spyropoulos P (1994) Spontaneous burst fracture of the thoracolumbar spine in osteoporosis associated with neurological impairment: a report of seven cases and review of the literature. Eur Spine J 3:286–288
78. Lamovec J, Rener M, Spiler M, et al (1999) Pseudosarcoma in Paget's disease of bone. Ann Diagn Pathol 3:99–100
79. Lander P, Hadjipavlou A (1986) A dynamic classification in Paget's. J Bone Joint Surg Br 68:431–438
80. Lander P, Hadjipavlou A (1991) Intradiscal invasion of Paget's disease of the spine. Spine 16:46–51
81. Lee KS, McWhorter JM, Angelo JN (1988) Spinal epidural hematoma associated with Paget's disease. Surg Neurol 30:131–134
82. Leech JA, Dulberg C, Kellie S, Pattie L, Gay J (1999) Relationship of lung function to severity of osteoporosis in women. Am Ref Respir Dis 141:68–71
83. Lieberman (2001) Initial outcome and efficacy of kyphopasty in the treatment of osteoporotic VCFs. Spine 26: 1631–1638
84. Linville DA (2002) Vertebroplasty and kyphoplasty. South Med J 95: 583–587
85. Lotz JC, Hu SS, Chiu DFM, Yu M, Colliou O, Poser RD (1997) Cardonated apatite cement augmentation of pedicle screw fixation in the lumbar spine. Spine 22:2716–2723
86. Lowe TG, Kasten MD (1994) An analysis of sagittal curves and balance after Cotrel-Dubousset instrumentation for kyphosis secondary to Scheuermann's disease. Spine 19:1680–1685
87. Lyles (1993) Association of osteoporotic vertebral compression fractures with impaired functional status. Am J Med 94:595–601
88. Manolagas SC (1999) Advances in the treatment of osteoporosis. Presented at the 21st Annual Meeting of the American Society for Bone Mineral Research. 30 September–4 October. Conference Report. Medscape Diabetes and Endocrinology, 1999
89. Marcelli C, Yates AJ, Barjon MC, Pansard E, Angelloz-Pessey L, Simon L (1995) Pagetic vertebral ankylosis and diffuse idiopathic skeletal hyperostosis. Spine 20:454–459
90. Maruo S, Tatekawa F, Nakano K (1987) Paraplegia caused by vertebral compression fractures in senile osteoporosis. Z Orthop Ihre Grenzgeb 125: 320–323
91. Mathe JF, Delobel R, Resche F, et al (1976) Syndromes medullaire au cours de la maladie De Paget: role du facteur vasculaire. Nouv Presse Med 5: 2619–2621
92. McLain RF (1997) Point of view: an experimental study of combination method using a pedicle screw and laminar hook for the osteoporotic spine. Spine 22:963
93. Mee AP (1999) Paramyxoviruses and Paget's disease: the affirmative view. Bone 24 [5 Suppl]:19–21
94. Melton LJ III, Riggs BL (1987) Epidemiology of age-related fractures. In: Avioli LV (ed) The osteoporotic syndrome. Grune & Stratton, New York, pp 1–30
95. Meunier PJ, Salson C, Mathieu L, et al (1987) Skeletal distribution and biochemical parameters of Paget's disease. Clin Orthop 217:37–44
96. Moore DC, Maitra RS, Farjo LA, Graziano GP, Goldstein SA (1997) Restoration of pedicle screw fixation with in situ setting calcium phosphate cement. Spine 22:1696–1705
97. Nguyen HV, Ludwig S, Gelb D (2003) Osteoporotic vertebral burst fractures with neurologic compromise. J Spinal Disord Techniques 16:10–19
98. O'Connor PA, Eustace S, O'Byrne J (2002) Spinal cord injury following osteoporotic vertebral fracture: case report. Spine 27:E413–415
99. Okuyama K, Sato K, Abe E, et al (1993) Stability of transpedicle screwing for the osteoporotic spine: an in vitro study of the mechanical stability. Spine 19:2240–2245
100. Paget J (1877) On a form of chronic inflammation of bone (osteitis deformans). Trans R Med Chir Soc London 60:36–43
101. Parfitt AM, Duncan H (1982) Metabolic bone disease affecting the spine. In: Rothman RH, Simone FA (eds) The spine, vol 2, 2nd edn. Saunders, Philadelphia, pp 828–830
102. Phillips FM, Todd Wetzel F, Lieberman I, Campell-Hupp M (2002) An in vivo comparison of the potential for extravertebral cement leak after vertebroplasty and kyphoplasty. Spine 27: 2173–2178
103. Porrini AA, Maldonado-Cocco JA, Morteo GO (1987) Spinal artery steal syndrome in Paget's disease of bone. Clin Exp Rheumatol 5:377–378
104. Pygott F (1957) Paget's disease of bone: the radiological incidence. Lancet 1:1170–1179
105. Radi I, Epiney J, Reiner M (1970) Chondrocalcinose et maladie asseuse de Paget. Rev Rheum 37:385–388
106. Ramussen H, Bordier P (1973) The physiological cellular basis of metabolic bone disease. N Engl Med 184: 25–29
107. Ravichandran G (1979) Neurologic recovery of paraplegia following use of salmon calcitonin in a patient with Paget's disease of the spine. Spine 4:37–40
108. Reginster JY, Lecart MP (1995) Efficacy and safety of drugs for Paget's disease of bone. Bone 17 [5 Suppl]: 485–488
109. Reid IR, Nicholson GC, Weinstein RS, et al (1996) Biochemical and radiologic improvement in Paget's disease of bone treated with alendronate: a randomized, placebo-controlled trial. Am J Med 101:341–348
110. Richter RL, Semble EL, Turner RA, et al (1990) An unusual manifestation of Paget's disease of bone: spinal epidural hematoma presenting as acute cauda equina syndrome. J Rheumatol 17:975–978
111. Riggs BL, Melton LJ (1995) The worldwide problem of osteoporosis: insights afforded by epidemiology. Bone 17 [5 Suppl]:505–511
112. Riggs BL, Melton LJ III (1986). Involutional osteoporosis. N Engl J Med 314:1676
113. Rosenkrantz JA, Wolf J, Kaicher JJ (1952) Paget's disease (osteitis deformans). Arch Intern Med 90:610–615

114. Ross PD, Davia JW, Epstein RS, Wasnich RD (1991) Pre-existing fractures and bone mass predict vertebral fracture incidence in women. Ann Intern Med 114:919–923
115. Ryan WG (1977) Treatment of Paget's disease of bone with mithramycin. Clin Orthop 127:106–110
116. Ryan MD, Taylor TKF (1992) Spinal manifestations of Paget's disease. Aust N Z J Surg 62:33–38
117. Sadar SE, Walton RJ, Grossman HH (1972) Neurological dysfunction in Paget's disease of the vertebral column. J Neurosurg 37:661–665
118. Saita K, Hoshino Y, Kikkawa I, et al (2000) Posterior spinal shortening for paraplegia after vertebral collapse caused by osteoporosis. Spine 25: 2832–2835
119. Salomon C, Chopin D, Benoist M (1988) Spinal cord compression: an exceptional complication of spinal osteoporosis. Spine 13:222–224
120. Schajowicz F, Araujo SE, Berestein M (1983) Sarcoma complicating Paget's disease of bone: a clinicopathology study of 62 cases. J Bone Joint Surg Br 65:299–307
121. Schlaich C (1998) Reduced pulmonary function in patients with spinal osteoporotic fractures. Osteoporosis Int 8:261–267
122. Schlaich C, Minnie HW, Bruckner T, et al (1998) Reduced pulmonary function in patients with spinal osteoporotic fractures. Osteoporosis Int 8: 261–267
123. Schmorl G (1932) Uber osteitis deformans Paget. Virchows Arch Anat Physiol 183:694–701
124. Schwarz GA, Reback S (1939) Compression of the spinal cord in osteitis deformans (Paget's disease of the vertebrae). Am Roentgenol Radium Ther 42:345–347
125. Shikata J, Yamamuro T, Iida I, Shimizu K, Yoshikawa J (1990) Surgical treatment for paraplegia resulting from vertebral fractures in senile osteoporosis. Spine 15:485–489
126. Siegelman SS, Levine SA, Walpin L (1968) Paget's disease with spinal cord compression. Clin Radiol 19: 421–425
127. Silverman SL (1992) The clinical consequences of vertebral compression fracture. Bone 13 [Suppl 2]: S27–S31
128. Singer RF, Millis BG (1977) The etiology of Paget's disease of bone. Clin Orthop 127:37–41
129. Siris ES, Kelsey JL, Flaster E, et al (1990) Paget's disease of bone and previous pet ownership in the United States: dogs exonerated. Intern J Epidemol 19:455–458
130. Smidt WR, Hadjipavlou AG, Lander P, Dzioba RB (1994) An algorithmic approach to the treatment of Paget's disease of the spine. Orthop Rev 23: 715–724
131. Soshi S, Shiba R, Kondo H, et al (1991) An experimental study on transpedicular screw fixation in relation to osteoporosis in the lumbar spine. Spine 16:1335–1341
132. Tanaka S, Kubota M, Fujimoto Y, Hayashi J, Nishikawa K (1993) Conus medullaris syndrome secondary to an L1 burst fracture in osteoporosis. A case report. Spine 18:2131–2134
133. Tiegs RD (1997) Paget's disease of bone: indications for treatment and goals of therapy. Clin Ther 19:1309–1329
134. Turner JWA (1940) Spinal complications of Paget's disease (osteiti deformans). Brain 63:321–327
135. Whalley N (1946) Paget's disease of the atlas and axis. J Neurol Neurosurg Psychiatry 9:84–91
136. Wyllie WG (1923) The occurrence in osteiti deformans of lesion of the central nervous system with a report of four cases. Brain 46:336–342
137. Zlatkin MB, Lander PH, Hadjipavlou A, Levine JS (1986) Paget's disease of the spine: CT with clinical correlation. Radiology 160:155–159

K. Lippuner

Medical treatment of vertebral osteoporosis

Abstract Although osteoporosis is a systemic disease, vertebral fractures due to spinal bone loss are a frequent, sometimes early and often neglected complication of the disease, generally associated with considerable disability and pain. As osteoporotic vertebral fractures are an important predictor of future fracture risk, including at the hip, medical management is targeted at reducing fracture risk. A literature search for randomized, double-blind, prospective, controlled clinical studies addressing medical treatment possibilities of vertebral fractures in postmenopausal Caucasian women was performed on the leading medical databases. For each publication, the number of patients with at least one new vertebral fracture and the number of randomized patients by treatment arm was retrieved. The relative risk (RR) and the number needed to treat (NNT, i.e. the number of patients to be treated to avoid one radiological vertebral fracture over the duration of the study), together with the respective 95% confidence intervals (95%CI) were calculated for each study. Treatment of steroid-induced osteoporosis and treatment of osteoporosis in men were reviewed separately, based on the low number of publications available. Forty-five publications matched with the search criteria, allowing for analysis of 15 different substances tested regarding their anti-fracture efficacy at the vertebral level. Bisphosphonates, mainly alendronate and risedronate, were reported to have consistently reduced the risk of a vertebral fracture over up to 50 months of treatment in four (alendronate) and two (risedronate) publications. Raloxifene reduced vertebral fracture risk in one study over 36 months, which was confirmed by 48 months' follow-up data. Parathormone (PTH) showed a drastic reduction in vertebral fracture risk in early studies, while calcitonin may also be a treatment option to reduce fracture risk. For other substances published data are conflicting (calcitriol, fluoride) or insufficient to conclude about efficacy (calcium, clodronate, etidronate, hormone replacement therapy, pamidronate, strontium, tiludronate, vitamin D). The low NNTs for the leading substances (ranges: 15–64 for alendronate, 8–26 for risedronate, 23 for calcitonin and 28–31 for raloxifene) confirm that effective and efficient drug interventions for treatment and prevention of osteoporotic vertebral fractures are available. Bisphosphonates have demonstrated similar efficacy in treatment and prevention of steroid-induced and male osteoporosis as in postmenopausal osteoporosis. The selection of the appropriate drug for treatment of vertebral osteoporosis from among a bisphosphonate (alendronate or risedronate), PTH, calcitonin or raloxifene will mainly depend on the effi-

The author has no conflict of interest

K. Lippuner (✉)
Osteoporosis Policlinic,
University Hospital of Berne,
3010 Berne, Switzerland
Tel.: +41-31-6323185,
Fax: +41-31-6329596,
e-mail: kurt.lippuner@insel.ch

cacy, tolerability and safety profile, together with the patient's willingness to comply with a long-term treatment. Although reduction of vertebral fracture risk is an important criterion for decision making, drugs with proven additional fracture risk reduction at all clinically relevant sites (especially at the hip) should be the preferred options.

Keywords Review · Medical treatment · Vertebral fractures · Osteoporosis · Relative risk reduction · Number needed to treat

Introduction

Osteoporosis was defined at a 1993 consensus conference as "a systemic skeletal disease characterized by low bone mass and micro-architectural deterioration of bone tissue with a resultant increase in fragility and risk of fracture" [24]. As bone quality cannot be evaluated easily in daily practice, the diagnosis of osteoporosis is made on low bone mineral density (BMD), expressed as the number of standard deviations above or below BMD for normal young adults (T-score). The World Health Organization study group's definition of osteoporosis is a T-score below –2.5 SD. Patients with a T-score below –2.5 who also have suffered a fragility fracture have severe osteoporosis [91].

Although a number of risk factors for osteoporotic fractures have been identified [26, 35], a history of previous vertebral fracture is a particularly important risk factor for future fractures. Postmenopausal women with radiographically detected vertebral fractures are at increased risk for new fractures, independently of bone mass [9, 17, 79]. In addition, vertebral fractures are common: 5% of Caucasian women aged 50 and 25% of those aged 80 have one or more fractures [58], and as many as 11–56% of patients on long-term steroids are estimated to have prevalent vertebral fragility fractures [3, 52, 60]. Vertebral fractures, even those not recognized clinically, are associated with substantial increases in back pain, functional limitation, disability, and with an excess mortality risk [44, 63]. However, physicians frequently do not diagnose osteoporosis in primary care patients with vertebral fractures, thereby missing an important preventive opportunity for patients at highest risk for future fractures: in a recently published study from Neuner et al., only 38% of subjects with vertebral compression fractures noted on routine radiographs (46% of women and 19% of men) were diagnosed with osteoporosis, and only 32% received prescription medication for osteoporosis [62].

Effective medical treatments of osteoporosis have increasingly become available over the last decade and their efficacy in reducing fracture risk, including at the spine, has been reviewed thoroughly in several recent publications [39, 45, 65].

The aim of this publication is to review the available data on drug treatment options in women with postmenopausal osteoporosis, with special focus on vertebral fracture risk reduction, and to briefly comment on steroid-induced osteoporosis and osteoporosis in men.

Materials and methods

We searched Medline, Embase and Current Contents from 1980 to 2002 for randomized controlled trials with drug treatment intervention in Caucasian *women with postmenopausal osteoporosis* (defined as T-score below –2SD at inclusion and/or prevalent anamnestic fracture) and reporting vertebral fracture data (either as a primary or secondary endpoint or as an adverse event). Duplicates, abstracts, and posters were eliminated by manual selection.

All definitions of radiological vertebral fractures (anterior, middle, or posterior vertebral height loss defined as any % loss and/or as any absolute value in millimeters), as chosen by the authors, were accepted for inclusion in the final analysis. Published results on risk reduction of clinically symptomatic vertebral fractures and risk reduction of multiple fractures were recorded separately.

Studies reporting on the number of patients who suffered at least one fracture were retained. Studies reporting on total number of fractures (i.e., fracture rates in patient-years) per treatment group without mentioning the number of patients with fractures were excluded from the analysis. Counting events instead of patients has been criticized as violating basic statistical assumptions and invalidating the use of common statistical tests as well as cross comparisons [93].

Studies of less than 36 months' duration were eliminated. The minimum required duration for a phase III trial for development of anti-osteoporotic drugs is usually specified at 3 years in Europe and in the US, the European CPMP regulations being the most stringent, requiring demonstrated anti-fracture efficacy prior to registration of an osteoporosis drug [14].

For each publication, the number of patients with a at least one new vertebral fracture and the number of randomized patients by treatment arm was recorded. The relative risk (RR) and the number needed to treat (NNT, i.e. the number of patients to be treated to avoid one radiological vertebral fracture over the duration of the study) as well as the respective 95% confidence intervals were calculated. When different dosages were used in different treatment arms, the results were pooled (active vs control) and dosage-specific comments as stated in the original publication were reported if appropriate.

For *steroid-induced osteoporosis* and *osteoporosis in men*, an overview is given based on selected publications.

Results

Forty-five publications resulted from the search of the medical databases. Six publications were excluded because they reported on total number of fractures and the number of patients with at least one fracture was not published and could not be derived from published data [34, 46, 73, 76, 80, 85]. Sixteen publications were excluded because the duration of observation was less than 36 months [5, 7, 15, 21, 29, 32, 33, 36, 41, 53, 55, 59, 66, 67, 90, 92]. Twenty-three publications matched all selection criteria: four with alendronate [10, 11, 27, 50], two with calcitriol [31, 86], one with calcium-vitamin D [69], one

Table 1 Calculated relative risk (RR), number needed to treat (NNT)[a] and respective 95% confidence intervals (CI) of radiological and clinical vertebral fractures in women with postmenopausal osteoporosis (*NPFx* number of patients with at least one vertebral fracture, *NPR* number of patients randomized, by treatment group, *bold type* indicates significant outcomes)

	Mths	Total no. of subjects	NPFx/NPR Active	NPFx/NPR Controls	RR (95%CI)	NNT (95%CI)
Radiological vertebral fractures						
Alendronate [27]	**50**	**4432**	**43/2214**	**78/2218**	**0.55 (0.38 to 0.79)**	**64 (38 to 152)**
Alendronate [11]	**48**	**3658**	**107/1841**	**197/1817**	**0.54 (0.43 to 0.67)**	**20 (14 to 31)**
Alendronate [10]	**36**	**2027**	**78/1022**	**145/1005**	**0.53 (0.41 to 0.68)**	**15 (10 to 24)**
Alendronate [50]	**36**	**994**	**17/597**	**22/397**	**0.51 (0.28 to 0.95)**	**38 (18 to 349)**
Calcitonin [20]	60	1255	171/944	70/311	0.81 (0.63 to 1.03)	23 (10 to –154)
Calcitriol [86]	**36**	**622**	**66/314**	**155/308**	**0.42 (0.33 to 0.52)**	**4 (2 to 5)**
Calcitriol [31]	36	86	10/47	6/39	1.38 (0.55 to 3.45)	–15 (12 to –3)
Calcium VitD [69]	52	191	27/91	34/100	0.87 (0.58 to 1.33)	24 (5 to –11)
Etidronate [37]	**36**	**380**	**28/196**	**51/184**	**0.55 (0.36 to 0.82)**	**8 (4 to 18)**
Etidronate [54]	48	100	4/50	9/50	0.44 (0.15 to 1.3)	11 (3 to –95)
Fluoride [71]	48	164	2/84	8/80	0.25 (0.6 to 1.01)	14 (6 to 67)
Fluoride [77]	**36**	**144**	**20/99**	**30/45**	**0.3 (0.2 to 0.47)**	**3 (1 to 4)**
Fluoride [68]	**48**	**110**	**7/54**	**22/56**	**0.33 (0.16 to 0.66)**	**4 (2 to 8)**
HRT [70]	42	128	3/64	4/64	0.75 (0.18 to 3.22)	65 (9 to –20)
Ipriflavone [6]	36	472	7/233	8/239	0.9 (0.33 to 2.44)	292 (25 to –40)
Pamidronate [16]	**36**	**91**	**5/46**	**15/45**	**0.33 (0.14 to 0.78)**	**5 (2 to 13)**
PTH [61]	**21**	**1637**	**41/1093**	**64/544**	**0.32 (0.22 to 0.46)**	**13 (9 to 20)**
PTH [51]	36	34	1/17	4/17	0.25 (0.04 to 1.67)	6 (2 to 213)
Raloxifene II [28]	**48**	**7705**	**278/5129**	**225/2576**	**0.62 (0.52 to 0.73)**	**31 (21 to 48)**
Raloxifene I [30]	**36**	**7705**	**272/5129**	**231/2576**	**0.59 (0.5 to 0.7)**	**28 (20 to 42)**
Risedronate [38]	**36**	**1641**	**61/821**	**93/820**	**0.66 (0.48 to 0.89)**	**26 (14 to 83)**
Risedronate [72]	**36**	**816**	**53/408**	**89/408**	**0.6 (0.44 to 0.81)**	**12 (7 to 26)**
Risedronate [22]	36	132	28/88	20/44	0.7 (0.44 to 1.11)	8 (3 to –42)
Clinical vertebral fractures						
Alendronate [11]	**48**	**3658**	**38/1841**	**67/1817**	**0.56 (0.38 to 0.82)**	**62 (36 to 169)**
Alendronate [10]	**36**	**2027**	**23/1022**	**50/1005**	**0.45 (0.28 to 0.73)**	**37 (22 to 84)**
Raloxifene [30]	**36**	**7705**	**86/5129**	**81/2576**	**0.53 (0.4 to 0.72)**	**69 (44 to 136)**

[a] The number of patients to be treated to avoid one radiological vertebral fracture over the duration of the study

with calcitonin [20], two with etidronate [37, 54], three with fluoride [68, 71, 77], one with hormone replacement therapy [70], one with ipriflavone [6], one with pamidronate [16], two with parathormone [51, 61], two with raloxifene [28, 30] and three with risedronate [22, 38, 72]. The study of Neer et al. with parathormone [61] had a median duration of only 21 months, but was kept in the final analysis as it was stopped early by the sponsor.

Radiological vertebral fractures

An overview of all calculated RR and NNT values with the respective 95% confidence interval (CI) by drug and by study is given in Table 1. Figure 1 shows the RR and 95%CI for selected drugs in alphabetical order (alendronate, calcitonin, parathormone (teriparatide, PTH), raloxifene and risedronate).

Alendronate

In three long-term endpoint trials [10, 27, 50] and in one published re-analysis of the anti-fracture efficacy in patients with osteoporosis as defined by the WHO [11], alendronate showed a consistent and significant reduction in vertebral fracture risk of between 45 and 49% across all studies. The calculated NNT ranged from 15 (95%CI 10 to 24) to 64 (95%CI 38 to 152), depending on the patient population studied, patients with highest fracture risk having the lowest NNTs.

Calcitonin

Only one published clinical trial of more than 36 months' duration was retrieved [20]. Although the vertebral fracture risk is reported to be significantly reduced, by 33%, at the intranasal dose of 200 IU per day in the original publication, the risk reduction of the pooled dosages (100,

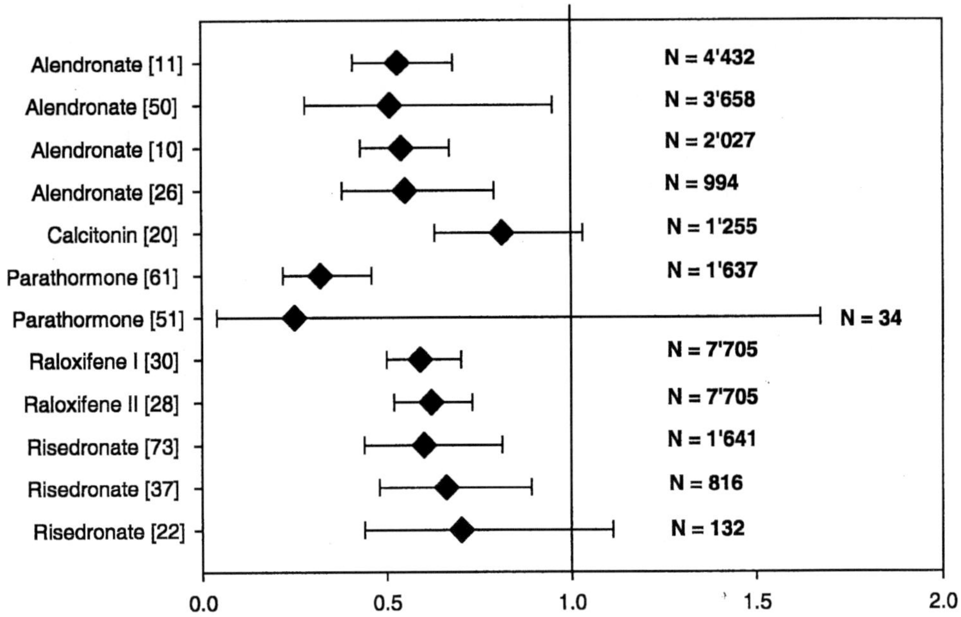

Fig. 1 Radiological vertebral fractures in women with postmenopausal osteoporosis: relative risks (*solid diamond*) and 95% confidence intervals following treatment with selected osteoporosis drugs

200 and 400 IU/day) reported here is not significant. Accordingly, the NNT is 23, with a 95% CI of 10 to –154.

Parathormone

Two published studies were eligible [51, 61]. Vertebral fracture risk was significantly reduced, by 68% (RR 0.32, 95%CI 0.22 to 0.46) in the endpoint trial [61], with an NNT of 13 (95%CI 9 to 20). In the other smaller trial, the risk reduction was not significant [51].

Raloxifene

Two publications report vertebral fracture data with raloxifene at 36 months [30] and in the 12 months extension [28]. The calculated vertebral fracture risk is significantly reduced, by 41% after 3 years and 38% after 4 years. The calculated NNTs are 28 (95%CI 20 to 42), and 31 (95%CI 21 to 48) respectively.

Risedronate

Risedronate significantly reduced calculated vertebral fracture risk, by 34% and 40% respectively, in two endpoint studies [38, 72]. In a third, smaller, study over 36 months, the risk reduction was not significant (RR 0.7, 95%CI 0.44 to 1.11) [22]. Calculated NNTs ranged from 8 (95%CI 3 to –42) to 26 (95%CI 14 to 83).

Other treatment options

Calcitriol, etidronate, fluoride and pamidronate showed calculated vertebral fracture risk reduction in single studies, while there is no publication demonstrating vertebral fracture risk reduction over 36 months for calcium-vitamin D, hormone replacement therapy or ipriflavone (Table 1).

Clinical (symptomatic) vertebral fractures

Clinical vertebral fractures were defined as clinically diagnosed and radiologically confirmed vertebral fractures, i.e. clinical fractures are usually symptomatic (back pain, height loss, kyphosis). Only two drugs had published data regarding risk reduction of symptomatic vertebral fractures. According to two reports, alendronate reduced the calculated risk for symptomatic vertebral fracture significantly, by 44% and 55% respectively (RR 0.56; 95%CI 0.38 to 0.82 and RR 0.45; 95%CI 0.28 to 0.73 respectively) [10, 11]. Raloxifene reduced the risk of clinical fracture by 47% (RR 0.53; 95%CI 0.4 to 0.72) [30] (Table 1).

Discussion

Postmenopausal osteoporosis

In women with postmenopausal osteoporosis, vertebral fractures can be prevented with efficacious drug treatments. Oral bisphosphonates (specific inhibitors of osteoclastic bone resorption: alendronate and risedronate), oral SERMs (selective estrogen receptor modulators: raloxifene) and subcutaneous PTH (amino-terminal parathyroid hormone 1–34: teriparatide) have demonstrated their clinical efficacy in large-scale trials with fractures as a primary endpoint. Calcium and vitamin D have no long-term clinical data to demonstrate their anti-fracture efficacy in the spine; however, calcium (500–1000 mg/day) and/or vitamin D substitution (400–800 IU/day) were always given to all patients in all treatment groups of all published clinical trials. Therefore, calcium and/or vitamin D substitution has to be considered as the established standard of all drug interventions against osteoporosis, even in the absence of conclusive fracture reduction endpoint data. Hormone replacement therapy (HRT) has not shown documented vertebral fracture risk reduction in large-scale trials to date. However, the effect of HRT on fracture risk (hip fractures and all clinical fractures) has been extensively studied. Hormones have systemic effects, some of which may be expected to be beneficial, others less so. Two recently published studies in 2,763 and 16,608 postmenopausal women respectively have shed a new light on the antifracture efficacy of HRT and its systemic effects. In the HERS trial, a randomized, double-blind, placebo-controlled secondary cardio-vascular prevention trial with combined estrogens and progestin in 2,763 postmenopausal women with documented coronary heart disease, where less than 15% of the women had osteoporosis at inclusion [19, 42, 43], HRT had no significant effect on clinical fractures (RR 0.95, 95%CI 0.75 to 1.21) nor on hip fractures (RR 1.10; 95%CI 0.49 to 2.5) nor on breast cancer incidence, nor on coronary heart disease, nor on stroke. Risk for venous thrombotic disease was significantly greater with HRT (RR 2.89; 95%CI 1.50 to 5.58) [42]. In the WHI trial, a randomized, double-blind, placebo-controlled trial with combined estrogens and progestin designed to assess the major health benefits and risks of combined HRT in 16,608 postmenopausal women who had not undergone hysterectomy, clinical and hip fracture risk was significantly reduced, by 24 and 34% respectively. However, risk for breast cancer, coronary heart disease, venous thrombotic disease and stroke was significantly increased with HRT [95]. The authors concluded that, in this trial, health risks exceeded the benefits from use of combined estrogen plus progestin in healthy postmenopausal women over a 5.2-year period of observation [95]. Therefore, HRT should be reserved for short-term treatment of postmenopausal symptoms and other drug alternatives considered for treatment or prevention of osteoporosis.

Osteoporosis is a systemic disease. Therefore, drugs that have been shown to reduce the risk of fracture at all clinically relevant sites, especially at the hip, should become preferred treatment options. Based on published data to date in postmenopausal women with osteoporosis, alendronate significantly reduced hip fracture risk, by 51% [10, 11], risedronate by 30% [56], while calcitonin [20], raloxifene [28, 30] and PTH [61] had no significant effect. The calculated numbers needed to treat, i.e. the number of patients to be treated to avoid one radiological vertebral fracture over the duration of the study, are comparable with NNTs calculated in other therapeutic fields for interventions usually considered as being good medical practice. The NNT of gemfibrozil in male patients with high cholesterol is 71 over 5 years to avoid one coronary event [40], the NNT to avoid one myocardial infarction with aspirin in healthy males is 111 over 5 years [84], and the NNT to avoid one serious gastrointestinal complication with misoprostol in rheumatoid arthritis patients is 263 over 6 months [83]. If taking additionally the fracture risk reductions achieved at all clinical fracture sites into

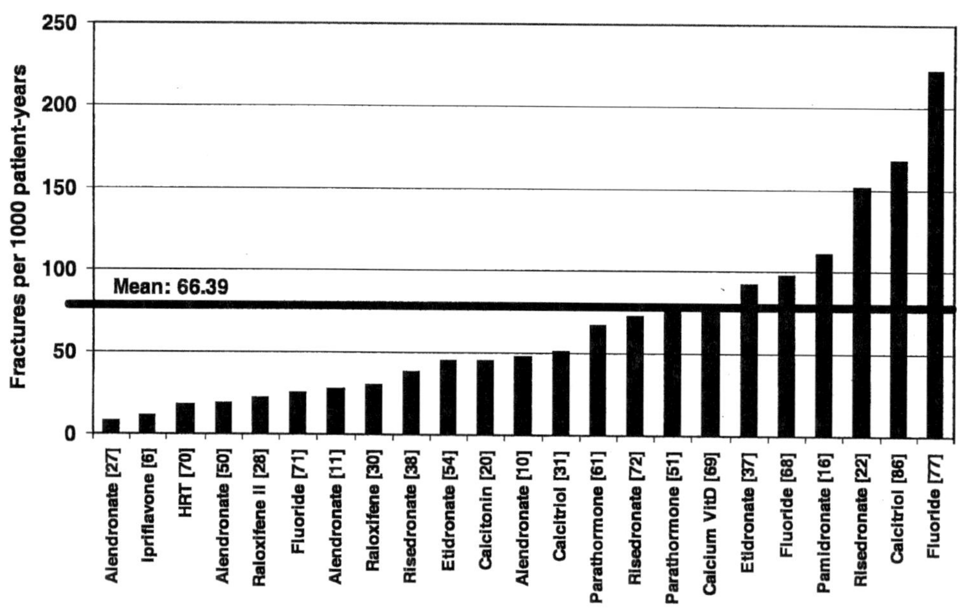

Fig. 2 Incidences of radiological vertebral fractures in the control group of women with postmenopausal osteoporosis (fractures per 1000 patient-years)

account, the NNTs for a drug intervention in osteoporosis would be expected to be even lower. This supposes that patients are well diagnosed by DEXA bone mineral density measurement at the hip or the spine, showing a T-score lower than or equal to –2.5 SD with or without anamnestic fractures, before getting drug therapy. An interesting finding was the great disparity in fracture incidences in the control groups of the selected trials (Fig. 2). They reflect the differences in definitions of vertebral fractures on the one hand and the fracture risk of the analysed patient population on the other. The definitions of radiological vertebral fractures used in the different trials range from a 15% reduction in vertebral height, including worsening of pre-existing fractures, to 20% reduction in vertebral height *and* more than 4 mm. Therefore, an expected finding would be that the most stringent definition will result in fewer fractures being detected than the looser one, independently of the antifracture efficacy of the drug. Some studies have included patients with low BMD (T-score below –2 SD) and no fractures, while others included patients with up to five pre-existent vertebral fractures. Therefore, an expected finding would be that the studies including highest-risk patients would show a greater fracture incidence, including in the control group. However, these studies may fail to be representative of the patients in which the drug will be used later in daily practice. The calculated NNTs should therefore be interpreted in this light, considering that in some cases less efficacious drugs have the best NNTs.

This review has several limitations. Firstly, we excluded from the analysis all studies of less than 36 months' duration. However, osteoporosis is a chronic, slowly debilitating disease, and European CPMP and US American FDA regulations require 36 months' data for registration of an osteoporosis drug [14]. Our results are in line with those of an exhaustive meta-analysis [65] and a recent review [39], which reached similar conclusions. Secondly, we excluded all studies reporting fracture rates only, and considered only studies reporting patients with at least one vertebral fracture. However, the drawback of the loss of data of isolated studies was outweighed by far by the improved quality of the remaining data, especially as the present review focused on vertebral fractures. In fact, for statistical analysis, the basic assumption is that all events can be regarded as independent; a second event in the same patient being as likely as a first event in this or in another patient. Vertebral fractures are not independent events [93]. By considering only patients with fractures (i.e., the true fracture incidence and not the fracture rate), the information about the drug effect on the risk reduction of multiple fractures is lost, and separate analyses would be required to answer this question. One publication addresses the risk reduction for multiple symptomatic fractures with alendronate, showing a significant risk reduction, of 84% (RR 0.16; 95%CI 0.05 to 0.42) [49].

Osteoporosis in men

Osteoporosis in men is more often secondary than primary. Therefore, the underlying cause (drug-induced bone loss, gastro-intestinal diseases, hypercalciuria, endocrine disorders, etc) must be identified and treated first. The best documented drug intervention is with alendronate, which showed similar efficacy in men and in postmenopausal women with regard to achieved increases in BMD. The studies were not statistically powered to evaluate the efficacy on vertebral fracture risk reduction; however, both showed a trend in favor of alendronate [64, 78]. Pooled results of two studies with risedronate in 184 men receiving chronic steroid therapy showed a significant reduction in the risk of vertebral fracture over 1 year of treatment [75]. As is the case in women, calcium and vitamin D deficiency have been prevented by systematic calcium substitution.

Glucocorticosteroid-induced osteoporosis

Glucocorticosteroid-induced osteoporosis (GIO) is by far the most frequent cause of secondary osteoporosis [4, 89], and fracture incidence under corticosteroids may be as high as 50% [3]. The pathogenesis of GIO is complex: proposed mechanisms include decreased osteoblast proliferation and biosynthetic activity as well as increased bone resorption [18], sex-steroid deficiency, decreased intestinal calcium absorption and secondary hyperparathyroidism [47]. Fracture risk is dose dependent, rises within the first months under glucocorticoid treatment, and remains elevated over the entire duration of therapy [87]. However, even short courses of oral corticosteroids or inhaled corticosteroids may be deleterious to bone [87, 94].

The comparative efficacy with respect to bone mineral density of several therapeutic agents for the management of GIO has been recently determined using meta-regression models [8]. Bisphosphonates were the most effective of the evaluated agents, whereas calcitonin and vitamin D were more effective than no therapy or calcium. Promising data with respect to BMD have furthermore been obtained with PTH, which had not yet been included in that meta-analysis of 2002 [48]. However, for all mentioned therapeutic strategies in GIO, fracture data are scarce, since many of the trials had a preventive design and were of short duration (1 or 2 years), including only modest numbers of patients with small numbers of fractures [1, 2, 23, 25, 74, 75, 81, 82, 88].

Using cyclical etidronate in 141 men and women who had recently begun high-dose corticosteroid therapy, Adachi et al. found no significant reduction in vertebral fracture incidence compared with the placebo group overall after 12 months [1]. However, among postmenopausal women 1/31 in the etidronate group versus 7/32 women receiving placebo experienced new vertebral fractures, demonstrating an anti-fracture effect of marginal significance (P= 0.05). The combined results of two parallel 12-months trials (one conducted in the US, one in 15 other countries) using alendronate in a total of 477 men and women who had been under glucocorticoid therapy for a varying duration (34% for less than 4 months, 21% for 4–12 months, 45% for more than 12 months) were quite similar compared with those of the etidronate trial. Again they showed no significant difference in overall incidence between the bisphosphonate and placebo groups (P=0.18), but there was a borderline significance, of P=0.05, in postmenopausal women, when a post-hoc binary semiquantitative fracture assessment was used (7/54 patients with new vertebral fractures in the placebo versus 6/135 in the alendronate group) [81]. Although patients had a relatively low background prevalence of vertebral fractures (12–15%) the reduction in the incidence of vertebral fractures under alendronate became significant in a sample of patients (144 women, 66 men) in which that combined trial was extended to 24 months (overall 4/59 patients of the placebo group and 1/143 patients in the alendronate group experienced new morphometric fractures over 2 years, P=0.026) [2]. A recent comparative 2-years trial between calcitriol, vitamin D plus calcium and alendronate plus calcium in 195 subjects (134 women, 61 men) commencing or already taking glucocorticoids showed that alendronate was superior to the other two treatment regimens for glucocorticoid-induced bone loss, especially in the spine [82]. Six of 66 subjects treated with calcitriol, 1 of 61 treated with ergocalciferol, and 0 of 64 treated with alendronate sustained new vertebral fractures. That study was not powered for a fracture endpoint; however, it is interesting to note that, as in all the above-mentioned studies, no vertebral fractures occurred in premenopausal women.

The efficacy of risedronate was evaluated in two 1-year studies for prevention [23] and treatment [74]. The prevention trial included 224 men and women who had begun to take glucocorticoids within the previous 3 months. The treatment study included 285 men and women who had been under glucocorticoids for at least 6 months. Risedronate reduced the risk of new vertebral fractures by 71% (P=0.072) in the prevention trial and by 70% (P= 0.042) in the treatment trial. When data from these two studies were combined, risedronate led to a 70% (P=0.01) reduction in the risk of vertebral fracture relative to placebo [88]: after 1 year, 18/111 patients (16%) under placebo and 12/195 patients (6%) under risedronate experienced new morphometric vertebral fractures. The significant antifracture effect in that combined study was reached for all patients together and for postmenopausal women, only. A separate (post hoc) analysis of male data from these two parallel risedronate trials on an intent to treat basis revealed a significant antifracture efficacy also for men under glucocorticoid treatment (P=0.008) [75].

Although more effective than calcium alone in maintaining lumbar BMD [8], calcitonin failed to reduce fracture risk in the spine or femoral neck in GIO [25].

The antifracture efficacy of PTH in that special condition remains to be proven.

Management of acute and chronic pain

Most osteoporotic vertebral fractures are asymptomatic. In the clinical trials that analyzed radiological and clinical vertebral fractures, symptomatic fractures represented 35% of all radiological fractures [10, 11, 30]. However, even asymptomatic fractures lead to spine deformity with chronic back pain and progressive disability. The management of chronic back pain relies on analgesics (paracetamol), non steroidal anti-inflammatory drugs (NSAIDs), and, more recently, on selective COX-II inhibitors (coxibs), which have demonstrated equal efficacy in pain relief and an improved gastrointestinal safety profile as compared to NSAIDs [13, 57]. Calcitonin, administered subcutaneously or intranasally, has demonstrated excellent analgesic efficacy in some patients [12]. Additional non-pharmacologic interventions include physiotherapy, physical activity and fall prevention programs.

Conclusion

The selection of the appropriate drug for treatment of vertebral osteoporosis among a bisphosphonate (alendronate or risedronate), PTH, calcitonin or raloxifene will mainly depend on its efficacy, tolerability and safety profile together with the patient's willingness to comply with a long-term treatment. Although reduction of vertebral fracture risk is an important criterion for decision-making, drugs with proven additional fracture risk reduction at all clinically relevant sites (especially at the hip) should be the preferred options.

References

1. Adachi JD, Bensen WG, Brown J, et al (1997) Intermittent etidronate therapy to prevent corticosteroid-induced osteoporosis. N Engl J Med 337:382–387
2. Adachi JD, Saag KG, Delmas PD, et al (2001) Two-year effects of alendronate on bone mineral density and vertebral fracture in patients receiving glucocorticoids. Arthritis Rheum 44:202–211
3. Adinoff AD, Hollister JR (1983) Steroid-induced fractures and bone loss in patients with asthma. New Engl J Med 309:265–268
4. Adler RA, Rosen CJ (1994) Glucocorticoids and osteoporosis. Endocrinol Metab Clin North Am 23:641–654

5. Alexandersen P, Riis BJ, Christiansen C (1999) Monofluorophosphate combined with hormone replacement therapy induces a synergistic effect on bone mass by dissociating bone formation and resorption in postmenopausal women: a randomized study. J Clin Endocrinol Metab 84:3013–3020
6. Alexandersen P, Toussaint A, Christiansen C, Devogelaer P, et al (2001) Ipriflavone in the treatment of postmenopausal osteoporosis: a randomized controlled trial. JAMA 285:1482–1488
7. Aloia JF, Vaswani A, Yeh JK, Ellis K, et al (1988) Calcitriol in the treatment of postmenopausal osteoporosis. Am J Med 84:401–408
8. Amin S, Lavalley M, Simms RW, Felson DT (2002) The comparative efficacy of drug therapies used for the management of corticosteroid-induced osteoporosis: a meta-regression. J Bone Miner Res 17:1512–1526
9. Black DM, Palermo L, Nevitt MC, et al (1995) Comparison of methods for defining prevalent vertebral deformities: the study of osteoporotic fractures. J Bone Miner Res 10:890–902
10. Black DM, Cummings SR, Karpf DB, Cauley JA, et al (1996) Randomised trial of effect of alendronate on risk of fracture in women with existing vertebral fractures. Lancet 348:1535–1541
11. Black DM, Thompson D, Bauer DC, Ensrud K, et al (2000) Fracture risk reduction with alendronate in women with osteoporosis: the Fracture Intervention Trial. J Clin Endocrinol Metab 85:4118–4124
12. Blau LA, Hoehns JD (2003) Analgesic efficacy of calcitonin for vertebral fracture pain. Ann Pharmacother 37:564–570
13. Bombardier C, Laine L, Reicin A, et al – VIGOR Study Group (2000) Comparison of upper gastrointestinal toxicity of rofecoxib and naproxen in patients with rheumatoid arthritis. N Engl J Med 343:1520–1528
14. Bone HG (2001) Development and evaluation of new drugs for osteoporosis. Osteoporosis (Second Edition) 2: 533–538
15. Bone HG, Downs RW, Tucci JR Harris ST, et al (1997) Dose-response relationships for alendronate treatment in osteoporotic elderly women. J Clin Endocrinol Metab 82:265–274
16. Brumsen C, Papapoulos SE, Lips P, Geelhoed-Duijvestijn P, et al (2002) Daily oral pamidronate in women and men with osteoporosis: a 3-year randomized placebo-controlled clinical trial with a 2-year open extension. J Bone Miner Res 17:1057–1064
17. Burger H, Van Daele PL, Algra D, et al (1994) Vertebral deformities as predictors of non-vertebral fractures. BMJ 309:991–992
18. Canalis E (2003) Mechanisms of glucocorticoid-induced osteoporosis. Curr Opin Rheumatol 15:454–457
19. Cauley JA, Black DM, Barrett-Connor E, Harris F, et al (2001) Effects of hormone replacement therapy on clinical fractures and height loss: the Heart and Estrogen/Progestin Replacement Study (HERS). Am J Med 110:442–450
20. Chesnut CH, Silverman S, Andriano K, Genant H, et al (2000) A randomized trial of nasal spray salmon calcitonin in postmenopausal women with established osteoporosis: the Prevent Recurrence Of Osteoporotic Fractures study. Am J Med 109:267–276
21. Chevalley T, Rizzoli R, Nydegger V, Slosman D, et al (1994) Effects of calcium supplements on femoral bone mineral density and vertebral fracture rate in vitamin-D-replete elderly patients. Osteoporos Int 4:245–252
22. Clemmesen B, Ravn P, Zegels B, Taquet AN, et al (1997) A 2-year phase II study with 1-year of follow-up of risedronate (NE-58095) in postmenopausal osteoporosis. Osteoporos Int 7:488–495
23. Cohen S, Levy RM, Keller M, Boling E, et al (1999) Risedronate therapy prevents corticosteroid-induced bone loss: a twelve-month, multicenter, randomized, double-blind, placebo-controlled, parallel-group study. Arthritis Rheum 42:2309–2318
24. Consensus Development Conference (1993) Diagnosis, prophylaxis and treatment of osteoporosis. Am J Med 94:646–650
25. Cranney A, Welch V, Adachi JD, Homik J, et al (2000) Calcitonin for the treatment and prevention of corticosteroid-induced osteoporosis. Cochrane Database Syst Rev 2:1983
26. Cummings SR, Nevitt MC, Browning WR, et al (1995) Risk factors for hip fracture in white women. N Engl J Med 322:767–773
27. Cummings SR, Black DM, Thompson DE, Applegate WB, et al (1998) Effect of alendronate on risk of fracture in women with low bone density but without vertebral fractures: results from the Fracture Intervention Trial. JAMA 280:2077–2082
28. Delmas PD, Ensrud KE, Adachi JD, Harper KD, et al (2002) Efficacy of raloxifene on vertebral fracture risk reduction in postmenopausal women with osteoporosis: four-year results from a randomized clinical trial. J Clin Endocrinol Metab 87:3609–3617
29. Dursun N, Dursun E, Yalcin S (2001) Comparison of alendronate, calcitonin and calcium treatments in postmenopausal osteoporosis. Int J Clin Pract 55:505–509
30. Ettinger B, Black DM, Mitlak BH, Knickerbocker RK, et al (1999) Reduction of vertebral fracture risk in postmenopausal women with osteoporosis treated with raloxifene: results from a 3-year randomized clinical trial. JAMA 282:637–645
31. Falch JA, Odegaard OR, Finnanger AM, Matheson I (1987) Postmenopausal osteoporosis: no effect of three years treatment with 1, 25-dihydroxycholecalciferol. Acta Med Scand 221: 199–204
32. Fogelman I, Ribot C, Smith R, Ethgen D, et al (2000) Risedronate reverses bone loss in postmenopausal women with low bone mass: results from a multinational, double-blind, placebo-controlled trial. J Clin Endocrinol Metab 85:1895–1900
33. Gallagher JC, Goldgar D (1990) Treatment of postmenopausal osteoporosis with high doses of synthetic calcitriol. A randomized controlled study. Ann Intern Med 113:649–655
34. Gallagher JC, Riggs BL, Recker RR, Goldgar D (1989) The effect of calcitriol on patients with postmenopausal osteoporosis with special reference to fracture frequency. Proc Soc Exp Biol Med 191:287–292
35. Greenspan S, Myers E, Maitland L, et al (1994) Fall severity and bone mineral density as risk factors for hip fracture in ambulatory elderly. JAMA 271: 128–133
36. Gutteridge DH, Stewart GO, Prince RL, Price RI et al. (2002) A randomized trial of sodium fluoride (60 mg) ± estrogen in postmenopausal osteoporotic vertebral fractures: increased vertebral fractures and peripheral bone loss with sodium fluoride; concurrent estrogen prevents peripheral loss, but not vertebral fractures. Osteoporos Int 13:158–170
37. Harris ST, Watts NB, Jackson RD, Genant HK, et al (1993) Four-year study of intermittent cyclic etidronate treatment of postmenopausal osteoporosis: three years of blinded therapy followed by one year of open therapy. Am J Med 95:557–567
38. Harris ST, Watts NB, Genant HK, McKeever CD, et al (1999) Effects of risedronate treatment on vertebral and nonvertebral fractures in women with postmenopausal osteoporosis: a randomized controlled trial. JAMA 282:1344–1352
39. Häuselmann HJ, Rizzoli R (2003) A comprehensive review of treatments for postmenopausal osteoporosis. Osteoporos Int 14:2–12

40. Heikki Frick M, Elo O, Haapa A, et al (1987) Helsinki Heart Study: primary prevention trial with gemfibrozil in middle-aged men with dyslipidemia. Safety of treatment, changes in risk factors and incidence of coronary heart disease. New Engl J Med 317:1237–1245
41. Hizmetli S, Elden H, Kaptanoglu E, Nacitarhan V, et al (1998) The effect of different doses of calcitonin on bone mineral density and fracture risk in postmenopausal osteoporosis. Int J Clin Pract 52:453–455
42. Hulley S, Grady D, Bush T, Furberg C, et al (1998) Randomized trial of estrogen plus progestin for secondary prevention of coronary heart disease in postmenopausal women. JAMA 280: 605–613
43. Hulley S, Furberg C, Barrett-Connor E, Cauley J, et al (2002) Noncardiovascular disease outcomes during 6.8 years of hormone therapy: Heart and Estrogen/progestin Replacement Study follow-up (HERS II). JAMA 288:58–66
44. Jalava T, Sarna S, Pylkkanen L, et al (2003) Association between vertebral fracture and increased mortality in osteoporotic patients. J Bone Miner Res 18:1254–1260
45. Kanis JA, Brazier JE, Stevenson M (2002) Treatment of established osteoporosis: a systematic review and cost-utility analysis. Health Technology Assessment 6(29)
46. Kleerekoper M, Peterson EL, Nelson DA, Phillips E, et al (1991) A randomized trial of sodium fluoride as a treatment for postmenopausal osteoporosis. Osteoporos Int 1:155–161
47. Lafague-Proust MH, Boudignon B, Thierry T (2003) Glucocorticoid-induced osteoporosis: pathophysiological data and recent treatments. Joint Bone Spine 70:109–118
48. Lane NE, Sanchez S, Modin GW, Genant HK, Pierini E, Arnaud CD (1998) Parathyroid hormone treatment can reverse corticosteroid-induced osteoporosis. J Clin Invest 102:1627–1633
49. Levis S, Quandt SA, Thompson D, Scott J, et al (2002) Alendronate reduces the risk of multiple symptomatic fractures: results from the fracture intervention trial. J Am Geriatr Soc 50:409–415
50. Liberman UA, Weiss SR, Bröll J, Minne HW, et al (1995) Effect of oral alendronate on bone mineral density and the incidence of fractures in postmenopausal osteoporosis. N Engl J Med 333:1437–1443
51. Lindsay R, Nieves J, Formica C, Henneman E, et al (1997) Randomised controlled study of effect of parathyroid hormone on vertebral-bone mass and fracture incidence among postmenopausal women on oestrogen with osteoporosis. Lancet 350:550–555
52. Luengo M, Picado C, Dei Rio L, et al (1991) Vertebral fractures in patients with rheumatoid arthritis treated with corticosteroids. Thorax 46:803–806
53. Lufkin EG, Wahner HW, O'Fallon WM, Hodgson SF, et al (1992) Treatment of postmenopausal osteoporosis with transdermal estrogen. Ann Intern Med 117:1–9
54. Lyritis GP, Tsakalakos N, Papspati I, Skarantavos G, et al (1997) The effect of a modified etidronate cyclical regimen on postmenopausal osteoporosis: a four-year study. Clin Rheumatol 16: 354–360
55. McCloskey E, Selby P, De Takats D, Bernard J, et al (2001) Effects of clodronate on vertebral fracture risk in osteoporosis: a 1-year interim analysis. Bone 28:310–315
56. McClung MR, Geusens P, Miller PD, Zippel H, et al (2001) Effect of risedronate on the risk of hip fracture in elderly women. N Engl J Med 344:333–340
57. McKeogh DF (2003) Celecoxib versus diclofenac and omeprazole to prevent recurrent ulcer bleeding. N Engl J Med 348:2464–2466
58. Melton LJ, Kan SH, Frye MA, et al (1989) Epidemiology of vertebral fractures in women. Am J Epidemiol 129: 1000–1011
59. Meunier PJ, Slosman DO, Delmas PD, Sebert JL, et al (2002) Strontium ranelate: dose-dependent effects in established postmenopausal vertebral osteoporosis – a 2-year randomized placebo-controlled trial. J Clin Endocrinol Metab 87:2060–2066
60. Naganathan V, Jones G, Nash P, et al (2000) Vertebral fracture risk with long-term corticosteroid therapy. Arch Intern Med 160:2917–2922
61. Neer RM, Arnaud CD, Zanchetta JR, Prince R, et al (2001) Effect of parathyroid hormone (1–34) on fractures and bone mineral density in postmenopausal women with osteoporosis. N Engl J Med 344:1434–1441
62. Neuner JM, Zimmer, JK, Hamel MB (2003) Diagnosis and treatment of osteoporosis in patients with vertebral compression fractures. J Am Geriatr Soc 51:483–491
63. Nevitt MC, Ettinger B, Black DM (1998) The association of radiographically detected vertebral fractures with back pain and function: a prospective study. Ann Intern Med 128:793–800
64. Orwoll E, Ettinger M, Weiss S, et al (2000) Alendronate for the treatment of osteoporosis in men. N Engl J Med 343:604–610
65. Osteoporosis Methodology Group and Osteoporosis Research Advisory Group (2002) Meta-analyses of therapies for postmenopausal osteoporosis. Endocrine Rev 23:495–578
66. Ott SM, Chesnut CH (1989) Calcitriol treatment is not effective in postmenopausal osteoporosis. Ann Intern Med 110:267–274
67. Overgaard K, Hansen MA, Jensen SB, Christiansen C (1992) Effect of salcatonin given intranasally on bone mass and fracture rates in established osteoporosis: a dose-response study. BMJ 305:556–561
68. Pak CY, Sakhaee K, Adams-Huet B, Piziak V, et al (1995) Treatment of postmenopausal osteoporosis with slow-release sodium fluoride. Final report of a randomized controlled trial. Ann Intern Med 123:401–408
69. Recker RR, Hinders S, Davies KM, Heaney RP, et al (1996) Correcting calcium nutritional deficiency prevents spine fractures in elderly women. J Bone Miner Res 11:1961–1966
70. Recker RR, Davies KM, Dowd RM, Heaney RP (1999) The effect of low-dose continuous estrogen and progesterone therapy with calcium and vitamin D on bone in elderly women. A randomized controlled trial. Ann Intern Med 130:897–904
71. Reginster JY, Meurmans L, Zegels B, Rovati LC, et al (1998) The effect of sodium monofluorophosphate plus calcium on vertebral fracture rate in postmenopausal women with moderate osteoporosis. A randomized, controlled trial. Ann Intern Med 129:1–8
72. Reginster JY, Minne HW, Sorensen OH, Hooper M, et al (2000) Randomized trial of the effects of risedronate on vertebral fractures in women with established postmenopausal osteoporosis. Osteoporos Int 11:83–91
73. Reginster JY, Christiansen C, Roux C, Fechtenbaum J, et al (2001) Intermittent cyclic tiludronate in the treatment of osteoporosis. Osteoporos Int 12: 169–177
74. Reid DM, Hughes RA, Laan RF, et al (2000) Efficacy and safety of daily risedronate in the treatment of corticosteroid-induced osteoporosis in men and women: a randomized trial. European Corticosteroid-Induced Osteoporosis Treatment Study. J Bone Miner Res 15:1006–1013
75. Reid DM, Adami S, Devogelaer JP, Chines AA (2001) Risedronate increases bone density and reduces vertebral fracture risk within one year in men on corticosteroid therapy, Calcif Tiss Int 69:242–247

76. Riggs BL, Hodgson SF, O'Fallon WM, Chao EYS, et al (1990) Effect of fluoride treatment on the fracture rate in postmenopausal women with osteoporosis. N Engl J Med 322:802–809
77. Ringe JD, Kipshoven C, Cöster A, Umbach R (1999) Therapy of established postmenopausal osteoporosis with monofluorophosphate plus calcium: dose-related effects on bone density and fracture rate. Osteoporos Int 9:171–178
78. Ringe JD, Faber H, Dorst A (2001) Alendronate treatment of established primary osteoporosis in men: results of a 2-year prospective study. J Clin Endocrinol Metab 86:5252–5255
79. Ross PD, Davis JW, Epstein RS, et al (1991) Pre-existing fractures and bone mass predict vertebral fracture incidence in women. Ann Intern Med 114: 919–923
80. Ryan PJ, Blake GM, Davie M, Haddaway M, et al (2000) Intermittent oral disodium pamidronate in established osteoporosis: A 2-year double-masked placebo-controlled study of efficacy and safety. Osteoporos Int 11:171–176
81. Saag KG, Emekey R, Schnitzer TJ, et al (1998) Alendronate for the prevention and treatment of glucocorticoid-induced osteoporosis. N Engl J Med 339:292–299
82. Sambrook PN, Kotowicz M, Hash P, et al (2003) Prevention and treatment of glucocorticoid-induced osteoporosis: a comparison of calcitriol, vitamin D plus calcium and alendronate plus calcium. J Bone Miner Res 18:919–924
83. Silverstein FE, Graham DY, Senior JR, et al (1995) Misoprostol reduces serious gastro-intestinal complications in patients with rheumatoid arthritis receiving non steroidal anti-inflammatory drugs. Ann Int Med 123:241–249
84. Steering Committee of the Physicians' Health Study Group (1989). Final report on the aspirin component of the ongoing Physicians' Health Study. N Engl J Med 321:129–135
85. Storm T, Thamsborg G, Steiniche T, Genant HK, et al (1990) Effect of intermittent cyclical etidronate therapy on bone mass and fracture rate in women with postmenopausal osteoporosis. N Engl J Med 322:1265–1271
86. Tilyard MW, Spears GFS, Thomson J, Dovey S, et al (1992) Treatment of postmenopausal osteoporosis with calcitriol or calcium. N Engl J Med 326: 357–362
87. van Staa TP, Leufkens HG, Cooper C (2001) Use of inhaled corticosteroids and risk of fractures. J Bone Miner Res 16:581–588
88. Wallach S, Cohen S, Reid DM, et al (2000) Effects of risedronate treatment on bone density and vertebral fracture in patients on corticosteroid therapy. Calcif Tissue Int 67:277–285
89. Walsh LJ, Wong CA, Pringle M, Tattersfield AE (1996) Use of oral corticosteroids in the community and the prevention of secondary osteoporosis: a cross-sectional study. BMJ 313:344–346
90. Watts NB, Harris ST, Genant HK, Wasnich RD, et al (1990) Intermittent cyclical etidronate treatment of postmenopausal osteoporosis. N Engl J Med 323:73–79
91. WHO study group (1994) Assessment of fracture risk and its application to screening for postmenopausal osteoporosis. WHO Technical Report series. WHO, Geneva
92. Wimalawansa SJ (1998) A four-year randomized controlled trial of hormone replacement and bisphosphonate, alone or in combination, in women with postmenopausal osteoporosis. Am J Med 104:219–226
93. Windeler J, Lange S (1995) Events per person year, a dubious concept. BMJ 310:454–456
94. Wong CA, Walsh LJ, Smith CJP, et al (2000) Inhaled corticosteroid use and bone mineral density in patients with asthma. Lancet 355:1399–1403
95. Writing Group for the Women's Health Initiative Investigators (2002) Risks and benefits of estrogen plus progestin in healthy postmenopausal women: principal results from the Women's Health Initiative randomized controlled trial. JAMA 288:321–333

H. Fleisch

Bisphosphonates in osteoporosis

Abstract Bisphosphonates are compounds characterized by a P-C-P structure. They act essentially on bone, inhibiting bone resorption. Through this mechanism they decrease bone loss, increase bone mineral density, and decrease bone turnover. They are therefore administered in diseases with elevated bone destruction, such as Paget's disease, metastatic bone disease, and osteoporosis. In the latter they diminish both vertebral and nonvertebral fractures. The adverse events are few, mostly gastrointestinal, and can be avoided to a large extent by correct administration. Since there are no other compounds available which have a similar profile, they represent today the drugs of choice in the treatment and the secondary prevention of osteoporosis.

Keywords Bisphosphonates · Etidronate · Alendronate · Risedronate · Osteoporosis

H. Fleisch (✉)
Av. Désertes 5, 1009 Pully, Switzerland
Tel.: +41-31-3899276,
Fax: +41-31-3899284,
e-mail: fleisch@bluewin.ch

Preclinical characteristics

Chemistry

The bisphosphonates used in clinical practice are compounds characterized by a P-C-P structure. This structure allows a great number of possible variations, especially by changing the two lateral chains in the carbon atom. These compounds have been known for a long time, the first bisphosphonates having been synthesized by German chemists as early as 1865. The bisphosphonates were first used only for a variety of industrial applications, among them as antiscaling agents. It was only in 1968–1969 that we showed these compounds also to have biological effects, more specifically on the calcified tissues [7, 8]. Each bisphosphonate has its own physicochemical and biological characteristics, and therefore each compound must be considered on its own, with respect to its action and behavior.

Biological actions

The bisphosphonates have been shown to have various physicochemical effects on bone salt crystals and biological effects on bone mineralization and bone resorption.

Physicochemical effects

Bisphosphonates inhibit the formation and aggregation and slow down the dissolution of calcium phosphate crystals. These effects are related to the marked affinity of these compounds for solid-phase calcium phosphate, on the surface of which they bind strongly. This property is the basis for the use of these compounds as skeletal markers in nuclear medicine and the basis for their selective pharmacological effects.

Inhibition of bone resorption

The main effect of the pharmacologically active bisphosphonates is to inhibit bone resorption [7]. This effect has been shown both in vitro culture and in intact animals. In growing rats bisphosphonates can block the degradation of both primary and secondary trabeculae, thus arresting the modeling and remodeling of the metaphysis. The latter therefore becomes club shaped and radiologically more dense than normal. This effect is often used as an experimental assay to determine the potency of new compounds (Schenk test) [22]. The inhibition of bone resorption by bisphosphonates has also been documented using ^{45}Ca kinetic studies, markers of bone resorption, and by other means. The effect occurs within 24–48 h and is therefore slower than that of calcitonin. The decrease in resorption is accompanied, at least in the growing animal, by a positive calcium balance, and an increase in the mineral content of bone and in bone mass. This is possible because of an increase in intestinal calcium absorption.

Bisphosphonates can also prevent an experimentally induced increase in bone resorption. Thus they impair resorption induced by many bone resorbing agents such as parathyroid hormone, $1,25(OH)_2D$ and retinoids, the latter effect having been used to develop a powerful and rapid screening assay for new compounds. They also inhibit bone loss induced by different procedures to induce experimental osteoporosis such as immobilization, the first model used [15], ovariectomy, corticosteroids, or lactation combined with a low calcium diet. When not given in excess, bisphosphonates have also a positive effect on mechanical characteristics both in normal animals and in various experimental osteoporosis models [25]. This effect seems to be due to alterations in bone mass, architecture and quality.

The activity of bisphosphonates on bone resorption varies greatly from compound to compound. For etidronate the dose required to inhibit resorption is relatively high, very near that which impairs normal mineralization. One of the aims of bisphosphonate research has therefore been to develop compounds with a more powerful antiresorptive activity, without a stronger inhibition of mineralization. This has proven to be possible. Compounds have been developed that are up to 10,000 times more powerful than etidronate in the inhibition of bone resorption in experimental animals without being more active in inhibiting mineralization.

Inhibition of mineralization

When given in larger amounts, bisphosphonates can inhibit normal mineralization of bone and cartilage as well as ectopic mineralization [22].

Mechanisms of action

While the effect on mineralization is due to the physicochemical inhibition of crystal growth, the action on bone resorption is mediated through mechanisms other than the physicochemical inhibition of crystal dissolution, as was initially postulated, namely by acting on the osteoclast. Four mechanisms appear to be probably involved: inhibition of osteoclast recruitment, inhibition of osteoclastic adhesion, shortening of the life span of osteoclasts due to earlier apoptosis, and inhibition of osteoclast activity. Very recently the cellular mechanism has been partially unraveled. It was found that nitrogen containing bisphosphonates can, by inhibiting farnesyl pyrophosphate synthase, decrease the formation of some compounds important for many cell functions, including cytoskeletal assembly and intracellular signaling, which leads eventually to apoptosis and death. In contrast, some non-nitrogen-containing bisphosphonates, such as clodronate, and etidronate, can be incorporated into the phosphate chain of ATP-containing compounds, which also impair cell function, leading to apoptosis and cell death. Thus the bisphosphonates can be classified into two major groups with different modes of action but the same final effect [19].

Pharmacokinetics

The bisphosphonates appear to be absorbed, stored, and excreted unaltered in the body. Therefore the bisphosphonates seem to be nonbiodegradable, at least with respect to their P-C-P bond. The bioavailability of an oral dose of a bisphosphonate both in animals and in humans lies between less than 1% and 10%. Absorption is substantially diminished when the drug is given with meals, especially in the presence of calcium and iron. Therefore bisphosphonates should never be given at mealtimes and never together with milk or dairy products. Between 20% and 80% of the absorbed bisphosphonate is taken up very rapidly by bone, the remainder being rapidly excreted in the urine. This rapid uptake by bone means that the soft tissues are exposed to bisphosphonates for only short periods, explaining why practically only bone is affected in vivo. The areas of deposition are mostly those of bone formation and destruction. Once deposited in the skeleton and covered under new layers of bone, the bisphosphonates are released to a large extent only when the bone in which they were deposited is resorbed. The half-life in bone bisphosphonates is therefore very long, for humans it can be over 10 years. The renal clearance of bisphosphonates is high, at least in animals higher than that of inulin, indicating active secretion.

Clinical use in osteoporosis

Bisphosphonates are today the most frequently used drug in metabolic bone disease. About ten are commercially available in the world, the conditions treated most frequently with these compounds being osteoporosis, Paget's disease and metastatic bone disease. This review deals only with osteoporosis. A more extended clinical and clinical information can be found in a book written for the practicing physician [6].

Definition and pathophysiology of osteoporosis

Osteoporosis is a disease characterized by a decrease in bone mass and a deterioration in the architecture of the bones, which leads to an enhanced fragility of the skeleton and therefore to a greater risk of fracture. It is defined as present in women when the bone mass is more than 2.5 SD below that of the young woman (*t* score). It is a very common disorder which will become even more common with the increase in life expectancy. It is also frequent in men, although less so than in women. Its main cause is the continuous loss during life of both cancellous and cortical bone, which is exacerbated in women after the menopause. The second contributory factor is failure to achieve adequate peak bone mass during adolescence. The causes of these changes are not yet clear, although genetic factors are involved, at least for the latter.

The clinical manifestations of osteoporosis are fractures, occurring often spontaneously or after minimal trauma, and their consequences. Osteoporosis is diagnosed and assessed quantitatively by techniques that measure bone mineral density (BMD), most commonly dual X-ray absorptiometry. Chemical analyses cannot be used to diagnose osteoporosis. Markers of bone turnover, however, are useful to determine bone turnover and consequently to identify those patients who are likely to be losing bone rapidly and to follow the effect of treatment.

Treatment of osteoporosis

Until recently the only mechanism by which to prevent or treat osteoporosis was to influence bone mass. It was also thought that the latter was reflected with fidelity by BMD. Both of these assumptions have proven to be wrong. Thus we do know today that bone mass is not the only parameter responsible for bone strength, but that bone architecture and bone turnover are also very important in the determination of fracture risk. Furthermore, BMD, although a good indicator of bone mass is not a perfect one since it is also influenced by the degree of mineralization of bone tissue [13]. This is especially true when inhibitors of bone resorption, such as bisphosphonates, are administered, in which case BMD as assessed by densitometry can increase without any change in the amount of bone [2].

The main future aim for therapy is still to try to increase bone mass by increasing bone formation. Unfortunately there was no way to do this until very recently. Fluoride does increase bone formation, but has not been shown to decrease the occurrence of fractures. However, it was shown recently that parathyroid hormone administered daily dramatically increases bone formation and bone mass and reduces the occurrence of fractures [16]. This therapy has just been commercialized in the United States and is now given in very advanced cases of osteoporosis. However, this treatment is not yet advocated for less disabling cases and for prevention. For these patients the decrease in bone resorption is still the pharmacological mechanism used.

For many years the most commonly used treatment acting through a decrease in bone resorption, apart of bisphosphonates, was estrogen replacement after the menopause. However, it has recently been shown that estrogens increase the risk of breast cancer, and increase instead of decrease cardiovascular insults [20]. Calcitonin is sometimes used, but parenteral administration can have unpleasant side effects, and the nasal form is relatively weak in its effect on BMD and fracture incidence. Calcium can also decrease bone turnover and diminish bone loss in certain conditions. It was found to diminish hip fractures when given with vitamin D in the elderly institutionalized patients [3]. This is why calcium, although it is not effective enough to affect strongly fractures in most patients with osteoporosis, is recommended at a dose of about 1 g daily in the elderly. Calcium is, however, an obligatory adjunction in all patients who receive an antiresorptive treatment. Vitamin D should be present in sufficient amounts, and the addition of 400–800 U are generally recommended in the elderly.

Treatment of osteoporosis with bisphosphonate

Although many bisphosphonates have been investigated in human osteoporosis, most of the studies have been carried out with alendronate, etidronate, and risedronate. These are the compounds which are commercialized in the greatest number of countries. Many well controlled studies have confirmed the efficacy of bisphosphonates in preventing the decrease in BMD, as assessed by dual X-ray absorptiometry first in not-menopausal osteoporosis and then in various other types of osteoporosis. Actually BMD was most often even increased. The first compound thoroughly investigated was etidronate [26]. This was then followed by alendronate [11] and later risedronate [14]. Bisphosphonates are active in whites, Asians, and black osteoporotic women. They are also effective in elderly women without osteoporosis [12] and in healthy women, as well as in men. They prevent and partially even reverse the bone loss in glucocorticoid-treated patients [4, 21] and are therefore a standard therapy in patients receiving this drug over longer time.

All the bisphosphonates induce a marked decrease in bone turnover when given in doses effective on BMD. Both bone formation and resorption are decreased. The important question to answer was whether bisphosphonates were also be able to decrease the fracture risk. Indeed an efficacious drug in osteoporosis should not be tested on BMD but on fracture risk, fractures, both vertebral and appendicular, being the key clinical problem. Both alendronate [1, 17] and risedronate [10, 18] decrease by about one-half the occurrence of vertebral and nonvertebral fractures in osteoporotic patients. Etidronate could not be proven to be efficacious on these parameters. This effect on fractures is probably due both to the increase in BMD and the decrease in bone turnover. It is not yet known which is the relative part played by each of them. However, the fact that the fractures decrease even after 6 months, when the effect on BMD is still very small, suggests that turnover is important. Lastly, bisphosphonates do reduce fractures also in children with osteogenesis imperfecta [9].

Only few studies have addressed what happens after the discontinuation of the drug. It seems that this depends of the duration of the previous treatment. After a short-term treatment of 1–2 years, turnover and bone loss pick up again to some extent, the latter less so than the former one. After long-term treatment such as 7 years bone turnover goes up only very slowly and BMD stay constant for at least 1–2 years [24].

The treatment regimens for the three main commercialized compounds are the following:

- Alendronate: The dose recommended by the producers is 10 mg orally daily, 5 mg in Japan. Since this compound has a similar effect on BMD when given once weekly at 70 mg [23], the weekly regimen is used today in the countries where this regimen is commercialized.
- Etidronate: The regimen recommended by the producer is 400 mg daily orally for 2 weeks every 3 months.
- Risedronate: The recommended regimen is 5 mg daily orally or 35 mg once weekly.

Adverse events

As is the case in animals, studies in humans have revealed only a few important adverse events. Oral administration of bisphosphonates, especially those containing a nitrogen atom, can be accompanied by digestive tract disturbances [5]. The latter can be substantially reduced by taking the drug with enough fluid, and by not reclining after the intake. It also seems that these disturbances are decreased when the compounds are administered once a week instead of daily, at the same total dose. The intravenous administration of N-containing compounds can induce a transient pyrexia of usually 1–2°C, accompanied by flulike symptoms, which resembles an acute-phase response. Until now no negative consequences of these episodes have been described. Lastly, compounds with little efficiency and which must administered in higher doses, such as etidronate, can inhibit normal skeletal mineralization. This can happen at doses of etidronate above 800 mg daily. Fracture healing or new orthopedic implants are no contraindication to the use of bisphosphonates provided they are not given in doses that inhibit mineralization. Lastly, bisphosphonates should not be given during pregnancy and lactation.

An important question is what happens after long-term treatment. A study of 7-years administration of alendronate did not show any adverse events. Actually the turnover stays at a constant level, the BMD still goes up, and the fracture rate remains low [24]. This course appears to continue up to 10 years of treatment. Similar results are seen with risedronate. Therefore there is until now no indication that one would have to stop the treatment because of an increase in osseous fragility. However, this issue has to be followed closely. Whether it would be of advantage to interrupt treatment for a certain time is not known.

References

1. Black DM, Cummings SR, Karpf DB, Cauley JA, Thompson DE, Nevitt MC, Bauer DC, Genant HK, Haskell WL, Marcus R, Ott SM, Torner JC, Quandt SA, Reiss TF, Ensrud KE (1996) Randomized trial of effect of alendronate on risk of fracture in women with existing vertebral fractures. Lancet 348: 1535–1541
2. Boivin GY, Chavassieux PM, Santora AC, Meunier PJ (2000) Alendronate increases bone strength by increasing the mean degree of mineralization of bone tissue in osteoporotic women. Bone 27:697–694
3. Chapuy MC, Arlot ME, Duboeuf F, Brun J, Crouzet B, Arnaud F, Delmas PD, Meunier PJ (1992) Vitamin D and calcium to prevent hip fractures in the elderly. N Engl J Med 327:1637–1642
4. Cohen S, Levy RM, Keller M, Boling E, Emkey RD, Greenwald M, Zizic TM, Wallach S, Sewell KL, Lukert BP, Axelrod DW, Chines AA (1999) Risedronate therapy prevents corticosteroid-induced bone loss. Arthritis Rheum 42: 2309–2318
5. De Groen PC, Lubbe DF, Hirsch LJ, Daifotis A, Stephenson W, Freedholm D, Pryor-Tillotson S, Seleznick MJ, Pinkas H, Wang KK (1996) Esophagitis associated with the use of alendronate. N Engl J Med 355:1016–1021
6. Fleisch H (2000) Bisphosphonates in bone disease – from the laboratory to the patient. Academic, San Diego
7. Fleisch H, Russell RGG, Francis MD (1969) Diphosphonates inhibit hydroxyapatite dissolution in vitro and bone resorption in tissue culture and in vivo. Science 165:1262–1264
8. Francis MD, Russell RGG, Fleisch H (1969) Diphosphonates inhibit formation of calcium phosphate crystals in vitro and pathological calcification in vivo. Science 165:1264–1256
9. Glorieux FH, Bishop NJ, Plotkin H, Chabot G, Lanogu G, Travers R (1998) Cyclic administration of pamidronate in children with severe osteogenesis imperfecta. N Engl J Med 339:947–952
10. Harris ST, Watts NB, Genant HK, McKeever CD, Hangartner D, Keller M, Chesnut CH, Brown J, Eriksen EF, Hoseyni MS, Axelrod DW, Miller, PD (1999) Effects of risedronate treatment on vertebral and nonvertebral fractures in women with postmenopausal osteoporosis. JAMA 14:1344–1352
11. Liberman UA, Weiss SR, Bröll J, Minne HW, Quan H, Bell NH, Rodriguez-Portales J, Downs RW Jr, Dequeker J, Favus M, Seeman E, Recker RR, Capizzi T, Santora AC II, Lombardi A, Shah RV, Hirsch LJ, Karpf DB (1995) Effect of oral alendronate on bone mineral density and the incidence of fractures in postmenopausal osteoporosis. N Engl J Med 333:1437–1443

12. McClung M, Clemmesen B, Daifotis A, Gilchrist NL, Eisman J, Weinstein RS, El Hajj Fuleihan G, Reda C, Yates AJ, Ravn P (1998) Alendronate prevents postmenopausal bone loss in women without osteoporosis. Ann Intern Med 128:253–261
13. Meunier PJ, Boivin GY (1997) Bone mineral density reflects bone mass but also the degree of mineralization of bone: therapeutic implications. Bone 5: 373–377
14. Mortensen L, Charles P, Bekker PJ, Digennaro J, Johnston CC (1998) Risedronate increases bone mass in an early postmenopausal population: two years of treatment plus one year of follow-up. J Clin Endocrinol Metab 83:396–402
15. Mühlbauer RC, Russell RGG, Williams DA, Fleisch H (1971) The effects of diphosphonates, polyphosphates, and calcitonin on 'immobilisation' osteoporosis in rats. Eur J Clin Invest 1:336–344
16. Neer N, Arnaud CD, Zanchetta JR, Prince R, Gaich, GA, Reginster YI, Hodsman AB, Erichsen EF, Ish-Shalom S, Genant HK, Wang O, Mitlak, BH (2001) Effect of parathyroid hormone (1-34) on fractures and bone mineral density in postmenopausal women with osteoporosis. N Engl J Med 344:1434–1444
17. Pols HAP, Felsenberg D, Hanley DA, Stepan J, Munoz-Torres M, Wilkin TJ, Qin-sheng G, Galich AM, Vandormael K, Yates AJ, Stych B (1999) Multinational, placebo-controlled, randomized trial of the effects of alendronate on bone density and fracture risk in postmenopausal women with low bone mass: results of the FOSIT study. Osteoporos Int 9:461–468
18. Reginster JY, Minne HW, Sorensen OH, Hooper M, Roux C, Brandi ML, Lund B, Ethgen D, Pack S, Roumagnac I, Eastell R (2000) Randomized trial of the effects of risedronate on vertebral fractures in women with established postmenopausal osteoporosis. Osteoporosis Int 11:83–91
19. Rogers MJ (2003) New insights into the molecular mechanisms of action of bisphosphonates. Curr Pharmaceut Design (in press)
20. Roussouw JE, Anderson GL, Prentice RL, LaCroix AZ, Kooperberg C, Stefanick ML, Jackson RD, Beresford SA, Howard BV, Johnson KC, Kotchen JM, Ockene J, Writing Group for the Women's Health Initiative Investigators (2002) Risks and benefits of estrogen plus progestin in healthy postmenopausal women: principal results From the Women's Health Initiative randomized controlled trial. JAMA 288:321–333
21. Saag KG, Emkey R, Schnitzer TJ, Brown JP, Hawkins F, Goemaere F, Thamsborg G, Lieberman UA, Delmas PD, Malice M-P, Czachur M, Daifotis AG (1998) Alendronate for the prevention and treatment of glucocorticoid-induced osteoporosis. N Engl J Med 339:292–299
22. Schenk R, Merz WA, Mühlbauer R, Russell RGG, Fleisch H (1973) Effect of ethane-1-hydroxy-1:1-diphosphonate (EHDP) and dichloromethylene diphosphonate (Cl_2MDP) on the calcification and resorption of cartilage and bone in the tibial epiphysis and metaphysis of rats. Calcif Tissue Res 11:196–214
23. Schnitzer T, Bone HG, Crepaldi G, Adami S, McClung M, Kiel D, Felsenberg D, Recker RR, Tonino RP, Roux C, Pinchera A, Foldes AJ, Greenspan SL, Levine MA, Emkey R, Santora AC, Kaur A, Thompson DE, Yates J, Orloff JJ (2000) Therapeutic equivalence of alendronate 70\mg once-weekly and alendronate 10\mg daily in the treatment of osteoporosis. Aging Clin Exp Res 12:1–12
24. Tonino RP, Meunier PJ, Emkey RD, Rodriguez-Portales JA, Menkes CJ, Wasnich RD, Bone HG, Santora AC, Wu M, Desai R, Ross PD (2000) Skeletal benefits of alendronate: 7-year treatment postmenopausal osteoporotic women. Phase III osteoporosis treatment study group. J Clin Endocrinol Metab 85:3109–115
25. Toolan BC, Shea M, Myers ER, Borchers RE, Seedor JG, Quartuccio H, Rodan G, Hayes WC (1992) Effects of 4-amino-1-hydroxybutylidene bisphosphonate on bone biomechanics in rats. J Bone Miner Res 7:1399–1406
26. Watts NB, Harris ST, Genant HK, Wasnich RD, Miller PD, Jackson RD, Licata AA, Ross P, Woodson GC, Yanover MJ, Mysiw WJ, Kohse L, Rao MB, Steiger P, Richmond B, Chesnut CH III (1990) Intermittent cyclical etidronate treatment of postmenopausal osteoporosis. N Engl J Med 323:73–329

REVIEW

Joseph M. Lane
Michael J. Gardner
Julie T. Lin
Marjolein C. van der Meulen
Elizabeth Myers

The aging spine: new technologies and therapeutics for the osteoporotic spine

J. M. Lane (✉) · M. J. Gardner · J. T. Lin
M. C. van der Meulen · E. Myers
Metabolic Bone Disease Service,
Hospital for Special Surgery,
New York, New York, USA
e-mail: lanej@hss.edu

J. M. Lane
Department of Orthopaedic Surgery,
Hospital for Special Surgery,
535 East 70th Street,
NY 10021 New York, USA

Abstract Osteoporosis results in low-energy fractures of the spine. The load necessary to cause a vertebral fracture is determined by the characteristics related to the vertebral body structure, mineral content, and quality of bone. Radiographic techniques centered on dual X-ray absorptiometry (DXA) permit a determination of bone mass and fracture risk. Current medical therapies principally using bisphosphonate and pulsatile PTH profoundly decrease the risk of fracture (50+%). Fall prevention strategies can further decrease the possibility of fracture. A comprehensive approach to osteoporosis can favorably alter the disease.

Keywords Vertebral fracture · Osteoporosis · Bisphosphonates · PTH (1–34) · Falls

Introduction

Osteoporosis is a serious problem in the United States, affecting as many as 13–18% of women and 3–6% of men [49, 55, 64, 68, 89]. If untreated, it is estimated that more than half of all Caucasian white women will sustain an osteoporotic fracture during their lifetime [16, 89]. Approximately one-half of these fractures are related to the vertebral bodies, with two-thirds being silent and one-third symptomatic. Epidemiological studies have demonstrated that multiple vertebral fractures increase morbidity [67, 69], and the presence and increasing numbers of fractures significantly increase mortality rates [11, 23, 41, 48]. Despite the recognition that osteoporotic fractures increase the risk for additional vertebral fractures as well as hip fractures, the majority of individuals with these fractures remain undiagnosed and untreated [28, 31, 74].

Over the last ten years, great strides have been made in understanding the pathophysiology of osteoporotic vertebral fractures. Radiographic methods have been enhanced to aid in the diagnosis of osteoporosis. New therapeutics have been developed that may decrease the fragility fracture rate by up to 50% compared with controls treated only with calcium [7, 24, 40, 70, 79]. During the same time period, two minimally invasive procedures have been developed to rapidly address painful vertebral fractures – vertebroplasty and kyphoplasty. Details regarding these procedures are the subject of separate articles within this issue.

Fracture etiology: factor of risk

Vertebral bodies sustain fractures under two different mechanical environments: repetitive loading that fatigues the cancellous bone and leads to the accumulation of microfractures, or single traumatic events may overload the vertebral body and lead to fracture [58]. To understand the etiology of vertebral fracture, information about the loads imposed onto the vertebral body and the load-bearing capacity of the vertebrae at the time of risk need to be quantified. This concept has been defined as the factor of risk, and represents the ratio of the load applied to the bone over the load necessary to cause a fracture [42]. The load necessary to cause a vertebral fracture is determined by the characteristics related to the vertebral body structure and mineral content.

The determinants of bone failure load

The ability of the vertebral body to bear certain loads depends on both the material properties of the bone and on the geometrical distribution of the tissue components which are able to withstand load [39]. Vertebral fractures occur in cancellous bone, which has a complex microstructure. The volume of tissue contained within cancellous bone is the "bone volume fraction," and the mass of the bone tissue within a given volume is the "apparent density." The cancellous apparent density is directly related to the load-bearing capacity of the bone, and the ultimate stress which represents the failure load per cross-sectional area is proportional to the square of the apparent density [9]. However, two regions of apparent density can differ substantially in ultimate stress as a result of trabecular microarchitecture. The ultimate stress along the superior to inferior direction is twice that of the medial-lateral or anterior-posterior directions [30]. Presently, noninvasive methods to accurately characterize the trabecular morphology are in development.

The final contributor to bone strength is the material properties of the tissue. Local changes in collagen matrix cross-linking, such as occur in osteogenesis imperfecta, or changes in mineral content, such as occur in osteomalacia, are known to affect the material properties. While the altered bone material properties can be determined invasively through chemical analysis, they can often be implied by patient characteristics and clinical laboratory tests. Overall, the strength of the vertebral body is related to the bone mass, the macroscopic and microscopic distribution of the bone mass and the material properties of the composite bone.

Diagnosis of osteoporosis

Radiographic methods

Commonly used in vivo imaging techniques do not capture cancellous bone volume fraction and architecture. Therefore, assessment of bone density occurs at the whole bone level. Areal bone mineral density (g/cm^2), measured by dual x-ray absorptiometry (DXA), is a single measure that captures both mineral content and bone size [10]. Studies have reported good correlation between bone mineral density, as measured by DXA, and vertebral body failure load [71]. There is a higher risk factor of fracture for a similar load as the bone density decreases. Numerous clinical studies have demonstrated that low bone mineral density is associated with increased fracture rates for the spine [66].

The DXA scan can be performed in a lateral or anteroposterior (AP) mode. The sagittal view is highly accurate and correlates well with fracture risk [13, 93]. However, with the presence of osteophytes and scoliosis, the precision decreases and may be artificially elevated, particularly with osteosclerotic facet joints [62]. Above the age of 60, lateral DXA avoids the posterior elements of the spine, and may address this problem in patients typically with evidence of osteoarthritis of the spine. However, the overhanging ribs and the superior projection of the iliac wing often obscure the L1 and L2, and L4 and L5 vertebral bodies, respectively, leaving one or two vertebral bodies available for analysis. This may significantly decrease the precision of the methodology. As a consequence, in patients over 60, attention is often directed to the hip, where both the femoral neck and the total femur have excellent correlation with vertebral fracture risk [51]. Since the hip has a greater content of cortical bone, there may be a lag time between bone mineral density and recent bone loss [63, 76]. Similarly, a comparable lag time may occur in demonstrating improved bone stock as a consequence of medical interventions.

Vertebral morphometry, which involves quantification of the vertebral height and shape, has been used to evaluate early vertebral deformities. These measurements have traditionally been accomplished using lateral radiographs of the spine [36]. An important advance in DXA imaging includes the "instant vertebral assessment" (IVA) technique, also termed "morphometric X-ray absorptiometry" (MXA). This allows visualization of both the lateral and AP views of the spine from T4 to L4 [37, 26], and is a new method for quantifying vertebral deformities. There is a close correlation with radiographic evaluation of the spine, and this supplement may detect early fractures. Comparison with standard X-ray has shown a precision error of approximately 2–3% [3, 27, 86]. Vertebral height measurement is also significantly associated with bone mineral density [5]. The scoliosis and kyphosis angles can be measured for spinal segments, but placing the patient in the prone position can often lead to an underestimation of the true kyphosis. Scoliosis is affected to a lesser degree, particularly in the elderly. MXA is a relatively fast, low-radiation technique to identify prevalent vertebral deformities, particularly moderate to severe deformities of the middle thoracic to lumbar spine. It has a high correlation to the gold standard lateral X-ray, and can be obtained using a DXA machine with a single image [25, 26, 85].

Quantitative computed tomography (QCT) measures volumetric bone mineral density of trabecular bone [32, 46], but has poor precision due to increasing fat content in the marrow of older patients. This technique is also technologist-dependent, with high variability depending on the site chosen for analysis. It has twenty times the radiation of a DXA scan, and its current use is mainly in the research setting.

Laboratory measurements

Laboratory studies used to assess quality and quantity of bone tissue in the spine are centered on bone marrow abnormalities (complete blood count, sedimentation rate, serum and urine immunoelectrophoresis); endocrinopathies (hyperthyroidism, hyperparathyroidism, type I diabetes mellitus, Cushing's disease); and osteomalacia (25-hydroxyvitamin D, bone alkaline phosphatase, intact parathyroid hormone, serum calcium and serum phosphate) [4, 94]. This latter group represents bone collagen breakdown products and may be further evaluated using urinary N-telopeptide, pyridinoline peptide, dehydroxypyridinoline peptide, or serum c-terminal peptide. These markers identify elevated bone turnover, which directly increases fracture risk, and also screen for individuals with collagen variance, which often have very low parameters of bone turnover, such as osteogenesis imperfecta [2].

Treatment modalities

Osteoporosis has been divided into high-turnover and low-turnover osteoporosis. The most common form is high-turnover post-menopausal osteoporosis, in which osteoclast resorption is accelerated. Bone formation is compromised in low-turnover osteoporosis. Several families of agents have been suggested and developed to address the high-turnover state, including estrogen, selective estrogen receptor modulators (SERMs) such as raloxifene, calcitonin and bisphosphonates. Although calcium and vitamin D are not considered anti-resorptive agents, approximately half of patients presenting at hospitals with hip fractures show evidence of calcium deficiency and secondary hyperparathyroidism [75, 91]. Therapeutic physiologic levels of calcium and vitamin D (1500 mg of elemental calcium, 400–800 units of vitamin D) have been shown in a series of studies to significantly decrease osteoporotic fractures in the elderly population, primarily by reversing secondary hyperparathyroidism [19. 87].

Estrogen is an anti-osteoporotic agent, and has been shown to increase bone mass while effecting a decrease of vertebral fracture incidence by approximately 50% [54, 60]. Unfortunately, estrogen in combination with progesterone therapy is associated with increased cardiovascular disease, initiation of dementia and a small rise in the risk for breast cancer. As a consequence, estrogen is mainly used in the early post-menopausal period to treat post-menopausal symptomatology, and then lowered to the least effective dose to control symptomatology [54]. It is no longer recommended by the US Federal Government for the treatment of osteoporosis [96].

SERMs, particularly raloxifene, are anti-resorptive agents which have a significant anti-estrogen effect on breast tissue. However, osteoblasts are preferentially stimulated by SERMs and upregulate the rate of bone formation. Consequently, raloxifene has been shown to be an effective anti-resorptive agent in the treatment of osteoporosis [24]. Post-menopausal use decreases vertebral fractures by approximately 40% and increases spinal bone mass [92]. Unfortunately, similar protective effects have not been demonstrated in preventing hip fractures [20, 24]. Early data suggest that raloxifene decreases the risk of breast cancer by 70% [12, 21], which was an early indication for this agent. However, by stimulating estrogen receptors, raloxifene similarly increases the risk of pulmonary emboli and thrombophlebitis and may cause profound post-menopausal symptomatology. In light of the fact that it has no protection against hip fractures, raloxifene is not considered a primary treatment for osteoporosis.

Calcitonin is an intranasal agent which has shown moderate protection against spine fractures, with an incidence decrease of 33% in one series [15]. However, it has little to no effect on preventing hip fractures. There are some controversial data suggesting that calcitonin may relieve bone pain through an unknown mechanism. Its current use is in alleviating painful vertebral fractures as a consequence of osteoporosis, and only as a secondary antiresorptive agent. It should be terminated as soon as pain has been controlled, as other agents are much more successful.

Bisphosphonates include alendronate and risedronate, both oral agents, and zolendronic acid and pamidronate, given intravenously. These agents have been shown to be extremely efficacious in high-turnover osteoporosis [43]. Bone turnover is rapidly decreased within 6 weeks with the oral agents and within 3 days with the intravenous drugs. They increase bone mass at all measurable sites and decrease fracture incidence by 50%, including in the spine and the hip [7, 18, 57]. Bisphosphonates' mechanism of action involves interposition between osteoclasts and Howship's lacunae, thus interfering with resorption. The drug is then ingested by the osteoclast and disrupts cellular membrane synthesis pathways, leading to the osteoclasts' premature death [80]. Reported side effects of oral bisphosphonates include esophagitis and indigestion, but the once weekly regimen appears to be better tolerated and just as efficacious as daily dosing [65, 38]. Intravenous therapies, while not tested specifically for treatment in osteoporosis, appear to be efficacious, and once yearly zoledronate (Zometa) infusions appear to be just as effective as the oral dose of alendronate regarding bone mass [22]. Prospective fracture risk data are still lacking.

Bisphosphonates decrease bone turnover, and in very high dosages in canine models have been shown to cause fatigue fractures that are not actively repaired. Recent data indicate that patients on alendronate for 10 years have an 8.6% fracture rate in the first three years and 8.1% in the last five years, while the placebo group has a 19.6% fracture rate [61]. Patients stopping alendronate therapy after 5 years retain the decreased fracture risk. This suggests that bisphosphonates remain active for extended periods once the bone surface has been coated. The half-lives of alendronate and risedronate are at least 10 years and 1.5–3 years, respectively.

Fracture healing with bisphosphonates has been studied in animal models, and although callus remodeling was somewhat delayed, the ultimate mechanical strength of the repaired bone was unchanged compared to the controls [84]. There are no published data reporting the effects of bisphosphonates on spinal fusions. Overall, bisphosphonates are extremely effective in the prevention of osteoporotic fragility fractures. In addition, bisphosphonates are just as efficacious in men as in women [1, 35, 78], and are particularly effective in preventing steroid-induced osteoporosis [14, 90].

The medications discussed to this point are aimed at inhibition of osteoclastic bone resorption, and fracture protection is afforded by the avoidance of significant bone mass loss. However, in low-turnover osteoporosis, the primary disturbance is ineffective osteoblast activity. Anabolic agents lead to bone mass accretion at a high rate. Parathyroid hormone (PTH 1–34) has been recently released for the treatment of osteoporosis. It can lead to up to a 13% increase in bone mass within a year of therapy, and appears to have protection against fractures, although possibly slightly later than the bisphosphonates [8, 17, 27, 29, 45, 73]. PTH is given by a self-administered subcutaneous dose. Appropriate serum levels of PTH stimulate osteoblasts preferentially, and do not lead to increased osteoclastic resorption.

As the cellular and genetic pathways activated by PTH are elucidated, other benefits of PTH have been proposed. Several articles report on the possible benefits of PTH on augmentation of fracture healing [44, 47, 72, 77]. Callus formation was accelerated by the early stimulation of proliferation and differentiation of osteoprogenitor cells and increases in production of bone matrix proteins [72]. There are no data at this time answering the question of whether PTH will play a role in enhancing spine fusion, though similar mechanisms may be involved. For high-turnover states, controversy exists as to the indications of PTH versus the bisphosphonates. Currently, we recommend bisphosphonates within the 1st year to impede the high osteoclast activity. Patients with low-turnover states, patients who have been on bisphosphonates and have further fragility fractures, or patients who have radiographic evidence of loss of bone mass would be candidates for PTH. Parathyroid hormone is acceptable in women of child-bearing age. Concerns of osteogenic sarcoma have been voiced regarding PTH due to PTH-like receptors on osteosarcoma cells. Therefore, PTH is not recommended for patients with higher rates of osteoblast activity, such as children, patients who have undergone radiation, or patients with Paget's disease [6, 34, 83].

Fall prevention

Patients with osteoporosis who sustain one or more falls within a year have a 25-fold higher risk of fracture [33]. Though hip fractures are typically considered the greatest cause of morbidity in osteoporotic patients following a fall, up to 15% of vertebral fractures are associated with falls and account for significant morbidity [50]. Therapeutic medications do not completely eliminate fractures, and furthermore these often take between 6 months to 1 year to become effective. Therefore, fall prevention becomes a critical factor in fracture prevention [81, 98]. Fall history can be determined through a complete patient interview, as can the inability to rise from a chair without using the hands, poor eye sight and neuromuscular impairment. Osteoporotic individuals without vertebral compression fractures have single-limb stance times ranging from 13 to 15 s [59]. Another easily administered and highly informative test is the heel-toe straight line walk. When considering the etiology for increased falls, a wide variety of factors must be considered, including neurologic, metabolic, ophthalmologic, vascular and cardiac contributors. The interplay of these factors to cause increased falling may best be evaluated in the hands of a neurologist, physiatrist, or a clinician with similar interests.

Fall prevention is achieved by balance training [98]. While therapeutic exercises for bone mass accretion focus on load bearing exercises [95], balance training utilizes a different array of activities. Enhancement of muscle coordination through water therapy and games, particularly racquet games, which require movement in different directions, have been successful. Tai Chi programs for fall prevention were first described by Wolf et al., who reported a decrease in falls by 47.5% and a similar subsequent decrease in fracture risk [100]. Its efficacy has been confirmed more recently [53, 101]. At the Hospital for Special Surgery, our Tai Chi program has been extremely well received, and 1-year follow-up has indicated that the majority of patients continue to perform Tai Chi after they graduate from the class. Regarding the fracture risk with exercise programs, as bone mass decreases, loads applied anterior to the center of gravity become more deleterious. Relatively heavy weight-lifting should be discouraged in patients with osteoporosis, and sit-ups or crunches should be avoided. Patients should rely on isometric exercises to strengthen abdominal musculature.

The characteristics of surfaces are extremely important, as many vertebral fractures occur with falls. Carpets and soft surfaces are suggested for individuals with a predisposition for falling. In addition, for nursing home patients with dementia or who are otherwise disoriented, floor surfaces adjacent to their beds must be closely scrutinized.

Future interventions

Recent investigations have suggested several local and systemic procedures that may lead to rapid restoration of vertebral body bone mass and architecture. The first group includes direct intervention in a high-risk vertebral body, such as a vertebral body adjacent to a fusion, between two vertebral fractures, or at a site of acute kyphosis. Potential agents include the bone morphogenetic proteins (BMPs), which have been demonstrated to lead to rapid bone augmentation, specifically BMP-2 and its analog receptor agonists[82, 102]. These agents may be placed directly in trabecular bone and can rapidly lead to enhanced bone mass, possibly by up to 30% within 6 weeks. The mechanical properties of this bone, however, will be shaped by the mechanical load applied to that vertebral body in the following weeks to months. Local bone regeneration using this technique can be maintained by systemic agents, including bisphosphonates and PTH.

The second area involves the use of gene therapy. Most growth factors and medications, even with slow release, are metabolized and excreted within a relatively short period of time. Lieberman and others have demonstrated that the utilization of a BMP gene can continue the production of BMP-2 over a long period of time, controlled by the promoters within the inserted gene [56]. Whether the gene is ideally transduced through a viral vector or through ex-vivo insertion into appropriate cells is uncertain, but this technique appears promising [88, 99]. It may be possible to insert cells containing gene therapeutics which will preferentially direct bone metabolism in osteoporotic vertebral sites. There is preliminary evidence in animal models that intravenous injection of specialized cells can be targeted to the site of the fracture and then allow the incorporated genes to produce their bone augmentation products.

Aside from activating biological systems to stimulate bone formation in vivo, a family of biodegradable ceramics has been established that can lead to mechanical bone augmentation. They may be injected into vertebral bodies, and because the size of their trabecular structure is similar to human bone, they are gradually resorbed and replaced by native bone over time [52, 97]. The calcium sulfate and tri-calcium phosphate classes are more resorbable than bone cements such as polymethylmethacrylate, but will still lead to mechanical protection for a period of years.

Osteoporotic vertebral fractures occur commonly and lead to long-term morbidity and mortality. Biomechanically, they result from the structure, mass and material quality of cancellous bone. There are diagnostic tools available which allow the clinician to recognize osteoporosis and to further classify the underlying etiologies. Many US Food and Drug Administration (FDA) approved agents now exist to address either the high-resorptive rate or the low-formation state successfully, and have been shown to decrease the vertebral fracture rate. Patients presenting with a fragility vertebral fracture require osteoporosis evaluation and treatment, because further fractures in both the spine and the hip will occur in the majority of individuals who remain untreated. New methodologies on the horizon include local and systemically administered substances, including cements, proteins and genes which may rapidly augment vertebral bone quality.

References

1. Adami S, Prizzi R, Colapietro F (2001). Alendronate for the treatment of osteoporosis in men. Calcif Tissue Int 69:239–241
2. Arnaud CD (1996) Osteoporosis: using 'bone markers' for diagnosis and monitoring. Geriatrics 51:24–30
3. Bagur A, Solis F, Di Gregorio S, Mautalen C (2000) Reference data of vertebral morphometry by X-ray absorptiometry (MXA) in Argentine women. Calcif Tissue Int 66:259–262
4. Baylink DJ (2000) The diagnosis and management of osteoporosis. J Rheumatol 59 [Suppl 1]:42–44
5. Bianco AC, Malvestiti LF, Gouveia CH, Wehba S, Lewin S, Marone MM (1999) Morphometric dual-energy X-ray absorptiometry of the spine: report of a large series and correlation with axial bone mineral density. J Bone Miner Res 14:1605–1613
6. Bidwell J, Feister H, Swartz D, Onyia J, Holden J, Hock J (1996) Parathyroid hormone regulates the expression of rat osteoblast and osteosarcoma nuclear matrix proteins. J Cell Biochem 63:374–383
7. Black DM, Cummings SR, Karpf DB, et al (1996) Randomised trial of effect of alendronate on risk of fracture in women with existing vertebral fractures. Fracture Intervention Trial Research Group. Lancet 348:1535–1541
8. Body JJ, Gaich GA, Scheele WH, et al (2002) A randomized double-blind trial to compare the efficacy of teriparatide [recombinant human parathyroid hormone (1–34)] with alendronate in postmenopausal women with osteoporosis. J Clin Endocrinol Metab 87:4528–4535
9. Carter DR, Hayes WC (1977) The compressive behavior of bone as a two-phase porous structure J Bone Joint Surg Am 59:954–962
10. Carter DR, Bouxsein ML, Marcus R (1992) New approaches for interpreting projected bone densitometry data. J Bone Miner Res 7:137–145
11. Cauley JA, Thompson DE, Ensrud KC, Scott JC, Black D (2000) Risk of mortality following clinical fractures. Osteoporos Int 11:556–561
12. Cauley JA, Norton L, Lippman ME, et al (2001) Continued breast cancer risk reduction in postmenopausal women treated with raloxifene: 4-year results from the MORE trial. Multiple outcomes of raloxifene evaluation. Breast Cancer Res Treat 65:125–134
13. Chausmer AB (2001) Bone density measurement techniques in the diagnosis and management of osteoporosi. J S C Med Assoc 97:106–110

14. Chavassieux PM, Arlot ME, Roux JP, et al (2000) Effects of alendronate on bone quality and remodeling in glucocorticoid-induced osteoporosis: a histomorphometric analysis of transiliac biopsies. J Bone Miner Res 15:754–762
15. Chestnut CH 3rd, Silverman S, Adriano K, Genant H (2002) A randomized trial of nasal spray salmon calcitonin in postmenopausal women with established osteoporosis: the Prevent Recurrence of Osteoporotic Fractures Study. PROOF Study Group. Am J Med 109:267–276
16. Cooper C (1997) The crippling consequences of fractures and their impact on quality of life. Am J Med 103:12S-17S; discussion 17S-19S
17. Crandall C (2002) Parathyroid hormone for treatment of osteoporosis. Arch Intern Med 162:2297–2309
18. Cummings SR, Black DM, Thompson DE, et al (1998) Effect of alendronate on risk of fracture in women with low bone density but without vertebral fractures: results from the Fracture Intervention Trial. JAMA 280:2077–2082
19. Dawson-Hughes B, Harris SS, Krall EA, Dallal GE (1997) Effect of calcium and vitamin D supplementation on bone density in men and women 65 years of age or older. N Engl J Med 337:670–676
20. Delmas PD, Ensrud KE, Adachi JD, et al (2002) Efficacy of raloxifene on vertebral fracture risk reduction in postmenopausal women with osteoporosis: four-year results from a randomized clinical trial. J Clin Endocrinol Metab 87:3609–3617
21. Dickler MN, Norton L (2001) The MORE trial: multiple outcomes for raloxifene evaluation – breast cancer as a secondary end point: implications for prevention. Ann N Y Acad Sci 949:134–142
22. Doggrell SA (2002) Zoledronate once-yearly increases bone mineral density – implications for osteoporosis. Expert Opin Pharmacother 3:1007–1009
23. Ensrud KE, Thompson DE, Cauley JA, et al (2000) Prevalent vertebral deformities predict mortality and hospitalization in older women with low bone mass. Fracture Intervention Trial Research Group. J Am Geriatr Soc 48:241–249
24. Ettinger B, Black DM, Mitlak BH, et al (1999) Reduction of vertebral fracture risk in postmenopausal women with osteoporosis treated with raloxifene: results from a 3-year randomized clinical trial. Multiple Outcomes of Raloxifene Evaluation (MORE) Investigators. JAMA 282:637–645
25. Ferrar L, Jiang G, Barrington NA, Eastell R (2000) Identification of vertebral deformities in women: comparison of radiological assessment and quantitative morphometry using morphometric radiography and morphometric X-ray absorptiometry. J Bone Miner Res 15:575–585
26. Ferrar L, Jiang G, Eastell R (2001) Longitudinal evaluation of morphometric X-ray absorptiometry for the identification of vertebral deformities. Osteoporos Int 12:661–671
27. Finkelstein JS, Klibanski A, Arnold AL, Toth TL, Hornstein MD, Neer RM (1998) Prevention of estrogen deficiency-related bone loss with human parathyroid hormone-(1–34): a randomized controlled trial. JAMA 280:1067–1073
28. Follin SL, Black JN, McDermott MT (2003) Lack of diagnosis and treatment of osteoporosis in men and women after hip fracture. Pharmacotherapy 23:190–198
29. Fujita T, Inoue T, Morii H, et al (1999) Effect of an intermittent weekly dose of human parathyroid hormone (1–34) on osteoporosis: a randomized double-masked prospective study using three dose levels. Osteoporos Int 9:296–306
30. Galante J, Rostoker W, Ray RD (1970) Physical properties of trabecular bone. Calcif Tis Res 5:236–246
31. Gardner MJ, Flik KR, Mooar P, Lane JM (2002) Improvement in the undertreatment of osteoporosis following hip fracture. J Bone Joint Surg Am 84:1342–1348
32. Gass R (2001) The early preclinical diagnosis of osteoporosis measuring the pure trabecular bone density. Eur J Med Res 6:228–230
33. Geusens P, Autier P, Boonen S, Vanhoof J, Declerck K, Raus JN (2002) The relationship among history of falls, osteoporosis, and fractures in postmenopausal women. Arch Phys Med Rehabil 83:903–906
34. Giannoukos G, Williams LJ, Chilco PJ, Abou-Samra AB (1999) Characterization of an element within the rat parathyroid hormone/parathyroid hormone-related peptide receptor gene promoter that enhances expression in osteoblastic osteosarcoma 17/2.8 cells. Biochem Biophys Res Commun 258:336–340
35. Gonnelli S, Cepollaro C, Montagnani A, et al (2003) Alendronate treatment in men with primary osteoporosis: a three-year longitudinal study. Calcif Tissue Int
36. Grados F, Fardellone P, Benammar M, Muller C, Roux C, Sebert JL (1999) Influence of age and sex on vertebral shape indices assessed by radiographic morphometry. Osteoporos Int 10:450–455
37. Greenspan SL, von Stetten E, Emond SK, Jones L, Parker RA (2001) Instant vertebral assessment: a noninvasive dual X-ray absorptiometry technique to avoid misclassification and clinical mismanagement of osteoporosis. J Clin Densitom 4:373–380
38. Greenspan SL, Bone G 3rd, Schnitzer TJ, et al (2002) Two-year results of once-weekly administration of alendronate 70 mg for the treatment of postmenopausal osteoporosis. J Bone Miner Res 17:1988–1996
39. Guermazi A, Mohr A, Grigorian M, Taouli B, Genant HK (2002) Identification of vertebral fractures in osteoporosis. Sem Musculoskeletal Radiol 6:241–252
40. Harris ST, Watts NB, Genant HK, et al (1999) Effects of risedronate treatment on vertebral and nonvertebral fractures in women with postmenopausal osteoporosis: a randomized controlled trial. Vertebral Efficacy With Risedronate Therapy (VERT) Study Group. JAMA 282:1344–1352
41. Hasserius R, Karlsson MK, Nilsson BE, Redlund-Johnell I, Johnell O (2003) Prevalent vertebral deformities predict increased mortality and increased fracture rate in both men and women: a 10-year population-based study of 598 individuals from the Swedish cohort in the European Vertebral Osteoporosis Study. Osteoporos Int 14:61–68
42. Hayes WC, Myers ER, Robinovitch SN, van den Kroonenberg A, Courtney A, McMahon T (1996) Etiology and prevention of age-related hip fractures
43. Heijckmann AC, Juttmann JR, Wolffenbuttel BH (2002) Intravenous pamidronate compared with oral alendronate for the treatment of postmenopausal osteoporosis. Neth J Med 60:315–319
44. Holzer G, Majeska RJ, Lundy MW, Hartke JR, Einhorn TA (1999) Parathyroid hormone enhances fracture healing. A preliminary report. Clin Orthop 258–263

45. Horwitz MJ, Tedesco MB, Gundberg C, Garcia-Ocana A, Stewart AF (2003) Short-term, high-dose parathyroid hormone-related protein as a skeletal anabolic agent for the treatment of postmenopausal osteoporosis. J Clin Endocrinol Metab 88:569–575
46. Ito M, Tsurusaki K, Hayashi K (1997) Peripheral QCT for the diagnosis of osteoporosis. Osteoporos Int 7 [Suppl 3]:120–127
47. Jahng JS, Kim HW (2000) Effect of intermittent administration of parathyroid hormone on fracture healing in ovariectomized rats. Orthopedics 23:1089–1094
48. Jalava T, Sarna S, Pylkkanen L, et al (2003) Association between vertebral fracture and increased mortality in osteoporotic patients. J Bone Miner Res 18:1254–1260
49. Jordan KM, Cooper C (2002) Epidemiology of osteoporosis Best Pract Res Clin Rheumatol 16:795–806
50. Kado DM, Duong T, Stone KL, Ensrud KE, et al (2003) Incident vertebral fractures and mortality in older women: a prospective study. Osteoporosis Int 14:589–594
51. Kanis JA (2002) Diagnosis of osteoporosis and assessment of fracture risk. Lancet 359:1929–1936
52. Kelly CM, Wilkins RM, Gitelis S, Hartjen C, Watson JT, Kim PT (2001) The use of a surgical grade calcium sulfate as a bone graft substitute: results of a multicenter trial. Clin Orthop 42–50
53. Kessenich CR (1998) Tai Chi as a method of fall prevention in the elderly. Orthop Nurs 17:27–29
54. Lane JM (1997) Osteoporosis. Medical prevention and treatment. Spine 22:32S-37S
55. Lane JM, Nydick M (1999) Osteoporosis: current modes of prevention and treatment. J Am Acad Orthop Surg 7:19–31
56. Lieberman JR, Le LQ, Wu L, et al (1998) Regional gene therapy with a BMP-2-producing murine stromal cell line induces heterotopic and orthotopic bone formation in rodents. J Orthop Res 16:330–339
57. Liberman UA, Weiss SR, Broll J, et al (1995) Effect of oral alendronate on bone mineral density and the incidence of fractures in postmenopausal osteoporosis. The Alendronate Phase III Osteoporosis Treatment Study Group. N Engl J Med 333:1437–1443
58. Lin JT, van der Meulen MCH, Myers ER, Lane JM (2003) Fracture evaluation and clinical complications. In: Favus MJ (ed) Primer on the metabolic bone diseases and disorders of mineral metabolism, 5th edn. (in press)
59. Lin JT, Backus S, Meyers E, Peterson M, Lane JM (2003) Six minute walk test: a new powerful predictor of functional dysfunction in osteoporotic patients with and without vertebral fractures (abstract). J Bone Min Res (in press)
60. Lindsay R, Hart DM, Forrest C, Baird C (1980) Prevention of spinal osteoporosis in oophorectomised women. Lancet 2:1151–1154
61. Lindsay R, Silverman SL, Cooper C, Hanley DA, et al (2002) Risk of new vertebral fracture in the year following fracture. JAMA 17:285:320–323
62. Liu G, Peacock M, Eilam O, Dorulla G, Braunstein E, Johnston CC (1997) Effect of osteoarthritis in the lumbar spine and hip on bone mineral density and diagnosis of osteoporosis in elderly men and women. Osteoporos Int 7:564–569
63. Lofman O, Larsson L, Toss G (2000) Bone mineral density in diagnosis of osteoporosis: reference population, definition of peak bone mass, and measured site determine prevalence. J Clin Densitom 3:177–186
64. Looker AC, Johnston CC Jr, Wahner HW, et al Prevalence of low femoral bone density in older US women from NHANES III (1995) J Bone Miner Res 10:796–802
65. Luckey MM, Gilchrist N, Bone HG, et al (2003) Therapeutic equivalence of alendronate 35 milligrams once weekly and 5 milligrams daily in the prevention of postmenopausal osteoporosis. Obstet Gynecol 101:711–721
66. Marshall D, Johnell O, Wedel H (1996) Meta-analysis of how well measures of bone density predict occurrence of osteoporotic fractures. BMJ 312:1254–1259
67. Matthis C, Weber U, O'Neill TW, Raspe H (1998) Health impact associated with vertebral deformities: results from the European Vertebral Osteoporosis Study (EVOS). Osteoporos Int 8:364–372
68. Melton LJ 3rd, Chrischilles EA, Cooper C, Lane AW, Riggs BL (1992) Perspective. How many women have osteoporosis? J Bone Miner Res 7:1005–1010
69. Melton LJ 3rd, Atkinson EJ, Cooper C, O'Fallon WM, Riggs BL (1999) Vertebral fractures predict subsequent fractures. Osteoporos Int 10:214–221
70. Miller PD (2001) New possibilities for diagnosis and treatment of osteoporosis. Int J Fertil Womens Med 46:215–221
71. Moro M, Hecker AT, Bouxsein ML, Myers ER (1995) Failure load of thoracic vertebrae correlates with lumbar bone mineral density measured by DXA. Calcif Tissue Int 56:206–209
72. Nakajima A, Shimoji N, Shiomi K, et al (2002) Mechanisms for the enhancement of fracture healing in rats treated with intermittent low-dose human parathyroid hormone (1–34). J Bone Miner Res 17:2038–2047
73. Neer RM, Arnaud CD, Zanchetta JR, et al (2001) Effect of parathyroid hormone (1–34) on fractures and bone mineral density in postmenopausal women with osteoporosis. N Engl J Med 344:1434–1441
74. Neuner JM, Zimmer JK, Hamel MB (2003) Diagnosis and treatment of osteoporosis in patients with vertebral compression fractures. J Am Geriatr Soc 51:483–491
75. Nordin BE, Morris HA (1989) The calcium deficiency model for osteoporosis. Nutr Rev 47:65–72
76. O'Gradaigh D, Debiram I, Love S, Richards HK, Compston JE (2003) A prospective study of discordance in diagnosis of osteoporosis using spine and proximal femur bone densitometry. Osteoporos Int 14:13–18
77. Okazaki K, Jingushi S, Ikenoue T, Urabe K, Sakai H, Iwamoto Y (2003) Expression of parathyroid hormone-related peptide and insulin-like growth factor I during rat fracture healing. J Orthop Res 21:511–520
78. Orwoll E, Ettinger M, Weiss S, et al (2000) Alendronate for the treatment of osteoporosis in men. N Engl J Med 343:604–610
79. Osteoporosis prevention, diagnosis, and therapy (2000) NIH Consensus Statement 17:1–45
80. Owens JM, Fuller K, Chambers TJ (1997) Osteoclast activation: potent inhibition by the bisphosphonate alendronate through a nonresorptive mechanism. J Cell Physiol 172:79–86
81. Paganini-Hill A, Chao A, Ross RK, Henderson BE (1991) Exercise and other factors in the prevention of hip fracture: the Leisure World study. Epidemiology 2:16–25
82. Park J, Ries J, Gelse K, et al (2003) Bone regeneration in critical size defects by cell-mediated BMP-2 gene transfer: a comparison of adenoviral vectors and liposomes. Gene Ther 10:1089–1098
83. Pasquini GM, Davey RA, Ho PW, et al (2002) Local secretion of parathyroid hormone-related protein by an osteoblastic osteosarcoma (UMR 106–01) cell line results in growth inhibition. Bone 31:598–605
84. Peter CP, Cook WO, Nunamaker DM, Provost MT, Seedor JG, Rodan GA (1996) Effect of alendronate on fracture healing and bone remodeling in dogs. J Orthop Res 14:74–79

85. Rea JA, Chen MB, Li J, et al (2000) Morphometric X-ray absorptiometry and morphometric radiography of the spine: a comparison of prevalent vertebral deformity identification. J Bone Miner Res 15:564–574
86. Rea JA, Chen MB, Li J, et al (2001) Vertebral morphometry: a comparison of long-term precision of morphometric X-ray absorptiometry and morphometric radiography in normal and osteoporotic subjects. Osteoporos Int 12:158–166
87. Recker RR, Hinders S, Davies KM, et al (1996) Correcting calcium nutritional deficiency prevents spine fractures in elderly women. J Bone Miner Res 11:1961–1966
88. Riew KD, Wright NM, Cheng S, Avioli LV, Lou J (1998) Induction of bone formation using a recombinant adenoviral vector carrying the human BMP-2 gene in a rabbit spinal fusion model. Calcif Tissue Int 63:357–360
89. Ross PD (1996) Osteoporosis. Frequency, consequences, and risk factors. Arch Intern Med 156:1399–1411
90. Saag KG, Emkey R, Schnitzer TJ, et al (1998) Alendronate for the prevention and treatment of glucocorticoid-induced osteoporosis. Glucocorticoid-Induced Osteoporosis Intervention Study Group. N Engl J Med 339:292–299
91. Sahota O(2000) Osteoporosis and the role of vitamin D and calcium-vitamin D deficiency, vitamin D insufficiency, and vitamin D sufficiency. Age Ageing 29:301–304
92. Sarkar S, Mitlak BH, Wong M, Stock JL, Black DM, Harper KD (2002) Relationships between bone mineral density and incident vertebral fracture risk with raloxifene therapy. J Bone Miner Res 17:1–10
93. Schousboe JT, DeBold CR, Bowles C, Glickstein S, Rubino RK (2002) Prevalence of vertebral compression fracture deformity by X-ray absorptiometry of lateral thoracic and lumbar spines in a population referred for bone densitometry. J Clin Densitom 5:239–246
94. Shields AT, Chesnut CH 3rd (2001) Diagnosis of postmenopausal osteoporosis: reviews in endocrine and metabolic disorders. Rev Endocr Metab Disord 2:23–33
95. Simkin A, Ayalon J, Leichter I (1987) Increased trabecular bone density due to bone-loading exercises in postmenopausal osteoporotic women. Calcif Tissue Int 40:59–63
96. Stephenson J (2003) FDA orders estrogen safety warnings: agency offers guidance for HRT use. JAMA 289: 537–538
97. Strocchi R, Orsini G, Iezzi G, et al (2002) Bone regeneration with calcium sulfate: evidence for increased angiogenesis in rabbits. J Oral Implantol 28:273–278
98. Tinetti ME, Baker DI, Garrett PA, Gottschalk M, Koch ML, Horwitz RI (1993) Yale FICSIT: risk factor abatement strategy for fall prevention. J Am Geriatr Soc 41:315–320
99. Varady P, Li JZ, Alden TD, Kallmes DF, Williams MB, Helm GA (2002) CT and radionuclide study of BMP-2 gene therapy-induced bone formation. Acad Radiol 9:632–637
100. Wolf SL, Barnhart HX, Kutner NG, McNeely E, Coogler C, Xu T (1996) Reducing frailty and falls in older persons: an investigation of Tai Chi and computerized balance training. Atlanta FICSIT Group. Frailty and injuries: cooperative studies of intervention techniques. J Am Geriatr Soc 44:489–497
101. Wu G (2002) Evaluation of the effectiveness of Tai Chi for improving balance and preventing falls in the older population – a review. J Am Geriatr Soc 50:746–754
102. Zerath E, Holy X, Noel B, Malouvier A, Hott M, Marie PJ (1998) Effects of BMP-2 on osteoblastic cells and on skeletal growth and bone formation in unloaded rats. Growth Horm IGF Res 8:141–149

A. Mehbod
S. Aunoble
J. C. Le Huec

Vertebroplasty for osteoporotic spine fracture: prevention and treatment

Abstract There is a relatively high prevalence of osteoporotic vertebral compression fractures (VCFs) in the elderly population, especially in women aged 50 or older. The result of these VCFs is increased morbidity and mortality in the short and long term. Medical treatment of these fractures includes bed rest, orthotics, analgesic medication and time. Percutaneous vertebroplasty (PVP) consists of percutaneous injection of biomaterial, such as methylmethacrylate, into the VCF to produce stability and pain relief. Biomechanical testing has shown that PVP can restore strength and stiffness of the vertebral body to the pre-fracture levels. Clinical results show immediate and maintained pain relief in 70–95% of the patients. Possible major complications include cement leakage into the spinal canal or into the venous system. Additionally, percutaneous vertebroplasty may alter the normal loading behavior of the adjacent vertebral body, and there is an increased risk of adjacent segment VCF. Kyphoplasty is a new technique, which introduces a balloon into the vertebral body transpedicularly to reduce the VCF while creating a cavity for the cement injection. This technique has the benefit of kyphosis reduction as well as less cement leakage. Research continues into the development of injectable biomaterials that are resorbable and allow for new bone formation. Vertebroplasty and kyphoplasty are safe and effective in the treatment of osteoporotic VCFs. They may allow for a faster return to function, and thus avoid the morbidity associated with medical treatment.

Keywords Vertebral compression fracture · Osteoporotic compression fracture · Percutaneous vertebroplasty · Vertebroplasty · Kyphoplasty

A. Mehbod
Twin Cities Spine Center,
Minneapolis, Minnesota, USA

S. Aunoble · J. C. Le Huec (✉)
Spine Unit, Bordeaux University Hospital,
CHU Pellegrin Tripode,
33076 Bordeaux, France
Fax: +33-5-56796089,
e-mail: j-c.lehuec@u-bordeaux2.fr

Introduction

Osteoporosis is a disorder of decreased bone mass, microstructural collapse, and fragility fractures. It can affect people of all ethnic backgrounds and can result in challenging complications, ranging from compression fractures of vertebral bodies to femoral neck fractures [59]. The geriatric population is especially at risk for such osteoporotic fractures, as bone mass decreases with age [53]. A loss of one standard deviation of bone mass doubles the risk of spine fractures [34, 56, 59]. It is estimated that 90% of hip and spine fractures occurring in the elderly are attributable to osteoporosis [45]. The consequences of such osteoporotic vertebral fractures are diverse and include back pain, functional limitations and impairment of mood [11, 37, 58].

A recent study in Canada examined the health-related quality of life (HRQL) in women aged 50 years and older with osteoporosis [1]. Subjects who had experienced a vertebral fracture had lower HRQL scores than participants without fracture in total score, symptoms, physical function, activities of daily living, and leisure. Acute complications of osteoporotic vertebral fractures include transient ileus, urinary retention, nausea, abdominal pain and chest pain [41, 49]. Long-term effects of osteoporotic fractures include increased kyphosis, deconditioning, insomnia and depression [14, 32, 41, 49]. Physiologic changes include significant diminution of pulmonary function in patients with spinal osteoporotic fractures and increased kyphosis. The degree of pulmonary function reduction correlates with the severity of the kyphosis [55]. In addition to the increased morbidity, mortality may also increase after osteoporotic vertebral fractures. A study from the Mayo Clinic found the estimated survival at 5 years after spine fractures in the elderly to be 61% compared with the expected value of 78% [12]. Treatment of osteoporosis to prevent such fractures is thus justified.

While physicians are aware of the risks of osteoporosis and fractures, the disease remains under-diagnosed and under-treated. A survey of physicians who treated elderly patients residing in long-term care facilities found that while the physicians are well aware of the prevalence of osteoporosis in their patients, 45% of the physicians did not routinely assess their patients for the disease and 26% did not routinely treat it [44]. One can only assume the use of preventive measures is even lower, which leads to a higher prevalence of osteoporotic vertebral compression fractures (VCFs). The prevalence of these fractures in women aged 50 or older has been estimated at 26% [58].

Historically, the painful VCF has been treated medically. Surgery in these patients has been limited because of its inherent risks, invasiveness and the poor quality of osteoporotic bone. However, surgery is indicated in patients with instability or neurological deficit [16]. The medical treatment of stable osteoporotic fractures without neurological involvement includes bed rest, orthotic management, narcotic analgesia, and time. Each of these modalities has side effects: bed rest over time results in loss of muscle mass, bone density and resultant deconditioning [10], braces are poorly tolerated [30], and narcotic medication can lead to mood or mental alteration. As a result, there has been a search for alternative ways to treat VCFs. Percutaneous vertebroplasty has become a very popular, safe, and effective treatment for this condition.

Percutaneous vertebroplasty (PVP) is a minimally invasive technique consisting of percutaneous injection of biomaterial, usually methylmethacrylate, into the pathologic fractured area, stabilizing the fracture and more importantly decreasing pain and improving function. It was first developed by Deramond in France in the late 1980s [19]. Initially it was used for treatment of aggressive hemangiomas and osteolytic neoplasms. However, as it proved successful with these lesions, the indications also expanded to include osteoporotic compression fractures refractory to medical treatment. The initial experience with vertebroplasty for the treatment of osteoporotic fractures has shown 70–95% pain relief [3, 13, 15, 18, 22, 23, 26, 28, 29, 31, 33, 46, 50, 51, 61]. The mechanism by which PVP achieves its palliative effect is not known. It may be due to the initial stability that it provides or due to neuronal damage caused by heat liberated during polymerization [17].

Vertebroplasty: technique with polymethylmethacrylate

PVP is performed under fluoroscopic guidance. The patient is under conscious sedation and is positioned prone on a radiolucent table. Adequate and clear pictures must be obtained prior to the start of the procedure, as it is crucial to be able to visualize the cement being injected into the vertebral body. The back is then prepped and local anesthetic is injected over the area of needle placement. Under fluoroscopic guidance, an 11-G bone marrow biopsy needle is introduced into the fractured vertebra via a transpedicular approach (Fig. 1a,b). In the thoracic spine, one can opt to enter the vertebral body extrapedicularly, between the rib head and the lateral aspect of the pedicle. The needle is then advanced to the anterior half of the vertebral body. At this point, an optional intraosseous venogram can be performed to aid in placement of the needle out of the venous flow path to avoid embolization to the lungs. Additionally, the intraosseous venogram can aid in determination of the flow pattern in the vertebral body, which may allow for cement leaks. Once the needle is in the correct position, the cement is injected. The cement should be radio opaque, with addition of barium powder or tungsten powder. Each kit of polymethylmethacrylate (PMMA) cement can be mixed with 5.0 g barium sulfate and 2.0 g tungsten powder [3]. The cement is allowed to achieve a paste-like consistency prior to injection. Using a 1-cc or

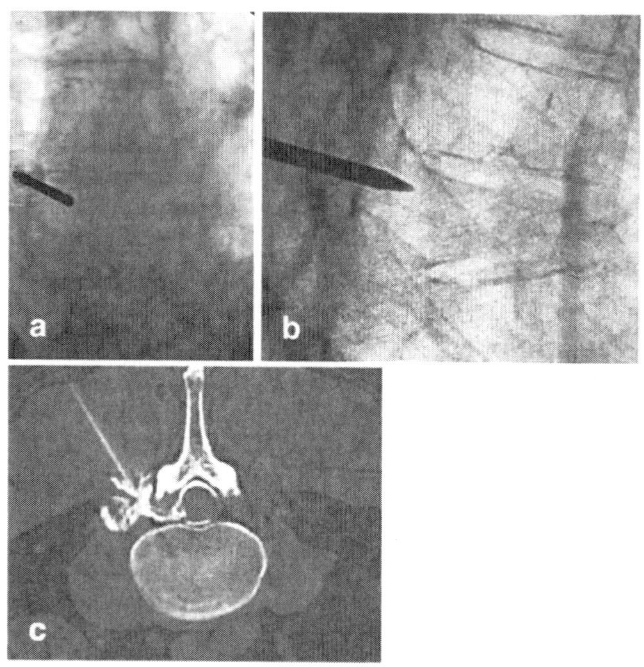

Fig. 1 a,b Radiograph of an osteoporotic fracture with a needle in the fractured vertebra. **c** Computed tomography scan showing needle positioning

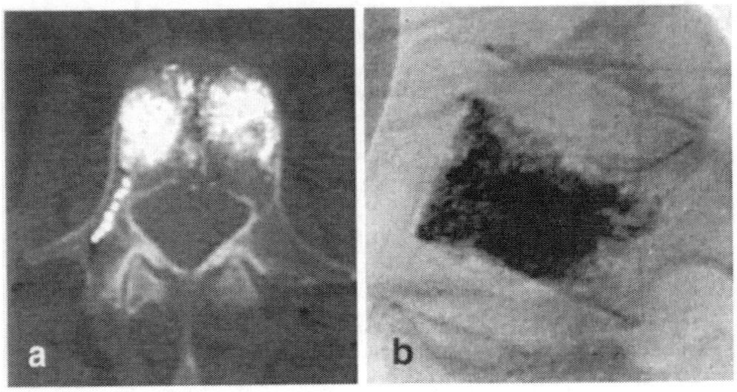

Fig. 2 **a** Computed tomography scan showing cement filling after bilateral needle injection. **b** Lateral view radiographic control

3-cc syringe, the cement is injected into the vertebral body under fluoroscopic guidance. Filling of the posterior one-third of the vertebral body should signal the end of the injection to avoid overfilling (Fig. 2). Typical volumes for cement injection are 2–3 cc for thoracic and 3–5 cc for lumbar vertebrae [3]. Usually there is symmetrical filling of the vertebral body, but if it is asymmetrical, then the contralateral pedicle can be used for further delivery of the cement. After the procedure, the patients are allowed to ambulate as tolerated.

Biomechanical considerations

There is a continual effort being made to optimize the technique of PVP. Biomechanical and clinical studies have been performed to determine the characteristics of different cements, the role of cement volume, and differences in the approach used (unipedicular vs bipedicular). Presently acrylic cement such as methylmethacrylate is used most frequently for PVP. Use of cement in a fractured vertebra has been shown to increase vertebral body strength and stiffness [4, 8, 25, 40]. Other materials, like glass-ceramic matrix [4], calcium phosphate [40], and hydroxyapatite [8, 25] have also been compared to methylmethacrylate and have shown similar biomechanical properties. The theoretical clinical benefit of using calcium phosphate or hydroxyapatite is that they are osteoconductive and can undergo remodeling, although the ability of pathologic osteoporotic bone to regenerate or, for that matter, to remodel is questionable.

The effect of different cement volumes on the biomechanical properties of the vertebrae depends on the type of cement used. Belkoff et al. [6] showed that when using Orthocomp, thoracic and thoracolumbar vertebrae needed 4 cc and lumbar vertebrae needed 6 cc to restore stiffness to the pre-fracture levels. For simplex P, the volumes needed were 6 cc and 8 cc, respectively. Using anatomically accurate finite-element models, it has been shown that approximately 15% volume fraction or approximately 3.5 cc is needed to restore stiffness of the vertebra to pre-fracture levels and that overfilling can increase the stiffness beyond that of the intact state. Overfilling has several other disadvantages: it can cause asymmetrical distribution and lead to single-sided load transfer and toggle, it can lead to leakage of cement into the epidural space [54], and in the long term it can cause increased stress on adjacent vertebrae, leading to increased risk of adjacent level fractures [9].

Whether to perform a bipedicular or unipedicular approach depends on the individual case. In biomechanical controlled studies, no significant difference has been found between the two techniques in terms of strength and stiffness [6, 39]. Further analysis, however, shows that while providing the same strength and stiffness, the use of a unipedicular approach leads to a medial-lateral bending motion or toggle toward the untreated side with uniform loading [39]. The clinical significance of this toggle is not known. Clinically, the two techniques have been shown to give similar results. The unipedicular approach can result in filling across the midline in 96% of cases [33]. The mean opacification of the vertebral body did not differ between the groups. More importantly, there was no difference in the amount of pain relief achieved with the two techniques.

Clinical results: literature review

The clinical results of PVP from the United States, Europe, and Asia show a 70–95% success rate in relieving pain. Most reports in the literature are retrospective, although a few prospective studies have been published. The main indication for the procedure is pain persisting despite non-operative treatment of osteoporotic compression fractures. One series bravely included four burst fractures treated with PVP [46]. The majority of the cases are around the thoracolumbar area. The largest retrospective study [18] was a collaboration between seven centers in the US, where 488 consecutive patients underwent PVP for vertebral compression fractures. A telephone questionnaire was conducted with 245 patients at median of 7 months' follow-up. Questions were designed to measure pain, ambulation, and ability to perform activities of daily living. The pain decreased from a mean of 8.9 pre PVP to 3.4 post PVP. Ability to ambulate was impaired in 72% pre PVP and in 28% post PVP. Ability to perform activities of daily living improved significantly post PVP. There was a 4.9% rate of minor complications.

In another study, Barr et al. [3] studied 38 patients with 70 symptomatic fractures who had failed to respond to medical treatment. After undergoing PVP, 63% reported marked to complete relief and 32% had moderate relief of pain. Peh et al. [50] retrospectively studied 37 patients with 48 compression fractures treated with PVP. At a mean follow-up of 11 months, pain relief was complete in 47% and partial in 50%.

More recently, prospective studies have shown similar success with PVP. The largest prospective study [43] reported on 100 patients who underwent PVP for vertebral compression fractures. At final follow-up averaging 21 months, 97% of the patients reported significant pain reduction, with the VAS improving from 8.9 to 2.0. Cortet et al. [13] added to the literature by reporting on 16 patients with 20 VCFs of more than 3 months' duration not responding to medical treatment. They all underwent PVP and showed a statistically significant improvement in VAS pain score immediately after the procedure, which remained at 30, 90, and 180 days after the procedure. Additionally, there was a significant improvement in the general health status as assessed by Nottingham Health Profile, which includes pain, mobility, emotional reaction, social isolation, and energy.

The longest follow-up has been reported by Perez-Higueras et al. [51], who followed 13 patients with VCFs for at least 5 years following PVP. The VAS improved significantly from a score of 9 pre PVP to 2 immediately post PVP, to 1 at 3 months. At 5 years, the VAS was 2.2. Significant improvement after treatment with PVP was also noted on the McGill Questionnaire.

The safety and efficacy of the procedure in the upper thoracic spine was reported by Kallmes et al. [29], who studied 41 patients with 63 vertebral compression fractures from T4 to T8. There was a significant pain reduction, as the mean VAS decreased from 9.7 pre PVP to 1.7 post PVP. There was one case of a pedicle fracture and no cases of pneumothorax.

The issue of timing of vertebroplasty was reviewed by Kaufman et al. [31]. Seventy-five patients with 122 VCFs underwent PVP. The age of the fracture at time of PVP was not independently associated with post PVP pain or activity. The procedure was efficacious in reducing pain and improving mobility in patients, regardless of the age of the fracture. However, the authors found that increasing age of the fracture was independently associated with increased needs of analgesia post PVP. Whether the delay in carrying out PVP leads to tolerance of and dependence on pain medication, leading to higher requirements post PVP, is not known.

Complications

While these clinical studies have shown good success rates in improving pain and function, the procedure is not without risks and complications. Most series report a complication rate of between 4 and 6% [3, 15, 18, 28]. Reported complications associated with the insertion of the needle include rib fractures [28], neuritis [3], pedicle fracture [29], and infection [29]. The most feared complication is the potential for leakage of cement into the spinal canal (Fig. 3) or into the venous system. Cement leakage into the spinal canal has been reported in a small number of patients without causing any clinical symptoms [46], while there have been reports of transient neuropathy [28] and one case of paraplegia associated with PVP of T11 [36]. We have consulted on a patient in whom PVP was performed for burst fracture of L2 with cement leakage into the spinal canal causing symptoms of spinal stenosis. The patient underwent a decompression and removal of cement from the spinal canal.

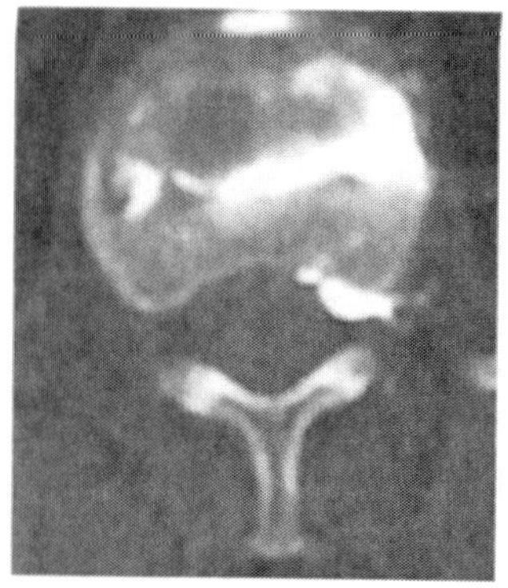

Fig. 3 Cement leakage in the foramen

Leakage of cement into the venous system can have a spectrum of clinical consequences, from being asymptomatic [51], causing pulmonary embolism [27, 47], or causing a paradoxical cerebral artery embolization in a patient with patent foramen ovale [57]. In a recent study [46], 17 patients had CT scans performed immediately after undergoing PVP. Cement in the epidural veins adjacent to the vertebra was found in 48% of the cases, with only one patient developing a transient neuritis. The risk of cement leakage into the spinal canal or venous system is increased with higher volumes of injected cement [54]. This problem is so feared that some have advocated the use of pre PVP venography to assess the risk of cement leakage.

Venography can document sites of potential leakage during cement injection [21, 42, 63]. In one study [42], venography was performed prior to vertebroplasty, and the results retrospectively reviewed. Venography could predict the flow characteristics of cement within the vertebral body and within the venous structures. While venography could predict cement leakage into endplates or central defects in 100% of cases, it could only predict leakage into the venous structures in 29% of the cases. Another study [63] specifically looked at 205 PVP procedures in 137 patients without antecedent venography, and found only one cement leakage causing symptoms of radiculopathy. The value of antecedent venography will need to be determined with prospective studies.

A topic of interest is the occurrence of new vertebral body fractures after PVP in patients with osteoporosis [2, 9, 62]. This was noted in a follow-up of 25 patients who underwent PVP. The average follow-up was 48 months. The authors found a significantly increased risk of vertebral fractures adjacent to a cemented vertebra, with the odds ratio of 2.27, whereas the odds ratio for sustaining a vertebral fracture next to an uncemented fracture was 1.44

[23]. In another report [62], 177 patients treated with PVP for osteoporotic fractures were followed for a minimum of 2 years. Twenty-two patients (12.4%) developed a total of 36 new vertebral body fractures. Two-thirds (67%) of the new fractures involved a vertebra adjacent to a previously treated vertebra.

New developments for treatment of osteoporotic spine

Kyphoplasty

Vertebroplasty carries its share of risks and complications, but it does lead to significant pain reduction and improved function. It does not, however, improve the sagittal balance or the kyphosis caused by the fracture. Kyphoplasty is a new technique, which tries to address this issue. Kyphoplasty is similar to vertebroplasty except that it calls for introduction of an inflatable bone tamp into the vertebral body which, when inflated, tries to restore the vertebral body height back to its original height while creating a cavity that can be filled with cement (Fig. 4). This technique is performed via a bipedicular approach for a uniform restoration of the compression. Why might reduction of the kyphosis be important in these patients? It has been shown that patients with spinal osteoporotic fractures have significantly diminished pulmonary function compared to those without fractures. More importantly, the reduction in the pulmonary functions has been shown to correlate significantly with severity of the spinal deformity [55]. Furthermore, it has been shown that, if left untreated, the thoracic compression fracture can lead to worsening of the kyphosis over 3 months and further deterioration at 3 years [14]. If the kyphosis can be corrected, pulmonary functions may improve and further collapse may be avoided.

An ex vivo biomechanical evaluation comparing vertebroplasty to kyphoplasty showed that both techniques result in significantly stronger vertebral bodies relative to the initial fractured state. Kyphoplasty was able to restore vertebral height to 97% of the original height. Vertebroplasty resulted in a significantly lower restoration of vertebral height, to 30% of the original height [5]. The ability to restore vertebral body height has been shown in other laboratory studies as well [7, 64]. Clinical studies have shown increased vertebral height, but not the level of increase obtained in the laboratory. Lieberman et al. [38] reported on 70 consecutive kyphoplasties performed on 30 patients for painful VCFs with a mean duration of symptoms of 5.9 months. The patients were followed prospectively for 3 months. In 70% of the patients, height was restored to 46.8% of predicted values. In 30% of the patients there was no restoration of height. Pain and physical functional scores significantly improved after kyphoplasty. Although no conclusions could be made with regards to the age of the fracture and the ability to regain height, the authors got the "impression" that they were able to restore height more predictably in fractures less than 3 months old. A balloon failure rate of 20% and cement leakage rate of 8.6% was also reported.

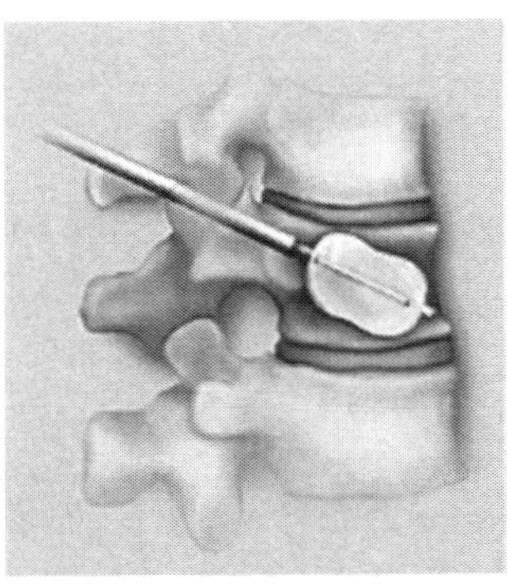

Fig. 4 The inflated balloon restores vertebral body height, while creating a cavity that can be filled with cement (kyphoplasty)

Since the approval of kyphoplasty by the FDA in 1998, a multi-center study in the US has been initiated, with results reported for 2,194 kyphoplasty procedures in 1,439 patients [20]. In fractures less than 3 months old, the average fractured vertebral body height improved from the 71% pre treatment to 92% after treatment. In fractures more than 3 months old, the height improved from 74% pre treatment to 84% after treatment. Ninety percent of the patients had relief of their pain as they returned to the pre-fracture level of pain medication use. There were three thoracic level parapareses related to instrument insertion through the medial wall of the seventh pedicle with cord injuries, and there was one case of epidural hematoma in a patient on anticoagulation medication. These complications occurred in the first 100 fractures treated. Since technique adjustment, no neurological complications have been reported.

Kyphoplasty has the added benefit of less cement leakage. When the balloon is inserted and inflated, it forms a contained cavity that can then be injected. As the cement travels along the path of less resistance, it will then fill this empty cavity rather than flowing into the surrounding osseous or venous structures. In an in vivo comparison of the potential for extravertebral cement leakage after vertebroplasty and kyphoplasty, there were significantly lower rates of leakage of contrast material with kyphoplasty [52]. In the recent US experience, there was only one cement embolus, without breathing consequences [20].

Vertebroplasty using Cortoss

Cortoss is a new synthetic bone void filler that contains bis glycidyl methyl-methacrylate, bisphenol, a polyethylene glycol diether dimethylacrylate, triethyleneglycol dimethylacrylate monomer and bioactive glass ceramic [60]. It is provided in a double lumen cartridge with specially designed tips for mixing. After the composite is expressed through these tips, polymerization begins and the material is ready for use. The monomer is not volatile and Cortoss polymerizes in a three-dimensional network, which minimizes the chances of leaking. After mixing, the material has the consistency of toothpaste, and stays that way until it polymerizes quickly, in a matter of seconds. This characteristic provides a consistent tactile feedback and allows for an even injection. The polymerization has a much lower exotherm than PMMA (63°C vs 84°C), which reduces the risk of thermal necrosis. The modulus of elasticity of Cortoss is close to that of bone [60]. This composite is bioactive, and in animal studies the cement-bone interface continues to be strengthened over time with bone apposition occurring at the interface without any fibrous interposition. Cortoss cement appears well suited for use in the treatment of VCFs. The aliquot delivery system allows for accurate amounts of cement to be injected directly into the region of interest.

A prospective clinical study has been conducted at our institution with Cortoss [48]. To participate, patients had to have fracture-related pain measuring at least 50/100 on the VAS, which also caused a change in lifestyle or disability. Patients were scheduled for follow-up at 4 days, 1 week, and 1, 3, and 6 months after the procedure. Two metal trocars of 10 G diameter were introduced through the pedicles at each level treated. Twenty-four patients with osteoporotic fractures were enrolled. The average pain scores were 69 preoperatively and 38 at 4 days postoperatively. The scores continued to decrease, to 33 at 1 week and 29 at 1 month, and then returned to 33 at 6 months. This represents a reduction of pain of 46% at 6 months. The quality of life has been evaluated with the short form 1 (SF-12) questionnaire. Ability to ambulate was impaired in 75% preoperatively and in 28% at 6 months postoperatively. Ability to perform activities of daily living improved significantly post PVP. There was a 3% rate of minor complications, and no leakage into the spinal canal. Results indicate that Cortoss addresses the shortcomings of PMMA for vertebroplasty augmentation. This cement is a fixed composition material with less variability than current variations of PMMA, and in conjunction with the Aliquot delivery system can be accurately delivered in incremental doses without excessive material waste.

Bone substitutes in vertebroplasty

As requested by Heini [24], bone substitutes for vertebroplasty need the following properties: injectability, radiopacity, adapted viscosity, long setting time, good mechanical properties for the load (compressive strength/stiffness), biocompatibility, bioactivity, and slow degradation. Calcium phosphate cement meets these criteria well. In their ceramic form they cannot be used as injectable device. Tetracalcium phosphate with dicalcium hydroxy apatite and amorphous calcium phosphate also meet the criteria and are readily available. They can be injected through a 10- or 11-G needle. The results of animal tests are very promising, and in vitro experimental studies have shown interesting resistance in compression, of around 45 MPa. As reported by Le Huec [35], these resorbable calcium phosphates provide the calcium for local bone formation and are of great interest for the treatment of osteoporotic fractures. Clinical applications on humans are in progress, but the results of these studies have not yet been published. Also yet to be reported on is the effect of combining the use of resorbable calcium phosphates with bone morphogenic protein as a carrier, which is a promising technique to promote bone healing in fracture cases.

Conclusion

Kyphoplasty and vertebroplasty are safe and effective in the treatment of osteoporotic VCFs that do not respond to conservative medical treatment. Kyphoplasty has the potential benefit of restoring the height of the vertebral body and reducing kyphosis, but the clinical benefit of this needs to be studied by prospective randomized trials comparing the two techniques. The other question remaining is whether we should perform vertebroplasty or kyphoplasty in patients with osteoporotic fractures in an acute setting, or wait until failure of medical treatment before carrying out the procedure. This question is also best addressed by conducting a prospective randomized trial comparing conservative treatment to vertebroplasty and kyphoplasty. Bone substitutes are promising devices to treat osteoporotic fractures, but more experimental and clinical data are required to assess their efficacy in this application.

References

1. Adachi J, Ioannidis G, Olszynski W, Brown J, Hanley D, Sebaldt Petrie A, Tenenhouse A, Stephenson G, Papaioannou A, Guyatt G, Goldsmith C (2002) The impact of incident vertebral and non-vertebral fractures of health related quality of life in postmenopausal women. BMC Musculoskeletal Disord 3:11
2. Aebli N, Krebs J, Davis G, Walton M, Williams M, Theis J (2002) Fat embolism and acute hypotension during vertebroplasty: an experimental study in sheep. Spine 27:460–466
3. Barr J, Barr M, TJ, McCann R (2000) Percutaneous vertebroplasty for pain relief and spinal stabilization. Spine 25:923–928
4. Belkoff S, Mathis J, Erbe E, Fenton D (2000) Biomechanical evaluation of a new bone cement for use in vertebroplasty. Spine 25:1061–1064
5. Belkoff S, Mathis J, Fenton D, et al (2001) An ex vivo biomechanical evaluation of an inflatable bone tamp used in the treatment of compression fracture. Spine 26:151–156

6. Belkoff S, Mathis J, Jasper L, Deramond H (2001) The biomechanics of vertebroplasty. The effect of cement volumes on mechanical behavior. Spine 26:1537–1541
7. Belkoff S, Jasper L, et al (2002) An ex vivo evaluation of an inflatable bone tamp used to reduce fractures within vertebral bodies under load. Spine 27: 1640–1643
8. Belkoff S, Mathis J, Jasper L (2002) Ex vivo biomechanical comparison of hydroxyapatite and polymethylmethacrylate cements for use with vertebroplasty. AJNR 23:1647–1651
9. Berlemann U, Ferguson S, Nolte L, Heini P (2002) Adjacent vertebral failure after vertebroplasty. A biomechanic investigation. J Bone Joint Surg 84:748–752
10. Convertino V, Bloomfield S, Greenleaf J (1997) An overview of the issues: physiological effects of bed rest and restricted physical activity. Med Sci Sports Exerc 29:187–190
11. Cook D, Guyatt G, Adachi J, Clifton J, Griffith L, Epstein R, Juniper E (1993) Quality of life issues in women with vertebral fractures due to osteoporosis. Arthritis Rheum 36:750–756
12. Cooper C, Atkinson E, Jacobsen S, O'Fallon W, Melton III L (1993) Population based study of survival after osteoporotic fractures. Am J Epidemiol 137:1001–1005
13. Cortet B, Cotten A, Boutry N, Flipo R, Duquesnoy B, Chastanet P, Delcambre B (1999) Percutaneous vertebroplasty in the treatment of osteoporotic vertebral compression fractures: an open prospective study. J Rheumatol 26: 2222–2228
14. Cortet B, Roches E, Logier R, Houvenagel E, Gaydier-Souquieres G, Puisieux F, Delcambre B (2002) Evaluation of spinal curvatures after a recent osteoporotic vertebral fracture. Joint Bone Spine 69:201–208
15. Cyteval C, Carrabere M, Roux J, Thomas E, Jorgensen C, Blotman F, Sany J, Taourel P (1999) Acute osteoporotic vertebral collapse: open study on percutaneous injection of acrylic surgical cement in 20 patients. AJR 173:1685–1690
16. Denis F (1983) The three column spine and its signifance in the classification of acute thoracolumbar spinal injuries. Spine 8:817–831
17. Deramond H, Wright N, Belkoff S (1999) Temperature elevation caused by bone cement polymerization during vertebroplasty. Bone 25:17S–21S
18. Evans A, Jensen M, Kip K, DeNardo A, Lawler G, Negin G, Remley K, Boutin S, Dunnagan S (2003) Vertebral compression fractures: pain reduction and improvement in functional mobility after percutaneous polymethylmethacrylate vertebroplasty: retrospective report of 245 cases. Radiology 226:366–372
19. Galibert P, Deramond H, Rosat P, Le Gars D (1987) Preliminary note on the treatment of vertebral angioma by percutaneous acrylic vertebroplasty. Neurochirurgie 33:166–168
20. Garfin S (2001) A retrospective review of early outcomes of balloon kyphoplasty. In: Proceedings of the North American Spine Society, Seattle, Washington
21. Gaughen JJ, Jensen M, Schweickert P, Kaufmann T, Marx W, Kallmes D (2002) Relevance of antecedent venography in percutaneous vertebroplasty for the treatment of osteoporotic compression fractures. AJNR 23:594–600
22. Gaughen JJ, Jensen M, Schweickert P, Marx W, Kallmes D (2002) The therapeutic benefit of repeat percutaneous vertebroplasty at previously treated vertebral levels. AJNR 23:1657–1661
23. Grados F, Depriester C, Cayrolle G, Hardy N, Deramond H, Fardellone P (2000) Long-term observations of vertebral osteoporotic fractures treated by percutaneous vertebroplasty. Rheumatology (Oxford) 39:1410–1414
24. Heini PF, et al (2001) Bone substitutes in vertebroplasty. Eur Spine J 10: S205–S213
25. Hitchon P, Goel V, Drake G, Taggard D, Berenton M, Rogge T, Torner J (2001) Comparison of the biomechanics of hydroxyapatite and polymethylmethacrylate vertebroplasty in a cadaveric spinal compression fracture model. J Neurosurg 95:215–220
26. Hiwatashi A, et al (2003) Increase in vertebral body height after vertebroplasty. AJNR 24:185–189
27. Jang J, Lee S, Jung S (2002) Pulmonary embolism of polymethylmethacrylate after percutaneous vertebroplasty: a report of three cases. Spine 27:E416–418
28. Jensen M, Evans A, Mathis J, Kallmes D, Cloft H, Dion J (1997) Percutaneous polymethylmethacrylate vertebroplasty in the treatment of osteoporotic vertebral body compression fractures: technical aspects. AJNR 18: 1897–1904
29. Kallmes D, Schweickert P, Marx W, Jensen M (2002) Vertebroplasty in the mid and upper thoracic spine. AJNR 23:1117–1120
30. Karjalainen M, Aho A, Katevuo K (1991) Painful spine after stable fractures of the thoracic and lumbar spine. What benefit from the use of extension brace? Ann Chir Gynaecol 80:45–48
31. Kaufmann T, Jensen M, Schweickert P, Marx W, Kallmes D (2001) Age of fracture and clinical outcomes of percutaneous vertebroplasty. AJNR 22: 1860–1863
32. Keller T, Harrison D, Colloca C, Harrison D, Janik T (2003) Prediction of osteoporotic spinal deformity. Spine 28: 455–462
33. Kim A, Jensen M, Dion J, Schweickert P, Kaufmann T, Kallmes D (2002) Unilateral transpedicular percutaneous vertebroplasty: initial experience. Radiology 222:737–741
34. Lane J, Russell L, Khan S (2000) Osteoporosis. Clin Orthop 372:139–150
35. Le Huec J (1998) Evolution of the local calcium content around irradiated beta-tricalcium phosphate ceramic implants. Biomaterials 733–738
36. Lee B, Lee S, Yoo T (2002) Paraplegia as a complication of percutaneous vertebroplasty with polymethylmethacrylate: a case report. Spine 27:E419–422
37. Leidig-Bruckner G, Minne H, Schlaich C, Wagner G, Sheidt-Nave C, Bruckner T, Gebest H, Ziegler R (1997) Clinical grading of spinal osteoporosis: quality of life component and spinal deformity in women with chronic low back pain and women with vertebral osteoporosis. J Bone Miner Res 12: 663–675
38. Lieberman I, et al (2001) Initial outcome and efficacy of "kyphoplasty" in the treatment painful osteoporotic vertebral compression fractures. Spine 26: 1631–1638
39. Liebschner M, Rosenberg W, Keaveny T (2001) Effects of bone cement volume and distribution on vertebral stiffnesss after vertebroplasty. Spine 26: 1547–1554
40. Lim T, Brebach G, Renner S, Kim W, Kim J, Lee R, Andersson G, An H (2002) Biomechanical evaluation of an injectable calcium phospate cement for vertebroplasty. Spine 27:1297–1302
41. Lukert B (1994) Vertebral compression fractures: how to manage pain, avoid disability. Geriatrics 49:22–26
42. McGraw J, et al (2002) Predictive value of intraosseous venography before percutaneous vertebroplasty. J Vasc Interv Radiol 13:149–153
43. McGraw J, Lippert J, Minkus K, Rami P, Davis T, Budzick R (2002) Prospective evaluation of pain relief in 100 patients undergoing percutaneous vertebroplasty: results and follow-up. J Vasc Interv Radiol 13:883–886

44. McKercher H, Crilly R, Kloseck M (2000) Osteoporosis management in long-term care. Survey of Ontario physicians. Can Fam Physician 46: 2228–2235
45. Melton III L, Thamer M, Ray N, Chan J, Chestnut III C, Einhor T, Johnston C, Raisz L, Silverman S, Siris E (1997) Fractures attributable to osteoporosis: Report from the national osteoporosis foundation. J Bone Miner Res 12:16–23
46. Nakano M, Hirano N, Matsuura K, Watanabe H, Kitagawa H, Ishihara H, Kawaguchi Y (2002) Percutaneous transpedicular vertebroplasty with calcium phosphate cement in the treatment of osteoporotic vertebral compression and burst fractures. J Neurosurg 97:287–293
47. Padovani B, et al (1999) Pulmonary embolism caused by acrylic cement: a rare complication of percutaneous vertebroplasty. AJNR 20:375–377
48. Palussiere (2003) The clinical use of Cortoss synthetic bone void filler in the repair of fractures of the vertebral body. In: Szpalski M, Gunzburg R (eds) Vertebral osteoporotic compression fractures. Lippincott Williams and Wilkins, pp 151–158
49. Patel U, Skingle S, Campbell G, Crisp A, Boyle I (1991) Clinical profile of acute vertebral compression fractures in osteoporosis. Br J Rheumatol 30: 418–421
50. Peh W, Gilula L, Peck D (2002) Percutaneous vertebroplasty for severe osteoporotic vertebral body compression fractures. Radiology 223:121–126
51. Perez-Higueras A, Alvarez L, Rossi R, Quinones D, Al-Assir I (2002) Percutaneous vertebroplasty: long-term clinical and radiologic outcome. Neuroradiology 44:950–954
52. Phillips F, Todd Wetzel F, Lieberman I, Campbell-Hupp M (2002) An in vivo comparison of the potential for extravertebral cement leak after vertebroplasty and kyphoplasty. Spine 27: 2173–2179
53. Ryan P, Blake G, Fogelman I (1992) Fracture thresholds in osteoporosis: implications for hormone replacement treatment. Ann Rheum Dis 51:1063–1065
54. Ryu K, Park C, Kim M, Kang J (2002) Dose-dependent epidural leakage of polymethylmethacrylate after percutaneous vertebroplasty in patients with osteoporotic vertebral compression fractures. J Neurosurg 96:56–61
55. Schlaich C, Minne H, Bruckner T, Wagner G, Gebest H, Grunze M, Ziegler R, Leidig-Bruckner G (1998) Reduced pulmonary function in patients with spinal osteoporotic fractures. Osteoporos Int 8:261–267
56. Schousboe J, DeBold C, Bowles C, Glickstein S, Rubino R (2002) Prevalence of vertebral compression fracture deformity by X-ray absorptiometry of lateral thoracic and lumbar spines in a population referred for bone densitometry. J Clin Densitom 5:239–246
57. Scroop R, et al (2002) Paradoxical cerebral arterial embolization of cement during intraoperative vertebroplasty: case report. AJNR 23:868–870
58. Silverman S (1992) The clinical consequences of vertebral compression fracture. Bone 13:S27–31
59. Sinaki M (1998) Musculoskeletal challenges of osteoporosis. Aging (Milano) 10:249–262
60. Szpalski M, Gunzburg R, Deramond H (2003) Percutaneous injection of Cortoss synthetic bone void filler in the repair of fractures in the vertebral body. In: Szpalski M, Gunzburg R (eds) Vertebral osteoporotic compression fractures. Lippincott Williams and Wilkins, pp 171–177
61. Tsou I, Goh P, Peh W, Goh L, Chee T (2002) Percutaneous vertebroplasty in the management of osteoporotic vertebral compression fractures: initial experience. Ann Acad Med Singapore 31: 15–20
62. Uppin A, et al (2003) Occurrence of new vertebral body fracture after percutaneous vertebroplasty in patients with osteoporosis. Radiology 226:119–124
63. Vasconcelos C, Gailloud P, Beauchamp N, Heck D, Murphy K (2002) Is percutaneous vertebroplasty without pretreatment venograph safe? Evaluation of 205 consecutive procedures. AJNR 23:913–917
64. Verlaan J, van Helden W, Oner F, Verbout A, Dhert W (2002) Balloon vertebroplasty with calcium phosphate cement augmentation for direct restoration of traumatic thoracolumbar vertebral fractures. Spine 27:543–548

REVIEW

Helmut Franck
Bronek M. Boszczyk
Michael Bierschneider
Hans Jaksche

Interdisciplinary approach to balloon kyphoplasty in the treatment of osteoporotic vertebral compression fractures

Abstract Osteoporotic vertebral compression fractures (VCFs) are associated with a series of clinical consequences leading to increased morbidity and even mortality. Early diagnosis and therapeutic intervention is desirable in order to remobilise patients and prevent further bone loss. Not all fractures are, however, sufficiently treatable by conservative measures. Here, vertebroplasty and kyphoplasty may provide immediate pain relief by minimally invasive fracture stabilisation. In cases of acute fractures, kyphoplasty has the potential to reduce kyphosis and restore the normal sagittal alignment of the spine. The complex nature of systemic osteoporosis, coupled with the intricate biomechanics of vertebral fractures, leads to a clinical setting which is ideally treated interdisciplinarily by the rheumatologist and spine surgeon.

Keywords Vertebral compression fracture · Osteoporosis · Kyphoplasty · Vertebroplasty

H. Franck (✉)
Center of Rheumatology,
Hubertusstr. 40 Oberammergau,
82487 Oberammergau, Germany
Tel.: +49-8822-914261,
Fax: +49-8822-914222,
e-mail: hfranck@wz-kliniken.de

B. M. Boszczyk · M. Bierschneider
H. Jaksche
Department of Neurosurgery,
Berufsgenossenschaftliche Unfallklinik
Murnau, Prof. Küntscher Str.8,
D-82418 Murnau, Germany

Introduction

Osteoporotic vertebral compression fractures (VCFs) are the most common type of fracture, followed by hip fractures. The incidence rate is 117 per 100,000 persons per year, but it accounts for 41,000 hospitalizations per year, with an average length of stay of 20 days [7, 10]. The European Commission estimates hospital expenditures in Europe to be greater than 340,000,000 Euro (almost 1,000 Euro per day) [10].

This economic burden [10] is partly the result of progressive kyphosis and chronic pain, often leading to significant morbidity in the elderly individual [19]. Pain can be caused by nociceptors in bone itself, the disc complex, the perivertebral structures, through nerve compression, joint or muscle pain. Although the majority of patients with this injury experience a benign and self-limited course of gradually resolving pain, a significant number continue to experience chronic pain, progressive kyphosis and disability. Long-term consequences include significantly decreased activities of daily living (ADL) amounting to five million limited activity days in the U.S. [28]. As a consequence, patients suffer from an increased dependence on others, sleeping disorders and clinical anxiety, including reduced mobility [13, 32]. Furthermore, VCF symptoms and consequent treatments may include overall inactivity, which leads to further bone loss and potential fracture. Patients treated for sleeping disorders with sedatives are less astute, which puts the patient at risk for falls. Decreased ADL with dependence on others further reduces the necessary activity level and strain on bone for healing processes [23]. Malnutrition from early satiety due to a compressed stomach results in poor calcium intake [32]. Finally, hyperkyphotic patients are at risk of reduced pulmonary function [30].

Diagnosis

VCF diagnosis requires a detailed history and physical examination. Investigations should be aimed at excluding other causes of back pain. In evaluating such a patient, the differential diagnosis must consider not only osteoporosis but also various causes of osteomalacia, endocrinopathy and malignancy. Sometimes further diagnostic tests, including psychology, physiotherapy and various medical specialities, are necessary to substantiate the need for therapeutic intervention. Magnetic resonance imaging is often helpful in excluding other causes of pathologic fracture and in distinguishing fresh from older fractures. For the latter, the STIR (Short Tau Inversion Recovery) imaging technique should be employed, which is very sensitive for osseous edema following a vertebral fracture.

High-risk patients need special attention. Patients with one or more vertebral fractures are five times more likely to have an additional VCF within the next year [22]. Some patients with secondary osteoporosis have multiple risk factors. In patients with rheumatoid arthritis, the inflammatory process itself, the physical inactivity and the necessary treatment with glucocorticoids also enhances the incidence of osteoporosis. These patients show a reduced bone volume and decreased bone turnover, which is further aggravated by microarchitectural deterioration stressing the severe osteoporosis associated with the disease. As a consequence, subjects with rheumatoid arthritis have reduced bone mineral density and at least a twofold increased risk of osteoporotic fractures [25].

Treatment options

An interdisciplinary approach is substantial not only in diagnostic, but also in therapeutic strategies. The aim of treatment of osteoporosis is to halt bone loss, to reduce pain and to prevent the occurrence of future fractures through osteoinduction. Pharmacological treatments for bone loss include the bisphosphonates, hormone replacement therapy, selective oestrogen receptor modulators, calcitonin, the 1–34 fragment of parathyroid hormone, calcium and vitamin D supplements, and calcitriol. Long acting strategies for patients with secondary osteoporosis must include effective treatment of the primary disease. In rheumatoid arthritis, this aims to reduce risk factors by inhibiting inflammatory activities of the disease by avoiding glucocorticoids and applying physical therapy.

However, these medications for osteoporosis alone cannot inhibit or reduce pain instantly or completely. Consequently, a conventional treatment for pain reduction including the WHO recommendations of staged pain treatment is necessary. Drugs for the treatment of pain should be prescribed cautiously if the drugs have side effects on the central nervous system that could potentially lead to falls.

Traditional treatment for these patients includes bed rest, analgesics and bracing, all of which are aimed toward pain management and remobilisation; however, none of these strategies address the immediate treatment of the local mechanical problem associated with the fracture itself. Furthermore, in most cases, early remobilisation is not initiated. Bed rest exasperates further bone loss, therefore increasing the risk of further fractures [14]. Lifestyle changes should also be encouraged in high-risk patients. Physical exercise is necessary, which includes site specific and weight-bearing loading, including muscle resistance. It should be performed two to three times per week, exceeding the normal daily loading with peak forces.

Interventional treatment options

With failure of conservative treatment, operative stabilisation should be considered. As vertebral fractures are biomechanically complex and surgical strategies vary according to the fracture type [24], the evaluation of the patient for surgery is ideally done in an interdisciplinary manner together with a spine surgeon. While taking the underlying medical condition into consideration, the surgeon's main focus is on the character of the fracture. Conventional reconstructive procedures involving implants are generally not a suitable option for this elderly population due to the poor bone quality and the reduced tolerance of operative trauma. Vertebroplasty and kyphoplasty pose minimally invasive alternatives for the direct stabilisation of the fracture. Both techniques may be performed under general or local anaesthesia using CT or biplanar fluoroscopy. The technique of vertebroplasty is well described in the literature [17]. Briefly, a needle (usually a bone biopsy needle) is percutaneously introduced into the affected vertebral body via a transpedicular or extrapedicular approach. Bone cement, polymethylmethacrylate (PMMA), is then injected directly into the vertebral body at moderate to high pressure at low viscosity in order to achieve trabecular filling. The fracture is stabilised once the PMMA is cured. Kyphoplasty employs the same approaches as vertebroplasty; however, working cannulae are bilaterally passed over initially placed guide pins and obturators, which allows inflatable balloons to be placed in the vertebral body (for detailed technique see Garfin et al. [11]). The balloon is slowly inflated under fluoroscopic guidance while carefully monitoring the balloon positioning in relation to the cortices. Once maximum fracture reduction and height restoration are achieved, both balloons are deflated and removed, leaving behind a defined cavity, which is then manually filled under low pressure with highly viscous, radiopaque PMMA cement. The dosage is regulated according to the end volume of the inflated balloon as noted on the inflation syringe. Biomechanically, both procedures are very efficient in restoring vertebral strength, both with regard to ultimate compressive strength [1, 36] and under cyclic loading [35]. As pain relief is similarly efficient for both procedures [11, 17], the choice of technique involves several factors.

Spinal deformity

The sagittal balance of the spine should be taken into account. As suggested by Keller et al. [20] in an example of a vertebral deformity model, kyphotic deformity in excess of 10° at T7 and T8 produces 15.1-cm anterior translation of the cervicothoracic spine with an increase of 19% compressive force and 40% increase in paraspinal extensor muscle force at these levels. While vertebroplasty essentially "freezes" the deformity, kyphoplasty has been found to reduce segmental kyphosis on average by 6–18° [11]. In fresh fractures, reduction reaches an average of 14° [11], with the possibility of near complete height restoration in the acute setting [4]. While vertebroplasty is an efficient stabilisation method when deformity is not of concern, kyphoplasty should be considered for fractures with kyphotic deformity, especially when treating acute fractures.

Fracture type

As vertebral augmentation procedures do not address flexion or rotation instability, the work-up of the patient should involve fracture classification according to Magerl et al. [24] in order to rule out type B and C injuries. When there is a doubt as to the fracture type, MRI should be performed to assess any injury of the discoligamentary structures. In type B or C injuries, posterior instrumentation remains a necessity. The vast majority of spontaneous fractures will be of the A1 type; however, more complex fractures can occur in trauma settings, e.g. from falling down stairs, off a bicycle or in motor vehicle accidents, as may occur infrequently in the more active, younger rheumatoid patients with secondary osteoporosis. Furthermore, assessment of the fracture type involves the fracture morphology of the vertebral body. Depending upon the degree of trabecular bone loss, failure of a severely osteoporotic vertebral body may result in complete collapse without significant fragmentation (type A1.3), while vertebral shattering (incomplete burst type A3.1, split burst type A3.2 and complete burst fracture type A3.3) generally occurs in less osteoporotic vertebra. The former fracture type is more common in the elderly patient with primary osteoporosis and is treatable by kyphoplasty, while the latter more often occurs in the younger patient with secondary osteoporosis in a trauma setting. These fractures must be evaluated carefully, as kyphoplasty in type A3.3 complete burst fractures may result in separation of the fragments rather than cavity formation if the osteoporosis is only mild. Although there is a theoretical risk of bone retropulsion through kyphoplasty in burst fractures, anterior placement of the balloon usually prevents expansion towards the posterior wall during inflation. Incomplete burst fractures of the type A3.1 have been treated successfully [4]. When treating burst fractures, the fissures in the posterior vertebral wall increase the risk of epidural cement leakage for all augmentation procedures, but especially for vertebroplasty due to the injection of PMMA at low viscosity and moderate to high pressure. Here, kyphoplasty increases operative safety, as PMMA is injected at high viscosity and low pressure into the cavity created during balloon inflation. Although minor leakage does not usually result in neurological impairment, several cases of severe neurological deficit and systemic embolism following vertebroplasty have been documented [2, 6, 15, 18, 21, 26, 27, 31, 33].

The potential for serious complications, however rare, require scrutinous intraoperative fluoroscopic monitoring for bone retropulsion or cement leakage and provisions should be made for potential conversion to open surgery and embolism management.

Neurological deficit

Severe vertebral collapse or posterior wall fragmentation, although rare, is able to induce neurological deficit due to nerve root compression. As neural decompression cannot be undertaken percutaneously, surgical decompression is required in addition to vertebral augmentation. Bilateral open decompression with transpedicular vertebroplasty and interlaminar microsurgical kyphoplasty have been described for the treatment of these severe fractures [34, 5].

Uncomplicated percutaneous vertebroplasty can usually be accomplished in approximately 15 min for a single level. For the same indication Kyphoplasty will need an additional 10–15 min. However, in fractures involving significant height loss, kyphotic deformity or fragmentation of the posterior vertebral wall, kyphoplasty should be considered despite the slightly prolonged operation time due to the potential for fracture reduction and lower cement leakage rate. Although the overall rate of serious complications is very low (under 2% in the kyphoplasty review by Garfin et al. [12]), precautions should be taken for the possibility of surgical decompression of the spinal canal, additional instrumentation and management of pulmonary embolism.

Post-operative management

Once the bone cement is cured, patients may be mobilised with full weight bearing. Application of an orthosis is not routinely recommended. While patients appear to benefit from this procedure, Kyphoplasty alone has not been shown to prevent further vertebral fractures. Hence, it is of utmost importance to inhibit the vetebral fracture rate in these patients. Pharmocotherapy should be continued for 2–3 years at least. Alendronat 10 mg/day or 70 mg/week [3], Raloxifen 60 mg/day [9] and Risedronat 5 mg/day [16] or 35 mg/week orally have been proven to reduce the fracture rate in patients with prevalent fractures. Calcium 500 mg and Vitamin D 400–800 IE should be taken daily. These medications have been shown to have an evidence based medicine grade A. If these drugs are not tolerated well, other medical treatments are recommended. This includes calcitonine spray, etidronate intermittently, estrogene/gestagene, fluoride or active vitamin D metabolites. Lifestyle changes should also be continued as described, with physiotherapy going ahead. Patients should be monitored every 3–6 months.

Discussion

Osteoporotic VCFs present a significant economic burden to society and result in severe clinical consequences leading to impaired physical function, reduced pulmonary function and overall increase in mortality. Traditional medical options, including bed rest, analgesics and bracing, have proven to be insufficient. Furthermore, the problem of osteoporosis is underestimated and often not diagnosed [10]. Therefore, an interdisciplinary approach that addresses both the underlying disease and the local mechanical problem of the fracture itself is recommended.

Geriatric patients treated with kyphoplasty in combination with pharmacologic and physical therapy quickly return to higher activity levels, leading to increased independence and quality of life. However, while the principle is innovative, the procedure deserves further investigation as a potentially effective means of correcting loss of vertebral height. Further light will be shed on the efficacy of this procedure by a recently initiated randomised multicentre study comparing conservative and operative treatment. A remaining matter of debate is the number of levels that should be treated and whether to prophylactically include unfractured levels between vertebrae that need stabilisation. As yet, the clinical and biomechanical literature is inconclusive on this topic. As patients with preexisting osteoporotic fractures have been shown to have a highly increased risk of developing new fractures (factor 7 with two fractures, factor 17 with multiple fractures) [29], especially of the thoracolumbar junction [8], augmentation of vertebrae adjacent to fractures in this high-risk zone should be considered on an individual basis. Further interdisciplinary investigations conducted by rheumatologists and surgeons are needed to determine the ideal treatment strategy for these patients.

References

1. Belkoff SM, Mathis JM, Fenton DC, Scribner RM, Reiley ME, Talmadge K (2001) An ex vivo biomechanical evaluation of an inflatable bone tamp used in the treatment of compression fracture. Spine 26:151–156
2. Bernhard J, Heini PF, Villiger PM (2003) Asymptomatic diffuse pulmonary embolism caused by acrylic cement: an unusual complication of percutaneous vertebroplasty. Ann Rheum Dis 62:85–86
3. Black DM, Thompson DE (1999) The effect of alendronate therapy on osteoporotic fracture in the vertebral fracture arm of the Fracture Intervention Trial. Int J Clin Pract Suppl 101:46–50
4. Boszczyk B, Bierschneider M, Potulski M, Robert B, Vastmans J, Jaksche H (2002) Erweitertes Anwendungsspektrum der Kyphoplastie zur Stabilisierung der osteoporotischen Wirbelfraktur. Unfallchirurg 105:952–957
5. Boszczyk BM, Bierschneider M, Robert B, Jaksche H (2003) Treatment of severe osteoporotic fractures through a microsurgical interlaminary approach. In: Szpalski M, Gunzburg R (eds) Vertebral osteoporotic compression fractures. Lippincott WW, Philadelphia, pp 179–188
6. Chen HL, Wong CS, Ho ST, Chang FL, Hsu CH, Wu CT (2002) A lethal pulmonary embolism during percutaneous vertebroplasty. Anesth Analg 95:1060–1062
7. Cooper C, Atkinson EJ, O'Fallon WM, Melton LJ III (1992) Incidence of clinically diagnosed vertebral fractures: a population-based study in Rochester, MN (1985–1989). J Bone Miner Res 7:221–227
8. Davis JW, Grove JS, Wasnich RD, Ross PD (1999) Spatial relationships between prevalent and incident spine fractures. Bone 24:261–264
9. Ettinger B, Black DM, Mitlak BH, Knickerbocker RK, Nickelsen T, Genant HK, Christiansen C, Delmas PD, Zanchetta JR, Stakkestad J, Gluer CC, Krueger K, Cohen FJ, Eckert S, Ensrud KE, Avioli LV, Lips P, Cummings (1999) Reduction of vertebral fracture risk in postmenopausal women with osteoporosis treated with raloxifene: results from a 3-year randomized clinical trial. Multiple Outcomes of Raloxifene Evaluation (MORE) Investigators. JAMA 282(7):637–645
10. European Commission (1998) Report on osteoporosis in the European Community, action for prevention.
11. Garfin SR, Hansen AY, Reiley MA (2001) Kyphoplasty and vertebroplasty for the treatment of painful osteoporotic compression fractures. Spine 26:1511–1515
12. Garfin SR, Lin G, Lieberman I, Phillips F, Truumees E (2001) Retrospective analysis of the outcomes of balloon kyphoplasty to treat vertebral body compression fracture refractory to medical management (Abstract). Eur Spine J 10: S7–S8
13. Gold DT (1996) The clinical impact of vertebral body fractures: quality of life in women with osteoporosis. Bone 3: S185–S189
14. Hansson T, Roos B, Naghemson A (1975) Development of osteopenia in the fourth lumbar vertebra during prolonged bed rest after operation for scoliosis. Acta Orthop Scand 46:621–30
15. Harrington KD (2001) Major neurological complications following percutaneous vertebroplasty with polymethylmethacrylate. J Bone Joint Surg 84-A: 1070–1073

16. Harris ST, Watts NB, Genant HK, McKeever CD, Hangartner T, Keller M, Chesnut CH 3rd, Brown J, Eriksen EF, Hoseyni MS, Axelrod DW, Miller PD (1999) Effects of risedronate treatment on vertebral and nonvertebral fractures in women with postmenopausal osteoporosis: a randomized controlled trial. Vertebral Efficacy With Risedronate Therapy (VERT) Study Group. JAMA 282(14):1344–1352
17. Heini PF, Wälchli B, Berlemann U (2000) Percutaneous transpedicular vertebroplasty with PMMA: operative technique and early results. Eur Spine J 9:445–450
18. Jang JS, Lee SH, Jung SK (2002) Pulmonary embolism of polymethylmethacrylate after percutaneous vertebroplasty. Spine 27: E416–E418
19. Kanis JA, Brazier JE, Stevenson M, Calvert NW, Lloyd Jones M (2002) Treatment of established osteoporosis: a systematic review and cost-utility analysis. Health Technol Assess 6(29): 1–146
20. Keller TS, Kosmopoulos V, Liebschner MA (2003) Modeling of bone damage and fracture in osteoporosis. In: Szpalski M, Gunzburg R (eds) Vertebral osteoporotic compression fractures. Lippincott WW, Philadelphia, pp 35–50
21. Lee BJ, Lee SR, Yoo TY (2002) Paraplegia as a complication of percutaneous vertebroplasty with polymethylmethacrylate. Spine 27: E419–E422
22. Lindsay R, Silverman SL, Cooper C, Hanley DA, Barton I, Broy SB, Licata A, Benhamou L, Geusens P, Flowers K, Stracke H, Seeman E (2001) Risk of new vertebral fracture in the year following a fracture. JAMA 285:320–323
23. Lyles KW, Gold DT, Shipp KM, Pieper CF, Martinez S, Mulhausen PL (1993) Association of osteoporotic vertebral body compression fractures with impaired functional status. Am J Med 94:595–601
24. Magerl F, Aebi M, Gertzbein SD, Harms J, Nazarian S (1994) A comprehensive classification of thoracic and lumbar injuries. Eur Spine J 3:184–201
25. Michel BA, Bloch DA, Wolfe F, Fries JF (1993) Fractures in rheumatoid arthritis: an evaluation of associated risk factors. J Rheumatol 10:1666–1669
26. Padovani B, Kasriel O, Brunner P, Peretti-Viton P (1999) Pulmonary embolism caused by acrylic cement: a rare complication of percutaneous vertebroplasty. Am J Neuroradiol 20:375–377
27. Ratliff J, Nguyen T, Heiss J (2001) Root and spinal cord compression from methylmethacrylate vertebroplasty. Spine 26:E300–E302
28. Riggs BL, Melton LJ III (1995) The worldwide problem of osteoporosis: insights afforded by epidemiology. Bone 5: S505–S511
29. Ross PD, Genant HK, Davis JW, Miller PD, Wasnich RD (1993) Predicting vertebral fracture incidence from prevalent fractures and bone density among none-black, osteoporotic women. Osteoporosis Int 3:120–126
30. Schlaich C, Minne HW, Bruckner T, Wagner G, Gebest HJ, Grunze M, Ziegler R, Leidig-Bruckner G (1998) Reduced pulmonary function in patients with spinal osteoporotic fractures. Osteoporosis Int 8:261–267
31. Scroop R, Eskridge J, Britz GW (2002) Paradoxical cerebral embolization of cement during intraoperative vertebroplasty: case report. Am J Neuroradiol 23:868–870
32. Silverman SL (1992) The clinical consequences of vertebral compression fractures. Bone 13: S27–S31
33. Tozzi P, Abdelmoumene Y, Corno AF, Gersbach PA, Hoogewoud HM, von Segesser LK (2002) Management of pulmonary embolism during acrylic vertebroplasty. Ann Thorac Surg 74: 1706–1708
34. Wenger W, Markwalder TM (1999) Surgically controlled, transpedicular methyl methacrylate vertebroplasty with flouroscopic guidance. Acta Neurochir 141:625–631
35. Wilke HJ, Mehnert U, Boszczyk B, Bierschneider M, Jaksche H, Claes LE (2002) Biomechanical evaluation of vertebro- and kyphoplasty under cyclic loading (Abstract). Eur Spine J 11:613
36. Wilson DR, Myers ER, Mathis JM, Scribner RM, Conta JA, Reiley MA, Talmadge KD, Hayes WC (2002) Effect of augmentation on the mechanics of vertebral wedge fractures. Spine 25: 158–165

Olof Johnell

Economic implication of osteoporotic spine disease: cost to society

Financial support was obtained from the Swedish Research Council (project no. K2003–73X-11610–08A), Greta and Johan Kock Foundation, and Albert Påhlsson Foundation

O. Johnell (✉)
Department of Orthopaedics, Malmö University Hospital, 205 02 Malmö, Sweden
Tel.: +46-40-332452,
Fax: +46-40-336227,
e-mail: olof.johnell@orto.mas.lu.se

Abstract The costs of vertebral fractures are less well defined than the costs of hip fractures. Large studies are urgently needed. From the data that exist, vertebral fractures have a higher cost than previously expected: for hospitalized fractures in a US study, USD 10 000 per year without rehabilitation costs, for all clinical fractures USD 2000 the first year, and in a Swedish study slightly more. These new data on the cost of vertebral fractures will have an impact on health economy calculations. In the future it may be be cost-effective only to prevent vertebral fractures.

Keywords Vertebral fractures · Spine fractures · Cost · Osteoporosis · Health economy

Vertebral fractures are one of the most important consequences of osteoporosis. Vertebral fractures can be divided into those detected radiologically in large populations and those that come to clinical attention. For the fractures detected in population surveys, the annual incidence at 65 years of age in the EPOS study is approximately 1% per year for women and 0.6% per year for men [2]. The figures for clinical fractures are roughly one-third of this, and a third of these are hospitalized. The reason for the difference is partly differences in pain, but also differences in attitudes in hospitals and by the patients, in that doctors sometimes do not take an X-ray of a woman over 50 years of age, if X-rays are taken some of them are misinterpreted [4], and the patients have learnt that very little can be done. To detect all vertebral fractures, we must have a campaign for the doctors to take more X-rays and for the patients to realize that we can do something about these fractures. Apart from the fact that they are common, they also reduce quality of life, as has been shown both for radiological vertebral fractures and for vertebral fractures that come to clinical attention [7]. This will of course have implications, in that the fractures will be costly.

There are numerous, well-performed studies on the cost of hip fractures. However, there are fewer studies on the cost of vertebral fractures.

Radiologically detected vertebral fractures in the population

The most cited study is from Rotterdam [1], which studied the additional cost of medical care (the incremental cost) caused by incident hip and vertebral fractures using a matched case–control design for the longitudinal follow-up. The incident vertebral fractures were recorded by morphometric comparison of spinal radiographs taken at an average interval of 2.2 years. The matched controls were randomly selected from other participants after the Rotterdam study. The cost for a vertebral fracture was USD 1000 per year. However, almost half of this difference was already present in patients before occurrence of the fracture. Thus, this incremental cost for radiographically detected vertebral fracture was approximately USD 500 per year [1].

Vertebral fractures which come to clinical attention

The cost of these fractures – i.e., those for which the patient visits a doctor because of pain – can be divided into those that lead to hospitalization and all clinical fractures.

Hospitalized vertebral fractures

Gehlbach et al. [5] studied the resource implications of hospitalization for osteoporosis-related vertebral fractures. They used data from national samples of patients with hospitalized fractures, mainly from discharge databases. Patients with metastatic cancer or severe trauma were excluded. The total charges averaged USD 8000–10 000 per hospitalization and were higher in men. The length of stay was just under 6 days, and more than 50% of discharged patients required some form of continuing care, indicating that the overall cost is much higher than just the hospitalization. These costs were gathered from a US database where vertebral fracture accounted for over 400 000 total hospital days and generated charges in excess of USD 500 million. In total, vertebral fractures were responsible for almost 70 000 annual hospitalizations, about one-fourth of the number due to hip fractures, and it was found that the average total charge for vertebral fracture hospitalization was about half of that of hospitalization due to hip fracture. However, the average length of stay was shorter for vertebral fracture than for hip fracture.

In a study from Europe the hospital cost of vertebral fractures was estimated using national data sets [3]. In that study there was a marked difference in length of stay, ranging from 0.3 days in Austria to 20.2 days in Spain. The total cost of vertebral fractures in the European Union was estimated at € 377 million per year, and across the European Union the hospital cost of vertebral fractures was on average 63% that of a hip fracture. The cost estimate was done using the average cost per day in hospital in the various countries. The hospitalization rate for vertebral fracture was estimated at 8%.

All clinical fractures

A pilot study for all vertebral fractures coming to clinical attention has been done in Sweden, where patients were followed prospectively for 1 year in order to assess the reduction in quality of life and also the costs [7]. The study included hip fractures, clinical vertebral fractures, wrist fractures, and shoulder fractures. At baseline there were only 42 vertebral fractures. The quality of life reduction was similar to that with hip fractures. The cost did not include all nursing home costs and therefore the total cost will be higher. The total costs for this small group of vertebral fractures were: direct costs SEK 30 000, and indirect costs SEK 31 000, i.e., an annual total cost of SEK 61 000. On the basis of this pilot study a large study has been started.

In a recent study from the Mayo clinic [6], the incremental cost in a case–control series was calculated for osteoporotic fractures. In this study, too, nursing home patients were not included. For 283 vertebral fractures, the incremental cost in the case–control study was almost USD 2000 per year.

Thus, the estimates of cost to society are only preliminary. The definitive data for vertebral fractures are still being acquired. It may be concluded that radiological fractures have an increased incremental cost of USD 500 per year. For hospitalized fractures, the cost is higher than expected – in a US study, up to USD 10 000 during the first year – and, surprisingly, this is roughly half the cost of a hip fracture. The rehabilitation cost is not included in this. In a European study it was also noted that the hospitalization cost of vertebral fractures was more than 50% of the average cost of a hip fracture, and that the total yearly cost of hospitalized vertebral fractures in the European Union was estimated at € 377 million per year. It is more difficult to estimate the total cost of all clinical vertebral fractures. A pilot study has shown a rather high amount in Sweden, with direct costs of SEK 30000 and indirect costs that are almost as high. A new large study has been started to verify this in a larger population. In a US study the incremental cost was USD 2000 per fracture per year. All this indicates that the cost of vertebral fractures has been underestimated; it is high, and is substantial even in compraison to hip fractures.

These new data showing a higher cost than expected, and also a greater loss of quality of life then previously calculated, will have an impact on health economy calculations. In the future, prevention of only vertebral fractures might be cost-effective on the basis of these data.

References

1. De Laet C, van Hout B, Burger H, Weel A, Hofman A, Pols H (1999) Incremental cost of medical care after hip fracture and first vertebral fracture: the Rotterdam study. Osteoporos Int 10:66–72
2. European Prospective Osteoporosis Study Working Group (2002) Incidence of vertebral fracture in Europe: results from the European Prospective Osteoporosis Study (EPOS). J Bone Miner Res 17:716–724
3. Finnern HW, Sykes DP (2003) The hospital cost of vertebral fractures in the EU: estimates using national datasets. Osteoporos Int 14:429-436 (electronic publication ahead of print)
4. Gehlbach SH, Bigelow C, Heimisdottir M, May S, Walker M, Kirkwood JR (2000) Recognition of vertebral fracture in a clinical setting. Osteoporos Int 11: 577–582
5. Gehlbach SH, Burge RT, Puleo E, Klar J (2003) Hospital care of osteoporosis-related vertebral fractures. Osteoporos Int 14:53–60
6. Melton III LJ, Gabriel SE, Crowson CS, Tosteson ANA, Johnell O, Kanis JA (2003) Cost-equivalence of different osteoporotic fractures. Osteoporos Int 14: 383–388 (electronic publication ahead of print)
7. Zethraeus N, Borgström F, Johnell O, Kanis J, Önnby K, Jönsson B. (2002) Costs and quality of life associated with osteoporosis related fractures – results from a Swedish survey. SSE/EFI Working Paper Series in Economics and Finance, no 512. http://swopec.hhs.se/hastef/abs/hastef0512.htm

Marek Szpalski
Robert Gunzburg

Lumbar spinal stenosis in the elderly: an overview

Abstract Lumbar spinal stenosis is a common condition in elderly patients and also one of the most common reasons to perform spinal surgery at an advanced age. Disc degeneration, facet degeneration and hypertrophy, and ligamentum flavum hypertrophy and calcification usually participate in the genesis of a stenotic condition in the elderly. These changes can lead to symptoms by themselves or decompensate a preexisting narrow canal. Although some lesions are more central or more lateral, this classic dichotomy is less present in the elderly patient, in whom the degenerative process usually encroaches both central and lateral pathways. Some less common causes of lumbar spinal stenosis are found in the aging subject, such as Paget's disease. However, it must be stressed that so-called stenotic images (sometimes severe) are present on imaging studies in a great number of symptom-free individuals, and that the relationship between degenerative lesions, importance of abnormal images, and complaints is still unclear. Lumbar stenosis is a very common reason for decompressive surgery and/or fusion. Various conditions can lead to a narrowing of the neural pathways and differential diagnosis with vascular troubles, also common in the elderly, can be challenging. The investigation of stenotic symptoms should be extremely careful and thorough and include a choice of technical examinations including vascular investigations. This is of utmost importance, especially if a surgical sanction is considered to avoid disappointing results.

Keywords Lumbar spinal stenosis · Elderly · Paget's disease

M. Szpalski (✉)
Department of Orthopedics,
Hôpitaux Iris Sud–Molière Longchamp,
142 rue Marconi, 1190 Brussels, Belgium
Fax: +32-2-3446606,
e-mail: mszp@win.be

R. Gunzburg
Department of Orthopedics,
Eeuwfeestkliniek,
Harmoniestraat 68, 2018 Antwerp,
Belgium

Introduction

Although stenosis and claudication were described as early as 1883 [14], the modern description of this pathology was performed by Verbiest [32] in the 1950s. Lumbar spinal stenosis is a common condition in elderly patients and also one of the most common reasons to perform spinal surgery at an advanced age [31]. Spinal stenosis leading to radiculopathy or neurogenic claudication can be caused by various factors, of which a number are related to degenerative processes. The real participation of so-called congenital stenosis is still subject of debate. Global degenerative changes in the osteoarticular system associated with aging causes similar lesions throughout the body. However, degeneration in the spine has some very specific characteristics. The three-joint nature of the functional unit and the intimate contact with neural structures as well as the existence of a large avascular structure (the intervertebral disc) account for this specificity. Degenerative disc disease is by far the most common cause of lumbar spinal stenosis. A bulging degenerated intervertebral disc anteriorly, combined with thickened infolding of ligamenta flava and hypertrophy of the facet joints posteriorly result in narrowing of the spinal canal. The site of compression may be central, lateral, or a combination of the two [36].

Also specific to spinal degeneration is the fact that although all elderly subjects do not present with osteoarthritis of peripheral joints such as hips or knees, nearly all exhibit radiological images of degeneration on spine imaging, as well in symptomatic than in symptom-free patients [3]. The latter observation is interesting, as most patients with severe osteoarthritis of knee or hip present complaints, but many with severe images of degeneration are symptom free [3]. Furthermore, abnormal images on magnetic resonance imaging (MRI) do not predict in any way the occurrence of spine-related complaints 7 years later [4]. Autopsy studies on large number of subjects have found disc degeneration, facet joints osteoarthritis, or osteophytes in 90–100% of subjects aged over 64 years [19, 34]. Identification of stenotic images in the middle and exit zones of the foramen have been made possible by MRI studies, and stenosis has been found in up to 80% of subjects aged over 70 years [25]. Furthermore, a poor correlation between radiological stenosis and symptoms has been reported [10]. This means that in many cases spinal degeneration cannot really be considered as a disease, and that the relationship between complaints and radiological changes must be very cautious.

As for many continuous characteristics, both canal size and dural sac size present a Gaussian distribution. When a canal size is too narrow for the dural sac size that it contains, stenosis occurs. An identical canal size can therefore be stenotic for one person but not for another who happens to have a smaller dural sac size. Lumbar spinal stenosis is therefore a clinical condition and not a radiological finding or diagnosis. In addition, a poor correlation between radiological stenosis and symptoms has been reported [11]. It must be stressed that stenosis is not a pathological entity per se as up to 21% of nonsymptomatic subjects over the age of 60 years demonstrate stenotic images on MRI [3]. This means that the size of the canal is only one component in the pathogenesis of symptomatic stenosis. Lumbar spinal stenosis refers to a pathological condition causing a compression of the contents of the canal, particularly the neural and vascular structures. If compression does not occur, the canal should be described as narrow but not stenotic [24]. The functional status of the spine has also been studied in relation to stenosis and the worsening of symptoms in extended position. It has been shown that subjects with degenerative changes inducing a borderline canal diameter but without complaints have abnormal patterns of motion in sagittal extension recalling those in stenotic patients [30]. This suggests a sort of proprioceptive protective behavior in the case of potentially stenotic movements.

Some definitions need to be clarified. The classic symptom characterizing spinal stenosis is neurogenic claudication. The pathophysiology of this phenomenon is not entirely understood. However, Porter [22] and Porter and Ward [23] have proposed an elegant theory. In this explanation claudication is caused by the venous pooling induced by the stenotic impairment of venous drainage at root level and occurs only if stenosis (central and/or lateral) is present at two adjacent levels. This situation is, however, not the rule and most stenotic patients do not present with true neurogenic claudication. In this review we consider as stenotic as stenosis all situations in which radiculopathy and/or claudication is present and compression of the dural sac and/or roots is found on imaging studies (with the exclusions of herniated discs, soft arthrosynovial cysts and tumors).

The participation of "congenital" stenosis to the later development of symptoms is controversial. It seems that, excluding the true severe achondroplasia and some other rare congenital conditions, the so-called congenital narrow canals are merely the extreme of the Gaussian distribution of normal subjects as described above. This is further stressed by the fact that these subjects rarely have any troubles unless they develop degenerative changes. The concomitant presence of degenerative changes appears to be a prerequisite to the development of symptomatic spinal stenosis [16]. Classically, central stenosis and lateral stenosis have been described as distinct entities. However, it appears that in the elderly with marked degenerative changes central and lateral lesions are linked in the genesis of complaints. These complaints linked to stenosis are sciatic pain due to the direct compression of neural structures and neurogenic claudication. The exact etiopathogenesis of the latter is still under debate, but the theory presented by Porter and Ward [22, 23] appears to explain (almost) the nature of this symptom. In elderly patients the differential diagnosis with claudication of vascular origin is of the utmost importance to find the adequate treatment and avoid useless surgical procedures.

Differential diagnosis

In elderly persons many concurrent pathologies are often present. Among these, vascular disorders can be a challenge in the differential diagnosis in both acute and chronic presentations of spinal stenosis. Among the acute conditions able to mimic a cauda equina syndrome are ruptured abdominal aortic or iliac aneurysms, acute aortic dissection, acute leg ischemia, and deep venous thrombosis. In the more frequent case of chronic conditions it is arterial insufficiency causing intermittent ischemia that most resembles neurogenic troubles. Presentation of intermittent leg pain and discomfort, usually during walking, shows, sometimes subtle, differences between the two pathologies. In both claudications walking becomes impossible but only in neurogenic is stooping or sitting necessary to alleviate the symptoms. Likewise, claudication appears in both cases during a walking test whereas cycling is interfered only by arterial problems. With advanced neurogenic claudication descending stairs becomes impossible obliging patients to walk downstairs backwards to adopt a forward flexed position, going upstairs is usually without problems, in contrast to arterial pathologies which all stair walking difficult.

Arterial claudication involves the posterior leg muscles only, sometimes the buttocks, perhaps the thighs, always the calf, but never the anterior muscles and the groin. Intermittent numbness (hypesthesia) in the sole of the foot may occur after exercise. This should not be confused with paresthesia (pins and needles). It is most likely to be confused with S1 root suffering [9]. In neurogenic claudication elements other than the leg pain are often present: sensory-motor disturbances and low back pain. The diagnosis is to be oriented by history (smoking, previous arterial disease, cold feet, previous lumbar problems, postural and occupation pain factors, walking stairs) and by a complete examination including appropriate orthopedic, neurological, and vascular tests. Given the age group involved, both pathologies may be present in the same patient. In these cases the differential diagnosis, especially if surgery is foreseen, may be a headache. Vascular and stenotic problems are maybe more frequently intercorrelated than generally assumed, and we advocate a basic vascular investigation prior to spinal stenosis surgery [8]. In diabetic patients it may be difficult to differentiate between lumbar stenosis and diabetic polyneuropathy as the latter is also common in older individuals. Electrophysiological investigations help to distinguish between these two pathologies although they are appear to be of more limited utility in the investigation of neurogenic claudication [1].

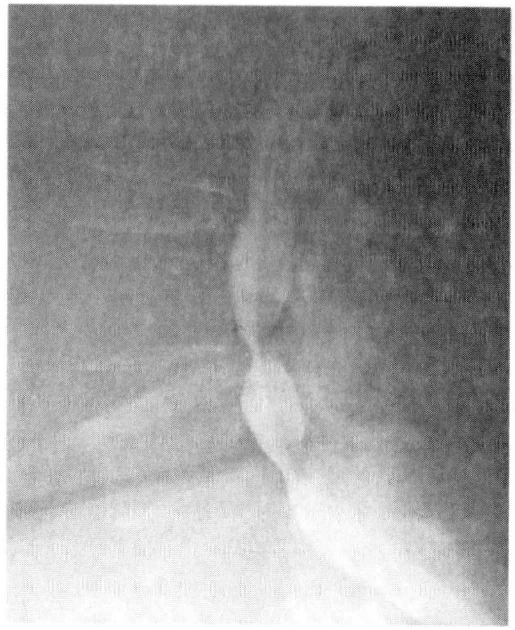

Fig. 1 Myelogram showing multilevel central degenerative stenosis. Myelography remains the only widely available examination enabling dynamic and upright assessment

Central stenosis

Central stenosis in the elderly is the result of a combination of factors. Disc degeneration and collapse of the disc results in a uniform bulging of the posterior annulus, which encroaches the neural canal surface. In some cases symptoms are present only in sagittal extension as a borderline stenosis may appear only in this position [30]. Dynamic assessment techniques are welcome in those cases (Fig. 1). Also as a result of disc collapse a secondary zygapophyseal arthrosis with facet hypertrophy occurs, further diminishing the central canal at the intervertebral level. Degenerated facet joint, when showing medial hypertrophic changes, may also participate in the canal stenosis (Fig. 2).

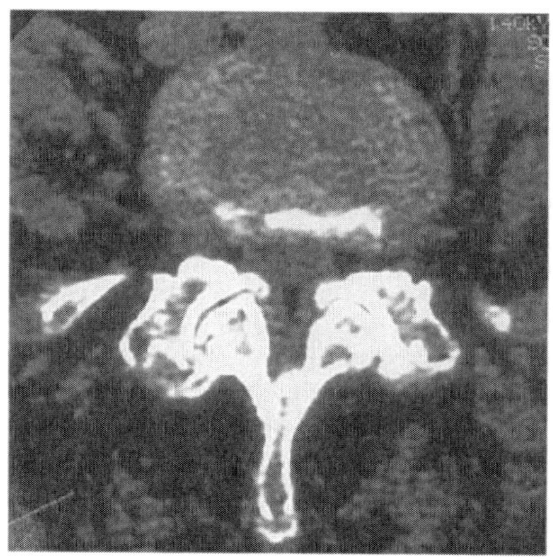

Fig. 2 Degenerative hypertrophy of joints narrowing central canal

Due to this disc collapse and decrease in intervertebral height the often thickened ligamentum flavum [27] may buckle [24], thus further decreasing canal space at the disc level. Furthermore, fibrotic chondrometaplasic changes and even ossification of the ligamentum flavum may also occur [20, 24, 28, 29]. This reduces the elasticity of the ligamentum, which may then bulge in the canal even if it keeps a normal thickness [24]. Several studies have shown a higher frequency of calcification of ligamentum flavum in stenotic than nonstenotic subjects [28]. The extent of these histological changes appears to be correlated with age [28]. It must, however, be stressed that in the elderly central and lateral lesions very often both participate in the stenostic pathology (Fig. 3).

Lateral or root canal stenosis

Lateral stenosis is defined as an entity in which a nerve root, dorsal root ganglion, or spinal nerve is entrapped in its pathway. In the case of degenerative changes the nerve

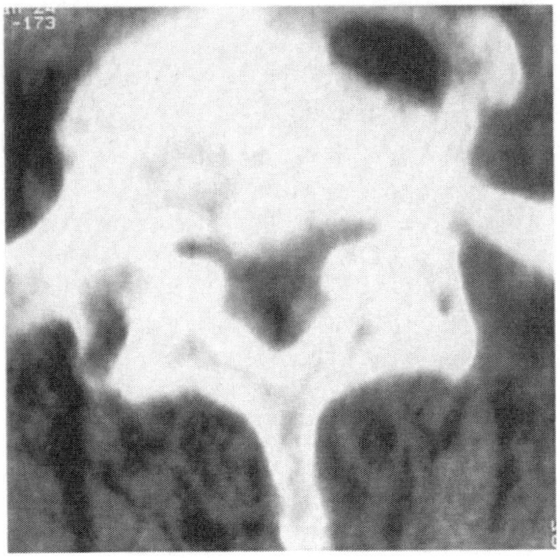

Fig. 3 Trefoil-shaped canal typical of combined central and lateral stenotic conditions

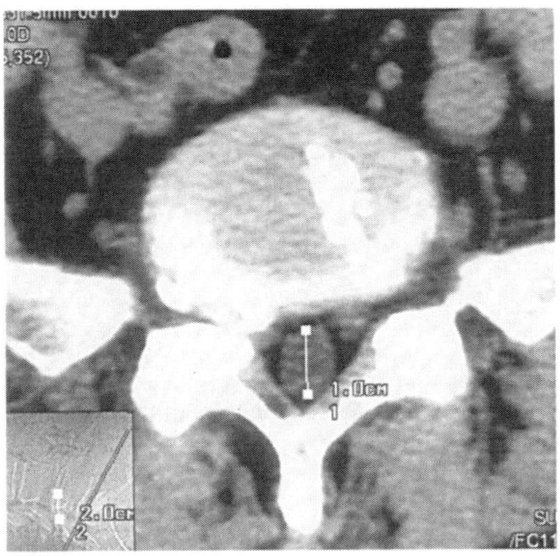

Fig. 4 Lateral stenosis with intraforaminal osteophyte causing nerve entrapment

root can be subject to compression secondary to the disc collapse by approximation of the pedicles due to the decrease in disc height. Furthermore, hypertrophy of the facet joint or other osteophytic changes can compress the root at its entrance in the foramen or in the foramen itself (Fig. 4). Whereas anteriorly McNab spurs (traction osteophytes at the insertion level of Sharpey fibers) are the rule in spondylosis, they seldom occur posteriorly. However, when present they participate in the narrowing the both the central and the lateral canal. Other osteophytes can be found such as those resulting from the calcification of an arthrosynovial cyst (Fig. 5). It appears that degenerative lesions are also often present in the middle zone or exit zone of the L4–L5 and L5–S1 foraminal pathways [25].

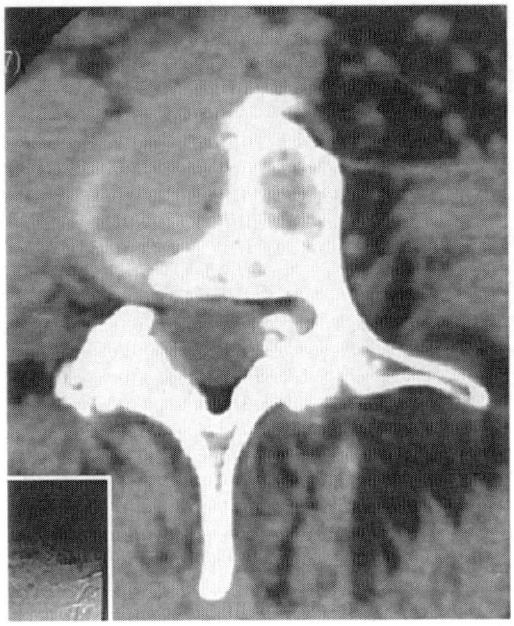

Fig. 5 Calcified arthrosynovial cyst causing root entrapment

Degenerative spondylolisthesis

Degenerative spondylolisthesis, described by McNab [18] as "spondylolisthesis with an intact neural arch," are most frequent at the L4–L5 level and may result in a stenotic condition. The term degenerative spondylolisthesis was coined by Newman [21]. The displacement due to facet hypertrophy can critically narrow the canal. In contrast to isthmic spondylolisthesis, degenerative spondylolisthesis is self-contained and rarely reaches grade II. Claudication, or much more often sciatic pain, are the encountered symptoms in stenosis secondary to degenerative spondylolisthesis. This is related to the fact that degenerative spondylolisthesis is usually at one level, and the two level pathogenesis described by Porter is not reached. Central stenosis is rare in lytic spondylolisthesis but in some cases of L5–S1 displacement the posterior element can be pulled forward against the body of S1, thus compressing the corda [35]. More often the loss of height of the disc induces a posterior bulging, which can trap the nerve root ion the foramen resulting in lateral stenosis. The osteofibrous callus present at the isthmic fracture level can exceptionally become hypertrophic (Gill's nodules) [7] and compress the neural canal. Although those conditions are usually discovered in younger patients, they are occasionally be a problem in the elderly.

Other conditions

Other conditions in the elderly can cause spinal stenosis. Neurological complications are common in Paget's dis-

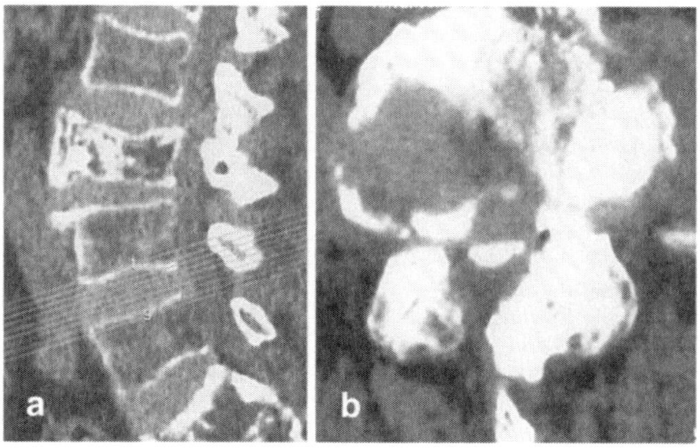

Fig. 6 **a** Lateral view of an enlarged Pagetic vertebra causing global stenosis. **b** Axial view

ease as the spine is one of the most common sites affected by the disease. The lumbar spine is involved in 50% of cases [12]. Enlargement of the vertebral body is common (Fig. 6), and this flattened body can compromise the integrity of the intervertebral foramina, interfere with the blood supply to the dura and nerve roots, or lead to spinal stenosis [26]. A single vertebra is usually involved; however, the frequency of neurological complications are rare compared with the high frequency of lumbar spine involvement in Paget's disease of bone. The vast majority of patients suffering of spinal Paget have no symptoms, yet when symptomatic, it is not necessarily at the level of Pagetic involvement. The Pagetic vertebra may favor disc prolapse, which in itself can cause nerve root entrapment. The increased vascularity of the Pagetic vertebrae may diminish the spinal cord or the nerve root blood supply, ultimately leading to a spinal artery steal syndrome [5]. The Pagetic process can involve the neural arches further reducing the diameter of the central or lateral canal.

Some cases of amyloidosis, associated with prolonged hemodialysis or amyloid tumors, and causing spinal stenosis or even cauda equina syndrome have been reported [15]. However, amyloid deposit in the ligamentum flavum have been reported in series of patients with spinal stenosis who did not present the amyloidosis conditions described higher. The presence and the abundance of those deposits are closely correlated to age [6]. The meaning of these deposits in the context of stenosis is, however, unclear. Rare cases of epidural gas leaks originating from the degenerative intradiscal space may cause compressive phenomena [13].

Iatrogenic stenosis

Iatrogenic stenoses are of course not specific to the elderly. They can happen after spinal surgery at any age (Fig. 7). However, some spinal disorders specific to the elderly are often treated in very aggressive way, and the generous use of instrumentation (or even abuse of it) may cause stenotic situations. One of these conditions is degenerative deformity, usually scoliosis.

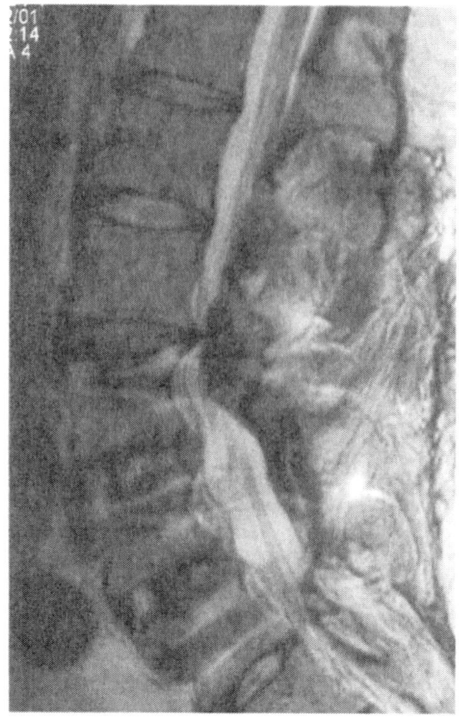

Fig. 7 Central stenosis above a fusion site. Fusion was performed with pedicular screws

Relationship of stenosis and heavy manual work

The relationship in elderly persons between back troubles and occupation is the subject of much discussion. Some authors have suggested a relationship between long-term heavy manual work and spinal stenosis [2]. Using ultrasound measurements McDonald et al. [17] showed that a narrower spinal canal is associated with increased back-related complaints in coal miners. There are conflicting reports about the relationship of long-term heavy physical labor and/or exposure to vibration and the appearance of spinal degeneration (disc degeneration and osteophytes). In very complete review Videman and Battié [33] found only a modest relation of occupational risk factors and spinal degeneration.

Conclusion

Lumbar spinal stenosis is a very common condition in the elderly. In most cases it is due to degenerative changes, the changes can lead to symptoms by themselves or decompensate a preexisting narrow canal. However, it must be stressed that so-called stenotic images (sometimes severe) are present on imaging studies in a great number of symptom-free individuals, and that the relationship between degenerative lesions, importance of abnormal images, and complaints is still unclear. Lumbar stenosis is also a very common reason for decompressive surgery and/or fusion. Various conditions can lead to a narrowing of the neural pathways and differential diagnosis with vascular troubles, also common in the elderly, can be challenging. The investigation of stenotic symptoms should be extremely careful and thorough and include a choice of technical examinations including vascular investigations. This is of utmost importance, especially if a surgical sanction is considered to avoid disappointing results.

References

1. Adamova B, Vohanka S, Dusek L (2003) Differential diagnosis in patients with mild lumbar spinal stenosis: the contributions and limits of various tests. Eur Spine J 12:190–196
2. Berney J (1994) Epidemiology of narrow spinal canal. Neurochirurgie 40: 174–178
3. Boden S, Davies DO, Dina TS et al (1990) Abnormal magnetic resonance scans of the lumbar spine in asymptomatic subjects. A positive investigation. J Bone Joint Surg Am 72:403–408
4. Borenstein DG, O'Mara JW Jr, Boden SD et al (2001) The value of magnetic resonance imaging of the lumbar spine to predict low-back pain in asymptomatic subjects: a seven-year follow-up study. J Bone Joint Surg Am 83:1306–1311
5. Douglas DL, Dugworth T, Kanis JA et al (1981) Spinal cord dysfunction in Paget's disease of bone. Has medical treatment a vascular basis. J Bone Joint Surg Br 63:495–503
6. Gagne F (1995) Intraligamentary amyloid deposits in spinal canal stenosis. Can J Neurol Sci 22:164–167
7. Gill GG, Manning JG, White HL (1955) Surgical treatment of spondylolisthesis without spine fusion. J Bone Joint Surg Am 37:493–520
8. GunzburgR, Keller TS, Szpalski M et al (2003) Clinical and psychofunctional measures of conservative decompression surgery for lumbar spinal stenosis: a prospective cohort study. Eur Spine J 12:197–204
9. Gutwirth P (2000) Distinguishing vascular disease from lumbar spinal stenosis. In: Gunzburg R, Szpalski M (eds) Lumbar spinal stenosis. Lippicott Williams & Wilkins, Philadelphia, pp 115–124
10. Herno A, Airaksinen O, Saari T (1994) Computed tomography after laminectomy for lumbar spinal stenosis. Spine 19:1975–1978
11. Herno A, Saari T, Suomalainen O et al (1999) The degree of decompressive relief and its relation to clinical outcome in patients undergoing surgery for lumbar spinal stenosis. Spine 24: 1010–1014
12. Kanis JA (1991) Pathophysiology and treatment of Paget disease of bone. Dunnitz, London
13. Kloc W, Wasilewski W, Imielinski BL, et al (1998) Epidural gas aggregation in the course of gaseous degeneration of lumbar intervertebral disk as a cause foot paresis. Neurol Neurochir Pol 32: 699–704
14. Lane WA (1893) Case of spondylolisthesis associated with progressive paraplegia: laminectomy. Lancet I:991
15. Marcelli C, Perennou D, Cyteval C et al (1996) Amyloidosis related cauda equina compression in long term hemodialysis patients. Three case reports. Spine 21:381–385
16. Martinelli TA, Wiesel SW (1992) Epidemiology of spinal stenosis. Instr Course Lect 41:179–181
17. McDonald EB, Porter R, Hibbert C et al (1984) The relationship between spinal canal diameter and back pain in coal miners. Ultrasonic measurement as a screening test. J Occup Med 26: 23–28
18. McNab I (1950) Spondylolisthesis with an intact neural arch: the so-called pseudo-spondylolisthesis. J Bone Joint Surg Br 32:325–333
19. Miller JAA, Schmatz C, Schultz AB (1988) Lumbar disc degeneration: correlation with age, sex and spine levels in 600 autopsy specimens. Spine 13: 173–178
20. Miyamoto S, Takaoka K, Yonenobu K et al (1992) Ossification of the ligamentum flavum induced by bone morphogenic protein. J Bone Joint Surg Br 74:279–283
21. Newman PH (1963) The aetiology of spondylolisthsesis. J Bone Joint Surg Br 45:39
22. Porter RW (2000) Vascular compression theory. In: Gunzburg R, Szpalski M (eds) Lumbar spinal stenosis. Lippincott Williams & Wilkins, Philadelphia, pp 159–162
23. Porter RW, Ward D (1992) cauda equina dysfunction: the significance of multiple level pathology. Spine 17:9–15
24. Postacchini F Gumina S, Cinotti G et al (1994) Ligamenta flava in lumbar disc herniation and spinal stenosis. Light and electron microscopic morphology. Spine 19:917–922
25. Sasaki K (1995) Magnetic resonance imaging findings of the lumbar nerve root pathway in patients over 50 years old. Eur Spine J 4:71–76
26. Schmidek HH (1977) Neurologic and neurosurgical sequalae of Paget disease of bone. Clin Orthop 127:70–77
27. Schonstron NR, Hansson GH (1991) Thickness of the human ligamentum flavum as a function of load: an in vitro experimental study. Clin Biomech 6:19–24
28. Schrader P, Grob D, Rahn BA (1993) Histological changes in the ligamentum flavum in patients with spinal stenosis. Orthopade 22:223–226
29. Schrader PK, Grob D, Rahm BA et al (1999) Histology of the ligamentum flavum in patients with degenerative lumbar spinal stenosis. Eur Spine J 8:323–328
30. Szpalski M, Michel F, Hayez JP (1996) Determination of trunk motion patterns associated with permanent or transient stenosis of the lumbar spine. Eur Spine J 5:332–337
31. Szpalski M, Gunzburg R (1998) The role of surgery in the management of low back pain. Baillieres Clin Rheumatol 12:141–159
32. Verbiest H (1954) A radicular symptom from developmental narrowing of the lumbar vertebral canal. J Bone Joint Surg Br 36:230–237
33. Videman T, Battié MC (1999) The influence of occupation on lumbar degeneration. Spine 24:1164–1168
34. Videman T, Nurminen M, Troup JDG (1990) Lumbar spinal pathology in cadaveric material in relation to history of back pain, occupation and physical loading. Spine 15:728–740
35. Wiltse LL, Rothman SLG (1996) Lumbar and lumbosacral spondylolisthesis. In: Wiesel SW, Weinstein JN, Herkowitz et al (eds) The lumbar spin. Saunders, Philadelphia, pp 621–654
36. Wong HK, Bose K (1992) Spinal stenosis–Result of surgical treatment. J Westn Pac Orthopaedic Assoc 29: 37–41

Robert Gunzburg
Marek Szpalski

The conservative surgical treatment of lumbar spinal stenosis in the elderly

R. Gunzburg (✉)
Department of Orthopaedics,
Eeuwfeestkliniek,
Harmoniestraat 68,
2018 Antwerp, Belgium
Tel.: +32-3-2402705,
Fax: +32-3-2402040,
e-mail: r.gunzburg@worldonline.be

M. Szpalski
Department of Orthopaedics,
Hôpitaux Iris Sud–Molière Longchamp,
142 rue Marconi,
1190 Brussels, Belgium

Abstract Canal stenosis is now the most common indication for lumbar spine surgery in elderly subjects. Degenerative disc disease is by far the most common cause of lumbar spinal stenosis. It is generally accepted that surgery is indicated if a well-conducted conservative management fails. A meta-analysis of the literature showed on average that 64% of surgically treated patients for lumbar spinal stenosis were reported to have good-to-excellent outcomes. In recent years, however, a growing tendency towards less invasive decompressive surgery has emerged. One such procedure, laminarthrectomy, refers to a surgical decompression involving a partial laminectomy of the vertebra above and below the stenotic level combined with a partial arthrectomy at that level. It can be performed through an approach which preserves a maximum of bony and ligamentous structures. Another principle of surgical treatment is interspinous process distraction This device is implanted between the spinous processes, thus reducing extension at the symptomatic level(s), yet allowing flexion and unrestricted axial rotation and lateral flexion. It limits the further narrowing of the canal in upright and extended position. In accordance with the current general tendency towards minimally invasive surgery, such techniques, which preserve much of the anatomy, and the biomechanical function of the lumbar spine may prove highly indicated in the surgical treatment of lumbar stenosis, especially in the elderly.

Keywords Lumbar spinal stenosis · Surgery

Introduction

Increasing numbers of patients, particularly the elderly, are undergoing surgery for lumbar stenosis. Indeed, canal stenosis is now the most common indication for lumbar spine surgery in elderly subjects. With the aging of the population the incidence of surgical decompressions will increase [6]. Verbiest [31] introduced the concept of spinal stenosis and brought the condition to the attention of the medical world. Lumbar spinal stenosis refers to a pathological condition causing a compression of the contents of the canal, particularly the neural structures. If compression does not occur, the canal should be described as narrow but not stenotic [26]. Degenerative disc disease is by far the most common cause of lumbar spinal stenosis. A bulging degenerated intervertebral disc anteriorly, combined with thickened infolding of ligamenta flava and hypertrophy of the facet joints posteriorly result in narrowing of the spinal canal. The site of compression may be central, lateral or a combination, of the two [33]. As for many continuous characteristics, both canal size and dural sac size present a Gaussian distribution. When a canal size is too narrow for the dural sac size that it contains, stenosis occurs. An identical canal size can therefore be stenotic for one person while not being stenotic for another who happens to have a smaller dural sac size. Lumbar spinal stenosis is therefore a clinical condition and not a radio-

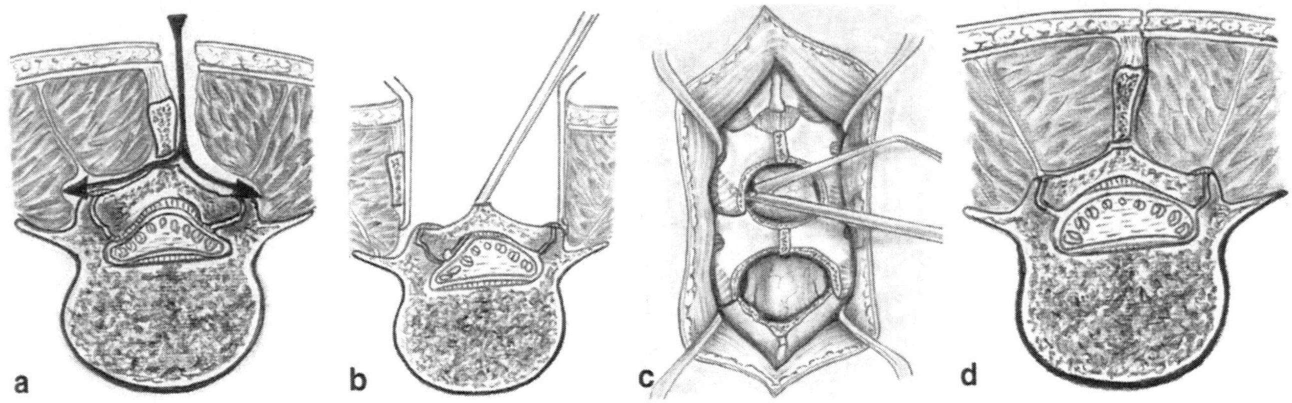

Fig. 1 **a** After a midline posterior skin and subcutaneous tissue incision, the dissection goes through the dorsolumbar fascia approximately 5 mm to the left of the midline, preserving the supraspinous ligamentous attachment to the lumbar fascia. The multifidus is detached from the left side of the spinous processes and laminar attachments. An osteotomy is performed with a curved chisel at the base of the spinous processes of the vertebrae above and below the stenotic levels. **b** Retractors are placed to keep the wound open and are being loosened at regular intervals to avoid damage to the retracted muscles. **c** The ligamentum flavum is detached with a freer elevator and then completely resected on both sides. The lower third of the upper laminae and the upper third of the lower laminae are resected using Kerrison rongeurs of varying widths and lengths. A plastic suction device, held in one hand, is also used as a retractor. With the other hand, the Kerrison rongeurs are used to remove the hypertrophic anterior portion of the facet joints and the overlying capsular tissues. The same instruments are used to partially undermine the roofs in the laminae while respecting the integrity of the laminae. The facet and lamina roof decompressions create a portal by which the neural foramina can be decompressed by means of an extralong (30-cm) Kerrison rongeur. The adequacy of decompression is checked with foraminal probes. **d** After removal of the retractors the supraspinous ligamentous/fascial complex with the osteotomized spinous processes regain their initial positions by resting on the remainder of the neural arches. Both the lumbar fascia and the subcutaneous tissue and skin are closed in a standard fashion. (With permission from [15])

logical finding or diagnosis. In addition, a poor correlation between radiological stenosis and symptoms has been reported [17].

Conservative treatment of lumbar spinal stenosis comprises physiotherapy, anti-inflammatory medications, lumbar corset, and epidural infiltration, and it is generally accepted that surgery is indicated if well-conducted conservative management fails. The aim of the operation is to improve quality of life. In recent publications from the Maine lumbar spine study Atlas et al. [3, 4]report a greater improvement in patient recorded outcomes in surgically treated patients than nonsurgically treated patients both at a 1- and at 4-year evaluation. In a prospective 10-year study Amundsen et al. [1] found considerably better treatment results in a group of patients randomized to surgical treatment that those receiving conservative treatment. A meta-analysis of the literature in 1991 showed on average that 64% of surgically treated patients for lumbar spinal stenosis were reported to have good-to-excellent outcomes [30]. It appears that the morbidity associated with surgical treatment of lumbar stenosis in the elderly is important as those patients often present with a number of preexisting endocrinological, cardiovascular, or pulmonary comorbidities [7, 20, 22]. An increased complication rate has also been shown to be associated with spinal fusion performed for lumbar stenosis in elderly patients [6]. Therefore less invasive surgical approaches are of particular interest. We describe two less invasive techniques which appear interesting in the surgical handling of spinal stenosis, particularly in the elderly.

Wide decompressive laminectomy, often combined with medial facetectomy and foraminotomy, was formerly the standard treatment. In recent years, however, a growing tendency towards less invasive decompressive surgery has emerged as a logical surgical treatment alternative, sparing anatomical structures and decreasing the risk for postoperative instability. Stenosis in the elderly is due mainly to a combination of facet hypertrophy and soft tissue buckling. It is therefore logical to limit the resection to the causative structures, thus limiting damage and instability. One such procedure, laminarthrectomy, refers to a surgical decompression involving a partial laminectomy of the vertebra above and below the stenotic level combined with a partial arthrectomy at that level. Other less invasive and destructive techniques have recently been proposed. Among these are devices inserted between the spinous processes and aiming at abolishing postural lordosis at the level of the narrowed functional unit.

Laminarthtrectomy

The partial laminectomy/arthrectomy or laminarthrectomy surgical procedure has been previously described in detail [9, 32]. Briefly, patients are placed in prone position with a padded support at the level of the iliac crests and sternum. A very slight flexion of hips and knees assures that the subjects lie in a lordotic position simulating the normal erect posture [14]. After a midline posterior skin and subcutaneous tissue incision the dissection goes through the dorsolumbar fascia approximately 5 mm to the left of the midline, preserving the supraspinous ligamentous attachment to the fascia. The multifidus is detached from the left side of the spinous processes and laminar attachments. An osteotomy is performed with a curved osteotome at the base of the spinous processes of the vertebrae above and below the stenotic levels, just superficially to their junction with the laminae. Flavectomies are carried out, and the superior and inferior laminae are partially resected. Partial facetectomies and foraminal decompressions are carried out under direct vision with the aid of Kerrisson rongeurs and/or a power drill. If needed, the remaining bridge of lamina is thinned. After completion of a thorough decompression the dorsolumbar fascia is resutured over a suction drain to the supraspinous ligamentous/fascial complex with the osteotomized spinous processes regaining their initial positions over the neural arches (Fig. 1). In a prospective study of 36 consecutive patients we observed a successful outcome of 58.3% at a minimum 1 year follow-up [16]. Successful surgical outcome was defined as an improvement in at least three of the following four criteria: self-reported pain on a visual analogue scale, self-reported functional status measured by low back outcome scale [12], reduction in pain during walking, and reduction in leg pain. Of the 15 patients (42%) who did not demonstrate sufficient improvement to be labeled a success 12 reported partial improvement.

Interspinous process distraction

One device aimed at obtaining an interspinous process distraction is the X-Stop (St. Francis Medical Technologies, San Francisco, Calif., USA) and is currently undergoing a prospective study for possible United States Food and Drug Administration approval. Biomechanical studies have shown an unloading of the disc at the instrumented level with no effect at adjacent levels [28]. This device is implanted between the spinous processes thus reducing extension at the symptomatic level(s) bt allows flexion and unrestricted axial rotation and lateral flexion (Fig. 2). The major portion of the interspinous ligament is preserved. It is indicated in patients in whom the symptoms are increased in extension. In a prospective, randomized, multicenter study Zuckerman et al. [35] showed a success rate at 1 year of 59% with X-Stop compared to 12% in the conservative treatment control group.

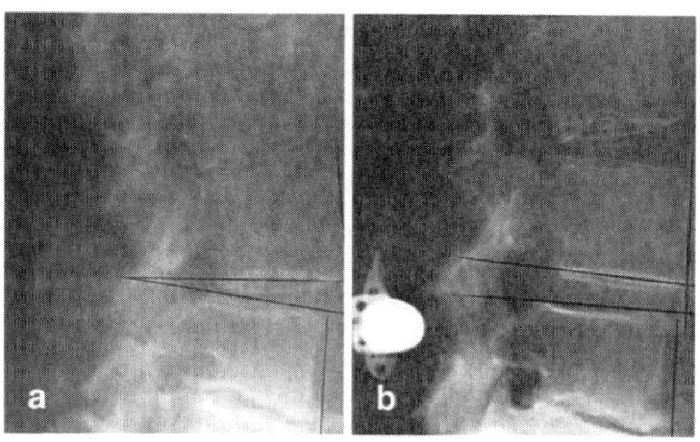

Fig. 2 **a** Preoperative standing upright lateral radiographic view of a degenerative spine. **b** Postoperative standing upright view with the X-Stop placed between the spinous processes. Note the enlarging of the foramen

Discussion

Surgery for lumbar spinal stenosis is generally accepted when conservative treatment has failed and aims at improving quality of life by reducing symptoms such as neurogenic claudication, restless legs, and radiating neurogenic pain. Surgery does not reduce low back pain, although most patients with lumbar spinal stenosis complain from low back pain [23]. Some recent publications have indicated that advanced age does not increase the morbidity, nor does it decrease patient satisfaction or lengthen return to activities [10, 27]. Other studies [6, 7] mention an increased mortality and complication rate with age and comorbidity. Postoperative complications increase with greater use of resources, particularly when arthrodesis is being performed [6]. In the light of the rapid increase in surgery rates in some areas these contradictions indicate the need for more information concerning the relative efficacy of surgical and nonsurgical treatments for spinal stenosis [6]. In a study on gender differences Katz et al. [21] found that women had a much worse functional status than men prior to laminectomy for spinal stenosis. However, women had a comparable or greater functional improvement following surgery.

The use of wide decompressive procedures for spinal stenosis, without regard for the integrity of the laminae and facet joints and without preservation of the spinous processes and interspinous ligaments, may lead to mechanical failure of the spine and chronic pain syndrome. Hence wide decompressive procedures are often combined with fusion. A number of recent studies have reported less aggressive surgical techniques that provide for adequate decompression [2, 5, 8, 19, 24, 25, 29, 34]. These procedures have been described as fenestration, laminotomy, selective decompression, and laminarthrectomy and are purported to improve postoperative morbidity, provide early mobility, and reduce hospital stay. Conservative surgical decompression allows spinal stability to be maintained since tissue disruption is minimized, and the decompression is carried out without violating the integrity of the laminae, facet joints, and interspinous ligaments. These considerations are particularly pertinent for elderly patients.

The need to achieve an adequate level of surgical decompression to obtain good results is important. However,

Herno et al. [18] found that patient satisfaction with the results of surgery is more important to a good surgical outcome than the degree of decompression determined by visually examining computed tomography scans. Comparison of pre- and postoperative scans or scans obtained on more than one occasion is complicated by a number of factors, however, including precise registration of the postoperative scans relative to the preoperative scans [13]. Greenough and Fraser [11] reported that the overall variation in vertebral morphology measurements was 2.8% in patients scanned on more than one occasion. We did find, however, that in the conservative laminarthrectomy technique the interfacet bony canal diameter was significantly increased postoperatively, and that the preoperative bony canal dimension was an important predictor of surgical outcome [15].

The interspinous process distraction device is little invasive, and the preliminary clinical results appear very satisfactory in those patients in whom symptoms are enhanced by extension. The operation is short and easy to perform and can even be carried out in lateral decubitus. For some elderly patients with important comorbidities this may be an additional advantage. The success rate obtained with these methods (58% with laminarthrectomy and 59% with the interspinous process distraction device) is similar to that generally reported for decompressive surgery [30]. If longer-term studies confirm these outcomes, in accordance with the current general tendency towards minimally invasive surgery such techniques which preserve much of the anatomy and the biomechanical function of the lumbar spine, may prove highly indicated in the surgical treatment of lumbar stenosis, especially in the elderly.

Acknowledgements The authors thank Prof. René Louis for preparation of the surgical drawings.

References

1. Amundsen T, Weber H, Nordal HJ et al (2000) Lumbar spinal stenosis: conservative or surgical management? A prospective 10-year study. Spine 25: 1424–1436
2. Aryanpur J, Ducker T (1990) Multilevel lumbar laminotomies: an alternative to laminectomy in the treatment of lumbar stenosis. Neurosurgery 26:429–432
3. Atlas SJ, Deyo RA, Keller RB et al (1996) The Maine lumbar spine study, part III. 1-year outcomes of surgical and nonsurgical management of lumbar spinal stenosis. Spine 21:1787–1795
4. Atlas SJ, Keller RB, Robson D et al (2000) Surgical and nonsurgical Management of lumbar spine stenosis. Four-year outcomes from the Maine lumbar spine study. Spine 25:556–562
5. Caspar W, Papavero L, Sayler MK et al (1994) Precise and limited decompression for lumbar spinal stenosis. Acta Neurochir (Wien) 131:130–136
6. Ciol MA, Deyo RA, Howell E et al (1996) An assessment of surgery for spinal stenosis: time trends, geographic variations, complications and re-operations. J Am Geriatr Soc 44:285–290
7. Deyo RA, Cherkin DC, Loeser JD et al (1992) Morbidity and mortality in association with operations on the lumbar spine: the influence of age, diagnosis, and procedure. J Bone Joint Surg Am 4:536–543
8. Epstein NE (1998) Decompression in the surgical management of degenerative spondylolisthesis: advantages of a conservative approach in 290 patients. J Spinal Disord 11:116–122
9. Fraser RD, Hall DJ (1992) Laminectomy combined with posterolateral stabilisation: a muscle-splitting approach to the lumbosacral spine. Eur Spine J 1:249–253
10. Fredman B, Arinzon Z, Zohar E et al (2002) Observations on the safety and efficacy of surgical decompression for lumbar spinal stenosis in geriatric patients. Eur Spine J 11:571–574
11. Greenough CG, Fraser RD (1992) Lumbar spinal canal morphometry from computed tomography scans: reproducibility, results and clinical implications. Eur Spine J 1:32–37
12. Greenough CG, Fraser RD (1992) Assessment of outcome in patients with low-back pain. Spine 17:36–41
13. Gunzburg R, Sandhu A, Fraser RD (1989) The value of computerized tomography in determining lumbar facet orientation. J Spinal Disord 2:170–175
14. Gunzburg R, Szpalski M, Hayez J-P (1996) The surgical approach to the lumbar spine. In: Szpalski M, Gunzburg R, Spengler D, Nachemson A (eds) Instrumented fusion of the lumbar spine: state of the art, questions and controversies. Lippincott-Raven, Philadelphia, pp 17–24
15. Gunzburg R, Keller TS, Szpalski M et al (2003) A prospective study on CT scan outcomes after conservative decompression surgery for lumbar spinal stenosis. J Spinal Disord Techn 16: 261–267:2003
16. GunzburgR, Keller TS, Szpalski M et al (2003) Clinical and psychofunctional measures of conservative decompression surgery for lumbar spinal stenosis: a prospective cohort study. Eur Spine J 12:197–204
17. Herno A, Airaksinen O, Saari T (1994) Computed tomography after laminectomy for lumbar spinal stenosis. Spine 19:1975–1978
18. Herno A, Saari T, Suomalainen O et al (1999) The degree of decompressive relief and its relation to clinical outcome in patients undergoing surgery for lumbar spinal stenosis. Spine 24: 1010–1014
19. Herron LD, Mangelsdorf C (1991) Lumbar spinal stenosis: results of surgical treatment. J Spinal Disord 4:26–33
20. Katz JN, Lipson SJ, Larson MG et al (1991) The outcome of decompressive laminectomy for degenerative lumbar stenosis. J Bone Joint Surg Am 73:809–816
21. Katz JN, Wright EA, Guadagnoli et al (1994) Differences between men and women undergoing major orthopaedic surgery for degenerative arthritis. Arthritis Rheum 37:687–694
22. Katz, JN, Lipson SL, Brick GW et al (1995) Clinical correlates of patient satisfaction after laminectomy for degenerative lumbar spinal stenosis. Spine 20:1155–1160
23. Katz JN, Lipson SL, Chang LC et al (1996) Seven to 10-year outcome of decompressive surgery for degenerative lumbar spinal stenosis. Spine 21: 92–98

24. Lin PM (1982) Internal decompression for multiple levels of lumbar spinal stenosis: a technical note. Neurosurgery 11:546–549
25. Munting E, Druez V, Tsoukas D (2000) Surgical decompression of lumbar spinal stenosis according to Senegas technique. In: Gunzburg R, Szpalski M (eds) Lumbar spinal stenosis. Lippincott-Williams & Wilkins, Philadelphia, pp 207–214
26. Postacchini F (1996) Management of lumbar spinal stenosis. J Bone Joint Surg Br 78:154–164
27. Ragab AA, Fye MA, Bohlman HH (2003) Surgery of the lumbar spine for spinal stenosis in 118 patients 70 years of age or older. Spine 28:348–353
28. Swanson KE, Lindsey DP, Hsu KY et al (2003) The effects of an interspinous implant on vertebral disc pressures. Spine 28:26–32
29. Tsai RY, Yaang R-S, Bray RS (1998) Microscopic laminotomies for degenerative lumbar spinal stenosis. J Spinal Disord 11:389–394
30. Turner JA, Ersek M, Herron L, Deyo R (1992) Surgery for lumbar stenosis: attempted meta-analysis of the literature. Spine 17:1–8
31. Verbiest H (1954) Radicular syndrome from developmental narrowing of the lumbar vertebral canal. J Bone Joint Surg Br 26:230–237
32. Weiner BK, Fraser RD, Peterson M (1999) Spinous process osteotomies to facilitate lumbar decompressive surgery. Spine 24:62–66
33. Wong HK, Bose K (1992) Spinal stenosis–Result of surgical treatment. J West Pac Orthop Assoc 29:37–41
34. Young S, Veerapen R, O'Laoire SA (1988) Relief of lumbar canal stenosis using multilevel subarticular fenestrations as an alternative to wide laminectomy: preliminary report. Neurosurgery 23:628–633
35. Zucherman JF, Hsu KY, Hartjen CA et al (2003) A prospective randomized multi-center study for the treatment of lumbar spinal stenosis with the X-STOP interspinous spacer: 1-year results. Eur Spine J (in press)

Jiri Dvorak
Martin Sutter
Joerg Herdmann

Cervical myelopathy: clinical and neurophysiological evaluation

J. Dvorak (✉)
Department of Neurology, Schulthess Clinic Spine Unit,
Lengghalde 2, 8008 Zürich, Switzerland
Tel.: +41-1-3857445,
Fax: +41-1-3857574,
e-mail: dvorak@kws.ch

M. Sutter
Department of Neurophysiology, Intraoperative Monitoring,
Schulthess Clinic Spine Unit,
Zürich, Switzerland

J. Herdmann
Department of Neurosurgery, SPINE Unit,
Heinrich-Heine-University,
Düsseldorf, Germany

Abstract The overall frequency of troublesome neck pain is estimated to be about 34%, and it was observed that the frequency of complaints lasting 1 month or longer was higher in women than in men. The prevalence increased with age, with regard to both pain duration and chronic pain. Approximately 14% of a randomly selected population meets the criterion for chronic neck pain: complaints lasting more than 6 months. Epidemiologic data substantiate the importance of morphologic, age-related changes of the cervical spine; however, the incidence and prevalence of cervical myelopathy is not known. It could be that the structural transformation of the intervertebral disc, the uncovertebral processes and the zygapophyseal joints is a process accompanied by disturbed function that ultimately not only induces pain, but can lead to narrowing of spinal canal, with symptoms and signs of cervical myelopathy. For a diagnosis of radicular and myelopathic syndromes, the functional and neurological examination is enhanced by neurophysiological assessment. Electromyography (EMG) performed with needle electrodes is the oldest method for diagnosing nerve root compression and anterior horn cell syndromes, and is claimed to have no false-positive results. For cervical myelopathy, as a routine examination sensory evoked potentials (SEPs) by stimulation of tibial nerve and motor evoked potentials (MEPs) from the upper and lower extremities are recommended.

Keywords Cervical spine · Myelopathy · Diagnosis · Evoked potentials

Introduction

Herbert von Luschka, a German anatomist, first pointed out the developmental changes of the cervical spine's anatomical structures, i.e., the uncovertebral joints, also commonly called Luschka's joints [21]. The processus articularis are covered by a thin layer of cartilage in healthy subjects, and the uneven surfaces in between the zygapophyseal processes are filled in by an infolding of the joint capsule described by Penning and Töndury as meniscoids [31]. These meniscoids consist of connective and fatty tissue, which is highly vascularized and innervated.

In healthy adults, the intervertebral discs in the cervical spine have a structure similar to that of the discs of the lumbar spine, consisting of the annulus fibrosus and nucleus pulposus. However, it has been observed that in the first and second decades of life, before complete ossification occurs, lateral tears do occur in the annulus fibrosus. The tears in the lateral part of the disc tend to enlarge towards the medial aspect of the intervertebral disc.

These anatomical observations by Töndury document the fact that, with increased age, the disc cannot bear or transfer load due to ongoing dehydration, medial splitting of the disc and the disappearance of the nucleus pulposus [40]. With the increased load on the uncovertebral processes, a new cow-horn-like uncovertebral flattening takes over the load bearing function of the intervertebral joint. It is obvious that such transformation of bony structures can lead to irritation or compression of the spinal nerve as well as the vertebral artery, which of course can cause not only intermittent or chronic pain and finally narrowing of the spinal canal due to bony growth, but also demyelisation of ascending and descending spinal pathways, due to a possible deficiency of blood supply to the spinal cord [9].

Those age-related, morphological changes, as described by Töndury, should be clearly differentiated from disc lesions due to trauma, where tears of the intervertebral disc at the vertebral body endplate have been documented [38].

Evidence of radiological degenerative changes of the cervical spine in the aging population are common. By the fourth decade of life, 30% of asymptomatic subjects show degenerative changes of the intervertebral discs, while by the seventh decade, up to 90% have developed degenerative alterations [39]. Similar findings were earlier presented by Kellgren and Lawrence [17, 19]. Therefore, it is always important to interpret these radiological findings in the light of the clinical picture. If symptoms and findings cannot be logically correlated, the presence of a different pathology should be suspected, and appropriate investigations are indicated.

Close collaboration between the orthopedic surgeon, the neurosurgeon and the neurologist is required in the assessment of the patient in the spine unit, in order to optimally indicate and analyze the clinical, radiological and laboratory findings, including neurophysiology, and relate them to the patient's symptoms.

Based on the history and the physical signs, a rational neurological work-up should be designed in order to confirm or reject the indication for spinal surgery. Patients with cervical spine disorders most commonly complain of local and referred pain, headache, dizziness or disturbance of the equilibrium, paresthesias, and weakness in the upper and lower extremities. In addition to the complete neurological assessment, which includes an examination of the cranial nerves and the upper and lower extremities, additional laboratory examinations may be required and may be helpful in the differential diagnosis, including:

- Analysis of cerebrospinal fluid (CSF)
- Electromyography (EMG)
- Electroneurography (ENG)
- Sensory evoked potentials (SEP)
- Motor evoked potentials (MEP)
- Computerized tomography (CT)
- Magnetic resonance imaging (MRI)

In the differential diagnosis of cervical spondylosis with involvement of neural structures leading to cervical spinal myelopathy, the following diseases should be considered:

- Multiple sclerosis
- Amyotrophic lateral sclerosis (ALS)
- Polyradiculitis (Landry-Guillain-Barré)
- Shoulder amyotrophy
- Borreliosis (Lyme disease)
- Syringomyelia
- "Double crush" lesion of the nerve root and peripheral nerve
- Rheumatoid arthritis with involvement of the cervical spine
- Psychogenic disorders (hysteria)

Neurological examination

The neurological examination aims to differentiate between nerve root and spinal cord compression. Examination of cranial nerves, especially the eye movements with the aid of Frentzel goggles, is useful. There is clear evidence showing interaction between the receptors of the cervical joint capsules and the vestibular organ [28, 29]. However, it is well established that the center projection of the cervical spine mechanoreceptors is close to the vestibular nuclei at the region of the brain stem, which makes the clinical differentiation (cervical vs vestibular origin of dizziness) very difficult [26, 27].

Neck pain may be the first clinical symptom of a slowly growing acusticus neurinoma, with absent corneal reflex being the first sign. Patients with referred pain in the region of trigeminus nerve pain commonly present an underlying pathology of the upper cervical spine, often observed in atlanto-axial instability due to rheumatoid arthritis [38, 42].

Electric pain along the spine irradiating to the extremities during maximal flexion and extension of the cervical spine has been described in patients with multiple sclerosis as the Lhermitte sign, but it is also generally observed in patients suffering from compression of the cervical spinal cord [20]. Radicular arm pain during ipsilateral sidebending rotation and manual compression of the head is described as the Spurling test, and expresses itself as a motion-induced radicular irritation/compression radiating pain along the involved dermatoma.

In patients where compression of the spinal cord is suspected, a neurological examination of the upper and lower extremities should be routinely performed.

According to the type of the lesion, the spinal cord will react primarily with demyelinisation of the descending and/or ascending pathways with the classical symptomatology of tetraspastics, pathologically increased muscle tendon reflexes, positive Babinski sign, absent abdominal reflexes and decreased vibratory sense on the lower extremities. It is not always appreciated, however well described by Ebara et al., that some patients with spinal cord compression will present atrophy of the small muscles of the hands, described as "myelopathic hand," as a result of segmental anterior horn cell necrosis [11, 30]. Shimizu et al. systematically observed the blind zone of the upper cervical spinal cord and analyzed the hyperactive scapulo-humeral reflex, which was described for the first time by Bechterev in 1900 [36]. Compression of the spinal cord at the level C2/C3 will result in hyperactive scapulo-humeral reflex.

One of the first symptoms and also signs of cervical myelopathy is gait disturbance, especially in dark surroundings, when the optical control should be compensated for by the proprioceptive receptors in the feet.

The European Myelopathy Score (EMS)

To asses the severity of cervical myelopathy, the European Myelopathy Score has been proposed [13], based upon the JOA (Japanese Orthopaedic Association) score.

The European Myelophathy Score has five subscores (Table 1). The significance of the each subscore is weighted by the maximal number of points that is achieved if the subscore is normal. All of these subscores are functional criteria that do not require formal testing. They can be obtained by taking the patient's history, or even by questionnaires filled in by the patients themselves. The upper motor neuron is critical in the control of lower limb function. Gait is of major importance for judgment of cervical myelopathy. It is the only subscore that can reach 5 points. Bladder and bowel function (3 points) depend on both motor and sensory integrity. In cervical myelopathy, however, bladder or bowel dysfunction is caused primarily by a bilateral upper motor neuron lesion. Cervical myelopathy is generally due to degenerative changes of the middle and lower cervical spine. Therefore, impairment of hand function can be attributed mainly to lower motor neuron function (4 points), although similar disturbances of precision movements are also seen in upper motor neuron function or cortical lesions. Proprioception and coordination depend on posterior column function (3 points). Posterior column function was included in the European Myelopathy Score instead of the JOA subscores for sensory function – a disturbance which is very difficult to classify into categories. Pain is not a major symptom in cervical myelopathy. Nevertheless, unpleasant sensations such as paresthesia or dysesthesia are often reported, and are mostly caused by a mechanical irritation of the afferent posterior cervical roots (3 points). The maximum number of points a normal subject can reach is 18.

Borrowing from the Glasgow Coma Scale, the worst result is rated with 1 point for each subscore. The minimum score is therefore 5. Depending on the sum reached in the score, cervical myelopathy is classified into three grades: grade III, 5–8 points; grade II, 9–12 points; and grade I, 13–16 points. Subjects with 17 or 18 points are considered free of signs of cervical myelopathy.

The functional character of the criteria used in the European Myelopathy Score allows a critical evaluation of cervical myelopathy from different centers and different countries. The European Myelopathy Score helps to judge the natural course of the disease and to determine the timing of surgery. It also allows a more objective control of postoperative outcome. The European Myelopathy Score is a valuable tool for the evaluation of all conditions involving cervical myelopathy. It will also allow for rapid communication when comparing radiological findings or neurophysiological results in patients with cervical myelopathy. Assessment of EMS on larger patient population with cervical myelopathy is needed.

Neurophysiological investigation of the cervical spine

Patients with spinal disorders, with or without sensorimotor symptoms and signs, often show discrepancies in clinical and neuroradiological (MRI, CT, myelogram) findings, which make it difficult to pinpoint the cause (i.e., particular nerve root or spinal cord segment) of the patient's complaints. Therefore, questions are raised as to which level or nerve root should be surgically approached.

Currently used electrodiagnostic techniques

The spectrum of neurophysiological assessment consists of electromyography (EMG), electroneurography (ENG), and evoked potentials. While somatosensory evoked potentials (SEPs) and motor evoked potentials (MEPs) are most helpful in the investigation of the central nervous system pathways, electromyography, conventional neurography and F-wave studies are more useful for evaluation of the peripheral segments of the sensory and motor pathways.

Somatosensory evoked potentials

For spinal cord evaluation, SEPs are relevant. These are potentials recorded from the lumbar and cervical spine as well as the first components of scalp recordings.

SEPs are generally recorded after electrical stimulation of peripheral nerves or skin. The nerves used are: the posterior tibial, sural, or common peroneal nerves of the lower limbs, and the median radial and the ulnar nerve for the upper limbs. In radicular and spinal disease, several nerves, supplied by different segments, must be stimulated for a level diagnosis. SEPs from tibialis nerve are recommended for the diagnosis of cervical myelopathy [41].

Motor evoked potentials

Somatosensory evoked potentials are delayed in cervical spondylosis and the latency of N11 is significantly delayed statistically. However, similar data have also been reported previously in electrical cortical stimulation studies [1, 12].

A method of painless magnetoelectric transcranial stimulation of the cerebral cortex was introduced in 1985 by Barker et al. [2, 3]. They applied short magnetic pulses, designed to stimulate peripheral nerves, to the scalp, and recorded muscle action potentials from upper and lower limb muscles.

The stimulating coil is placed in such a way as to stimulate the motor cortex, the cervical nerve roots, and the lumbar nerve roots. MEPs are generally recorded at the following muscles: abductor pollicis, adductor minimi, quadriceps, tibialis anterior, gastrocnemius, extensor hallucis, and abductor hallucis [8]. The segmental innervation of these muscles is used for a level diagnosis in analogy to the segmental distribution of the afferent nerves stimulated for SEPs. Surface recording electrodes are placed over the motor end plate [8].

For motor root stimulation over the cervical and lumbar spine, the intensity of the stimulator is adjusted so that a potential with a steep negative rise can be recorded. With this, the onset latency is not critically dependent on the positioning of the coil or the stimulation strength [6]. The excitation site of the nerve root is most likely in the region of the root exit from the intervertebral foramen, and does not differ from that suggested for electrical stimulation over the spine [6, 7, 23]. In patients diagnosed as having a lateral compression of the nerve root, the peripheral nerve latency is not delayed, whereas in patients with more medially localized herniations, a prolonged central motor latency (CML) is the most frequent finding [5].

M-wave and F-wave evaluation for the interpretation of MEPs

M-wave

In order to judge the MEP waveform it is also necessary to obtain an M-wave recording by means of conventional neurography. The M-wave is the response to a supramaximal stimulus of the peripheral nerve, and therefore an electric measure of muscle "size" [32]. It is used as a reference signal with which post transcranial stimulation MEP amplitude and duration are compared, i.e., MEP amplitude and duration are expressed as ratios of M-wave amplitude and duration respectively.

F-wave

F-wave recordings allow for the determination of a total peripheral conduction time (peripheral latency: PL) from the anterior horn cell to the muscle, which thus includes the conduction over the motor root to its exit from the intervertebral foramen. hnumber ="Sec12"

The F-wave is usually normal in mild cases of radiculopathy. Distinct delay of the F-wave or a reduced number of clearly distinguishable F-waves after a given number of supramaximal peripheral stimuli, in association with normal distal motor conduction, is a sign of a proximal lesion.

However, as the excitability of the spinal motor neuron fluctuates periodically, the appearance, latency, and amplitude of the F-wave changes in each record. In spite of these limitations, F-waves have a diagnostic value for anterior root lesions. When F-waves are recorded in a chronic neuropathic process, axonal reflexes must be differentiated [18, 33].

Electromyography (EMG)

Needle electromyography examines segmentally affected muscles, chosen based upon the clinical investigation. The needle is repositioned on ten different sites in a muscle in order not to miss denervated parts. Increased insertional activity, spontaneous activity (involuntary) such as sharp positive waves, fibrillations, fasciculations and diminished motor unit recruitment are considered signs of denervation due to deterioration of anterior horn cells (myelopathy hands), or due to compression of nerve root.

In normal muscles, motor unit action potentials (MUAPs) are elicited only in response to neural discharges. Denervated muscle fibers become unstable, as they are no longer under neural control, and individual muscle fibers will fire in the absence of neural stimuli. These signs of denervation in EMG can be spotted at the earliest about 8 days after the nerve lesion, and are termed acute signs of denervation.

EMG performed with needle concentric electrodes is the oldest neurophysiologic method for diagnosing nerve root compression syndrome [35]. EMG is claimed to have almost no false-positive results [43].

Diagnostic reliability

EMG is important in the differential diagnosis of cervical spondylosis. It shows degrees of denervation and the number of roots involved, but it has no prognostic value [25].

The increased latency of MEPs is a sensitive sign; however, the specificity is low. The increased CML can be found in not only degenerative but also inflammatory diseases of the central nervous system, such as multiple sclerosis. Kameyama examined 67 patients with clinically relevant cervical myelopathy, and 24 patients with cervical canal stenosis without myelopathy [15]. A positive correlation was found for the group of myelopathy patients. De Mattei found sensitivity of MEPs in patients with cervical compression myelopathy to be 70% for upper extremity muscles, and 95% for lower extremity muscles [10].

Tanaka et al.[37] examined MEPs in patients with clinically relevant cervical myelopathy who underwent decompressive surgery. Patients who presented a CML longer than 15 ms and/or polyphasic wave pattern of the potential had worse surgical results than the remaining patients.

A comparison of EMGs and SEPs in differentiating anterior horn cell disease from cervical spinal myelopathy showed dermatomal SEPs were clearly superior. They were found to be normal, as expected, in all 12 patients with amyotrophic lateral sclerosis, while in 19 out of 20 patients with cervical myelopathy, a pathological finding was observed.

For cervical myelopathy, Vohanka and Dvorak suggest, as a routine examination, SEPs by stimulation of the tibial nerve as well as MEPs from the upper and lower extremities [41].

The value of somatosensory and motor evoked potentials in predicting and monitoring the effect of therapy in spondylotic cervical myelopathy has been prospectively examined by Bednarik et al. [4]. The group changes of some SEP and MEP parameters correlated with the changes in clinical score, which means they could be used as an objective tool for the assessment of the results of therapy. In clinical "silent" cervical cord compression, abnormalities were found in half the subjects (*n*=91) and predicted clinical manifestation of myelopathy in one-third of them during a 2-year period.

Timing for surgery

Guidelines for treatment procedures, either conservative or surgical, in patients with cervical myelopathy do not exist. The literature in this respect presents controversial results. Increasing age, clinical, neurophysiological signs, and the general health condition are relevant factors in the decision-making process.

Sampath et al. [34] presented the results of 62 patients, at less than 1-year follow-up, who were treated for cervical myelopathy by 41 surgeons (members of CSRS), either surgically (*n*=31) or conservatively (*n*=31). Only 43 patients (69%!) were available for follow-up. When medical and surgical treatments are compared, surgically treated patients appeared to have a better outcome. This small, non-randomized study with a large number of surgeons has methodological flaws; the authors acknowledge the fact that randomized studies are necessary to validate the different treatment procedures.

Matsumoto et al. [22] analyzed the increased signal intensity (ISI) in MRI of spinal cord as a predictor for the outcome of conservative treatment in patients with mild myelopathy. Neither ISI nor spinal cord area was significantly associated with outcome. The authors conclude that early decompression for mild cervical myelopathy is not warranted either by ISI or reduced spinal cord area. Yonenobu [44] considers the transverse area of the spinal cord and duration of myelopathy as the most significant prognostic parameters for surgical outcome. Factors that are unchangeable by nature, such as developmental stenosis or progressive degenerative changes of the cervical spine, are parameters to consider or indicate surgical decompression.

A randomized controlled trial (RCT)on patients with mild cervical myelopathy comparing conservative versus surgical results with 3 years' follow-up (*n*=68) did not show surgery to be superior to conservative treatment [14]. The authors of this excellent study, which is the only RCT to have been conducted on cervical myelopathy, are aware of the difficulties and suggest a possible direction to developing this area of investigation:

> "The crucial question in the treatment of mild and moderate nonprogressing SCM is not whether 'to operate or not to operate' because both the conservative and the surgical treatments are potentially useful. The problem is to find the predictive factors for a satisfactory outcome either for the surgical or the nonsurgical approach. It would be desirable to arrange a multicenter study aimed at addressing these questions, as has been mentioned many times. First, however, it would be necessary to validate the scoring systems carefully, probably replacing those currently used to obtain more reliable and reproducible data.
>
> "The current results can serve as a contribution to the theory that conservative treatment has some advantages over surgery in a carefully selected group of patients. The most promising candidates for highly predicted good results from either conservative treatment or surgery could be the transverse area of the stenotic cord, duration of the disease [44], osseous or cartilaginous compression, developmental diameter of the canal, positivity of electrophysiologic findings, low-signal intensity changes on T1-weighted sequences [24], and severity of the neurologic deficit and its dynamics" [14].

The SPINE TANGO of the SSE might be the appropriate platform to search for the answer to this crucial question.

As the indications for surgical decompression of cervical myelopathy are the subject of ongoing discussion, at the authors' institution the following strategy for management of suspected or diagnosed cervical myelopathy has been adopted:

- Obtain a patient's history with respect to the development of symptoms and signs
- Improve awareness of the symptoms of cervical myelopathy among primary care physicians by continuous education
- Conduct a neurological assessment and diagnostic work out to exclude other systemic diseases
- If in doubt, "wait and see", but carry out regular controls
- Neurophysiology, including MEPs/SEPs/EMG, is the most useful way to monitor progression
- Surgery is indicated in progressive and/or severe forms of cervical myelopathy
- Multimodal intraoperative monitoring (MIOM) is required for demanding decompressive surgery, to optimize the surgical procedure

References

1. Abbruzzese G, Dall'Agata D, Morena M, Simonetti S, Spadavecchia L, Severi P, Andrioli GC, Favale E (1988) Electrical stimulation of the motor tracts in cervical spondylosis. J Neurol Neurosurg Psychiatry 51:796–802
2. Barker AT, Freeston IL, Alinous R, Merton PA, Morton HB (1985) Magnetic stimulation of the human brain. J Physiol 369:3
3. Barker AT, Jalinous R, Freeston IL (1985) Non-invasive magnetic stimulation of the human motor cortex. Lancet 1:1106–1107
4. Bednarik J, Kadanka Z, Vohanka S, Novotny O, Surelova D, Filipovicova D, Prokes B (1998) The value of somatosensory and motor evoked potentials in pre-clinical spondylotic cervical cord compression. Eur Spine J 7:493–500
5. Bischoff C, Meyer BU, Machetanz J, Conrad B (1993) The value of magnetic stimulation in the diagnosis of radiculopathies. Muscle Nerve 16:154–161
6. Britton TC, Meyer BU, Herdmann J, Benecke R (1990) Clinical use of the magnetic stimulator in the investigation of peripheral conduction time. Muscle Nerve 13:396–406
7. Cadwell J (1989) Principles of magnetoelectric stimulation. In: Chokroverty S (ed) Magnetic stimulation in clinical neurophysiology. Butterworths, Boston, pp 13–32
8. Chomiak J, Dvorak J, Antinnes J, Sandler A (1995) Motor evoked potentials: appropriate positioning of recording electrodes for diagnosis of spinal disorders. Eur Spine J 4:180–185
9. Crock HV, Yoshizawa H (1977) The blood supply of the vertebral column and spinal cord in man. Springer, Vienna New York
10. De Mattei M, Paschero B, Sciarretta A, Davini O, Cocito D (1993) Usefulness of motor evoked potentials in compressive myelopathy. Electromyogr Clin Neurophysiol 33:205–216
11. Ebara S, Yonenobu K, Fujiwara K, Yamashita K, Ono K (1988) Myelopathy hand characterized by muscle wasting. A different type of myelopathic hand in patients with cervical spondylosis. Spine 13:785–791
12. Esteban GR, Lagranja AR, Lopez MAC (1988) Delayed short-latency somatosensory evoked potentials in premature diagnosis of medullary disturbances in cervical spondylosis. Electromyogr Clin Neurophysiol 28:361–368
13. Herdmann J, Linzbach M, Krzan M, Dvorak J, Bock WJ (1994) The European Myelopathy Score. In: Bauer BL, Brock M, Klinger M (eds) Advances in neurosurgery. Springer, Berlin Heidelberg, pp 266–268
14. Kadanka Z, Mares M, Bednanik J, Smrcka V, Krbec M, Stejskal L, Chaloupka R, Surelova D, Novotny O, Urbanek I, Dusek L (2002) Approaches to spondylotic cervical myelopathy: conservative versus surgical results in a 3-year follow-up study. Spine 27:2205–2210; discussion 2210–2211
15. Kameyama O, Shibano K, Kawakita H, Ogawa R (1995) Transcranial magnetic stimulation of the motor cortex in cervical spondylosis and spinal canal stenosis. Spine 20:1004–1010
16. Deleted in production
17. Kellgren J, Lawrence J (1958) Osteoarthrosis and disc degeneration in an urban population. Ann Rheum Dis 17: 288–397
18. Kimura, J. (1974) F-wave velocity in the central segment of the median and ulnar nerves: a study in normal subjects and patients with Charcot-Marie-Tooth disease. Neurology 24:539–546
19. Lawrence J (1969) Disc degeneration: its frequency and relationship to symptoms. Ann Rheum Dis 28:121–136
20. Lhermitte F, Roullet E, Lyon-Caen O, Metrot J, Villey T, Bach MA, Tournier-Lasserve E, Chabassol E, Rascol A, Clanet M, et al (1986) [Double-blind treatment of 49 cases of chronic multiple sclerosis using hyperbaric oxygen]. Rev Neurol (Paris) 142: 201–206
21. Luschka H (1858) Die Halbgelenke des menschlichen Körpers. Reimers, Berlin
22. Matsumoto M, Toyama Y, Ishikawa M, Chiba K, Suzuki N, Fujimura Y (2000) Increased signal intensity of the spinal cord on magnetic resonance images in cervical compressive myelopathy. Does it predict the outcome of conservative treatment? Spine 25:677–682
23. Mills KR, Murray NMF (1986) Electrical stimulation over the human vertebral column: which neuronal elements are excited? Electroencephalogr Clin Neurophysiol 63:582–589
24. Morio Y, Teshima R, Nagashima H, Nawata K, Yamasaki D, Nanjo Y (2001) Correlation between operative outcomes of cervical compression myelopathy and MRI of the spinal cord. Spine 26:1238–1245
25. Negrin P, Lelli S, Fardin P (1991) Contribution of electromyography to the diagnosis, treatment and prognosis of cervical disc disease: a study of 114 patients. Electromyogr Clin Neurophysiol 31:173–179
26. Neuhuber WL, Zenker W (1989) Central distribution of cervical primary afferents in the rat, with emphasis on proprioceptive projections to vestibular, perihypoglossal, and upper thoracic spinal nuclei. J Comp Neurol 280:231–253
27. Neuhuber WL, Zenker W, Bankoul S (1990) Central projections of cervical primary afferents in the rat. Some general anatomical principles and their functional significance. In: Neuhuber WL, Zenker W (eds) The primary afferent neuron. Plenum, New York, pp 173–188
28. Norré ME (1979) Neck torsion nystagmus and neck motility. J Belg Med Phys 2:30–56
29. Norré ME (1985) Otoneurologischer Beitrag zum Problem des zervikalen Schwindels. In: Gutmann G (ed) Arteria vertebralis. Springer, Berlin Heidelberg New York, pp 123–131
30. Ono K (1987) Myelopathy hand. New clinical signs of cervical cord damage. J Bone Joint Surg Br 69:215–219
31. Penning L, Töndury G (1964) Entstehung, Bau und Funktion der meniskoiden Strukturen in den Halswirbelgelenken. Z Orthop Ihre Grenzgeb 98: 1–14
32. Reiners K, Herdmann J, Freund HJ (1989) Altered mechanisms of muscular force generation in lower motor neuron disease. Muscle Nerve 12:647–659
33. Roth G (1978) Intranervous regeneration of lower motor neuron. II. Study of 1153 motor axon reflexes. Second part: contralateral motor axon reflex crossed facial reinnervation. Electromyogr Clin Neurophysiol 18:311–350
34. Sampath P, Bendebba M, Davis JD, Ducker TB (2000) Outcome of patients treated for cervical myelopathy. A prospective, multicenter study with independent clinical review. Spine 25: 670–676
35. Shea P, Woods W, Werden D (1950) Electromyography in diagnosis of nerve root compression syndrome. Arch Neurol Psychiatry 64:93–104

36. Shimizu T, Shimada H, Shirakura K (1993) Scapulohumeral reflex (Shimizu). Its clinical significance and testing maneuver. Spine 18:2182–2190
37. Tanaka M, Dvorak J (1999) The evaluation of motor evoked potentials (MEPs) by magnetic stimulation in cervial spondylotic myelopathy. Neuroorthopedics 125:75–89
38. Taylor J, Tworney L (1993) Acute injuries to cervical joints: an autopsy study of neck sprain. Spine 18:1115–1122
39. Tepe HJ (1985) Die Häufigkeit osteochondrotischer Röntgenbefunde der Halswirbelsäule bei 400 symptomfreien Erwachsenen. Röfo 6:659–663
40. Töndury G, Theiler K (1990) Entwicklungsgeschichte und Fehlbildungen der Wirbelsäule, 2nd edn. Hippokrates-Verlag, Stuttgart
41. Vohanka S, Dvorak J (1993) Motor and somatosensory evoked potentials in cervical spinal stenosis. Presented at the 40th Congress of the Czech and Slovak Neurophysiology, Brno
42. Wälchli B, Dvorak J (1998) Axial symptoms including cervical migraine and cervical angina. In: Ono K, Dvorak J, Dunn E (eds) Cervical spondylosis and similar disorders. World Scientific, Singapore, New Jersey, London, pp 167–180
43. Wilbourn A, Aminoff M (1988) AAEE Mini Monograph 32. The electrophysiological examination in patients with radiculopathies. Muscle Nerve 11: 1011–1014
44. Yonenobu K (2000) Cervical radiculopathy and myelopathy: when and what can surgery contribute to treatment? Eur Spine J 9:1–7

P. W. Pavlov

Anterior decompression for cervical spondylotic myelopathy

P. W. Pavlov (✉)
Institute for Spine Surgery and Applied Research, St. Maartenskliniek, P.O. Box 9011, 6500 GM Nijmegen, The Netherlands
Tel.: +31-24-3659945,
Fax: +31-24-3659317,
e-mail: p.pavlov@maartenskliniek.nl

Abstract Cervical spondylotic myelopathy is a clinical entity that manifests itself due to compression and ischemia of the spinal cord. The goal of treatment is to decompress the spinal cord and stabilize the spine in neutral, anatomical position. Since the obstruction and compression of the cord are localized in front of the cord, it is obvious that an anterior surgical approach is the preferred one. The different surgical procedures, complications, and outcome are discussed here.

Keywords Cervical spondylotic myelopathy · Anterior surgery · Fusion · Decompression

Introduction

In cervical spondylotic myelopathy (CSM) there is dysfunction of the spinal cord because of degenerative changes in the spine. The pathophysiology of neural loss is still a subject of some debate. Essentially there are two major mechanisms which cause myelopathy: direct compression of the cord and ischemic changes because of alterations in the local blood flow [10, 14, 41, 42, 55]. Since studies have demonstrated that the pathology of CSM is located predominantly anteriorly [47], it seems logical to approach the spine where the lesion is and choose an anterior approach. Removal of extruding intervertebral disc, spurs, osteophytes and calcified posterior longitudinal ligament relieves the compression of the anterior cord and improves to some extent the blood supply to the cord. The surgical approach as described by Smith and Robinson [86] covers the area between the vertebral bodies of C2 and T1. In patients with long slender necks the vertebral body of T3 may be within reach by this approach. The Smith and Robinson approach allows atraumatic dissection of the anterior aspect of the cervical spine. There is a low potential risk for injuries of the esophagus, trachea, the recurrent laryngeal nerve, and the carotid artery. The direct visualization of the offending pathology allows atraumatic and extensive decompression.

Surgical strategy

The goal of surgical treatment is to achieve a maximum of decompression without compromising the spinal stability and respecting the sagittal profile of the spine. Depending on the affected area the decompression may be executed through a simple discectomy, with or without fusion, or through extensive vertebrectomy with grafting and internal fixation. There are reports in the literature, advocating a discectomy without fusion [60, 90], but the majority of patients included in those studies had disc herniation and not CSM. The nonfusion discectomy eliminates the radicular symptoms in most of the cases but results for a long time in axial neck pain and compromises the lordotic curvature of the spine. This is the reason why discectomy is predominantly combined with interbody fusion today.

In a systematic review covering the literature until 1996 we were not able to identify the anterior interbody fusion as a gold standard for the treatment of degenerative disc disease [56] Nevertheless, the anterior discectomy and interbody fusion is the time-honored procedure in treat-

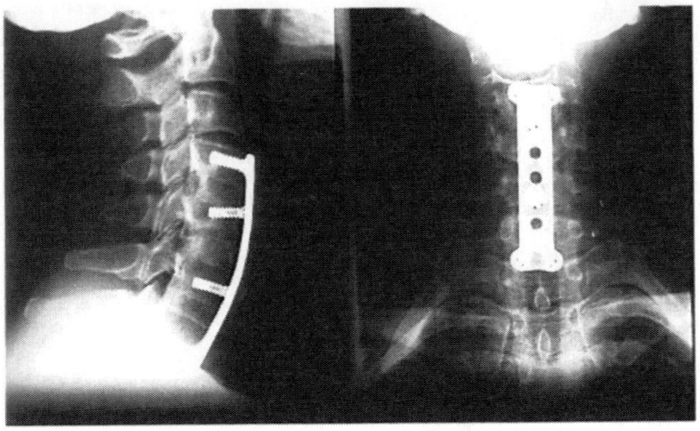

Fig. 1 Three level decompression and fusion with iliac crest grafts and internal fixation. Note the restoration of lordosis

ment of degenerative conditions of the cervical spine. This procedure is predictable with respect to decompression and symptom relief. It is suitable for addressing stenotic changes at single or multiple levels. Restoration of the intervertebral height and the lordotic curvature is possible when approaching each level separately (Fig. 1). On the other hand, this may result in increased risk for symptomatic pseudarthrosis because of the large number areas to fuse [39, 54, 83]. Since the degenerative changes in CSM cover a large area of the subaxial spine, corpectomy and grafting may be advocated [9, 10, 58]. Various terms have been adopted to describe the partial vertebral body resection, including complete or partial vertebrectomy, anterior corpectomy, and partial corpectomy. Basically all the terms refer to a partial resection of the vertebral body without removal of the transverse processes, pedicles, lateral masses, or other posterior elements. Resection of the lateral part of the uncovertebral joints must also be avoided to prevent injury of the vertebral artery. After decompression the spine must be reconstructed using strut grafts or artificial devices with or without internal fixation [21, 31, 36, 38, 44, 51, 63, 66, 94, 95].

Surgical technique

In monosegmental decompression and stabilization it is essential to have sufficient view of the posterior part of the intervertebral space. After excision of the intervertebral disc and resection of the posterior longitudinal ligament the osteophytes must be recognized and entirely removed. Use of the diamond bur is recommended, together with Kerrison rongeurs and curettes. To ensure sufficient distraction of the intervertebral space a strong interlaminar spreader may be used. Use of the Caspar distractor is also recommended. It must be recognized that this distractor has limited ability to mobilize collapsed segments. When performing partial vertebrectomy it is essential to have a wide trough, positioned symmetrically in the midline. The width of the trough is up to 18 mm and may include the medial part of the uncovertebral joints [65]. Some authors do not advocate entire removal of the midsection of the posterior wall of the vertebral body [33].

Grafts, bone substitutes, devices, internal fixation

Structural autografts harvested from the anterior iliac crest or from the fibula are used in anterior fusion of the cervical spine. The grafts must enhance stability and substitute for the regenerative capacity of bone. Fresh autologous grafts posess some osteogenic potential and have osteoinductive and osteoconductive properties [62]. Structural corticocancellous grafts from the anterior iliac crest are commonly used, and their mechanical strength is greater than that of the posterior crest [89]. Iliac crest grafts are used in mono- and bisegmental interbody fusion and also after corpectomy involving no more then two levels. They are considered the biological and biomechanical standard for mono- and bisegmental reconstruction of the anterior cervical spine [3, 11, 17, 73, 75, 86, 98, 102, 103, 107]. In longer fusions after corpectomies a structural fibula graft is appropriate. There are different techniques for stabilizing the strut graft within the decompressed site [7, 47, 78, 105, 106]. Vascularized fibula grafts may accelerate the process of fusion in the case of multiple vertebrectomies [80, 100]. Additional internal fixation may provide immediate intrinsic stability in long strut graft constructs [15, 16, 46, 67, 92]. There are disadvantages when using autologous grafts such as potential donor site morbidity, increased operative time, and hospital stay.

To avoid these disadvantages allografts may be considered. There are also disadvantages concerning the use of allografts, such as risk of transmitting infections from the donor, prolonged healing, and compatibility problems [26, 30, 34, 49, 74, 82, 88, 99, 107]. The use of allografts in multilevel reconstructions is associated with a nonunion rate up to 41%. This nonunion rate is significantly higher than that with autologous grafts, which is estimated at 27% [24]. Allografts may be preserved as fresh-frozen or freeze-dried [27, 52, 87]. Both processes are effective in suppressing antigenicity and retain some osteoinductive ability and osteoconductive properties [62]. Other methods, including sterilization with ethylene oxide gas and high-dose γ-irradiation are effective but decrease significantly the osteoinductive properties and mechanical integrity of the graft [69, 81].

Demineralized bone matrix is composed material, consisting from some collagen proteins and bone growth factors [45]. There are some osteoinductive and osteoconductive properties established [81]. Since demineralized bone matrix lacks mechanical properties that resist forces, it is not suitable for reconstruction of large defects in the cervical spine.

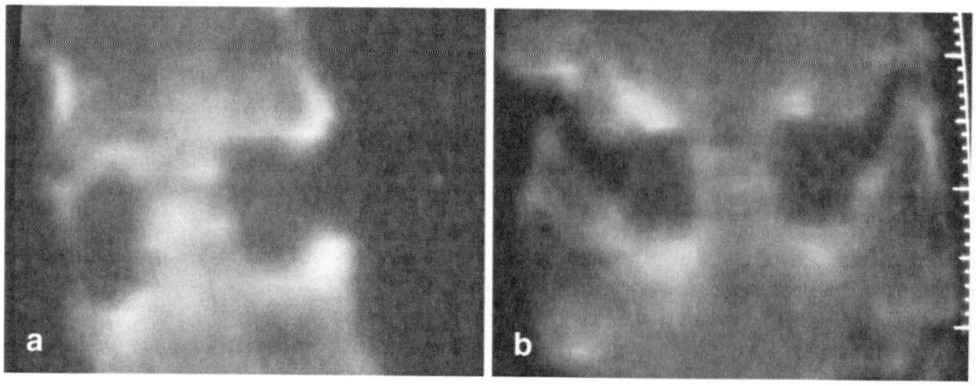

Fig. 2 Computed tomography 6 months after C5–C6 segmental fusion with cage (Cervios, Mathys, Bettlach, Switzerland) prefilled with β-tricalcium phosphate. Note the restitution of β-tricalcium phosphate by bone. **a** Sagittal plane. **b** Coronal plane

Bioceramics are calcium phosphate materials processed by sintering. Hydroxyapatite and β-tricalcium phosphate are examples of the ceramics which may be used in reconstructive surgery. Hydroxyapatite is almost unresorbable while β-tricalcium phosphate degrades and resorbs 6–12 weeks after surgery [40, 70]. The bioceramics are mechanically stable, but the material is brittle and not suitable for use as a stand-alone device. Combined with a rigid anterior fixation bioceramics may be very successful in anterior interbody fusion [91].

Interposition devices (cages)

The introduction of interbody spacers, so-called cages, is the answer to donor site morbidity and optimalization of the fusion construct. There are two major types of cages: threaded hollow cylinders and rectangular cages. There is a fundamental difference in mode of action. The threaded cages are introduced and screwed through the endplates of the vertrebral bodies, whereas the rectangular cages mimic the intervertebral space dimensions and are in accordance with the anatomy of the endplates. In long fusions cylindrical mesh cages are employed, filled with autologous bone. Most cages are made of titanium, carbon fiber of poly-ether-ether-keton. The cages may be used empty or filled with autologous bone or bone substitutes. Good results have been reported by different authors [35, 50]. Our experience with rectangular cages made of poly-ether-ether-keton and filled with β-tricalcium phosphate (Cervios and Chronos, Mathys Medical, Bettlach, Switzerland) is extremely good. In a study to be published, we report that the TCP inserts are resorbed and restored by trabecular bone within 9 months after surgery (Fig. 2).

Internal fixation

Internal fixation after decompression and fusion of the cervical spine provides high intrinsic stability of the construct, maintains alignment, and allows early functional recovery [2]. However, there is no substantial evidence to demonstrate higher fusion rates in plated fusion [1, 18, 96, 109, 110]. On the other hand, there are reports of improved maintenance of the sagittal profile of the spine after instrumented fusion [48, 93, 97]. Internal fixation is used by many surgeons today for mono- and bisegmental anterior interbody fusion [29, 76, 85]. In multilevel fusion after corpectomy (three or more levels), however, high rates of complications and pseudarthrosis have been reported [12, 20]. Di Angelo et al. [19] described the adverse effect of rigid anterior fixation on the stability of the construct. They concluded that the anterior plating reverses strut graft loading mechanics and excessively loads the graft in retroflexion. The stress shielding phenomenon has been observed by using rigid plates and screws with fixed angular orientation [108]. To improve some shortcomings of rigid fixation systems the concept of dynamic fixation has been introduced [1]. The "old" Caspar plates (Aesculaap, Braun, Tuttlingen, Germany) and Orozco (Synthes, Switzerland) are the first examples of noncontroled dynamic fixation on the cervical spine. Numerous different systems have been introduced to permit controlled dynamization of anterior fixation. Early reports are promising but not sufficiently convincing.

Complications

Mono- or bisegmental interbody fusion is usually not complication prone. The major complaints with autologous iliac crest grafts are from the donor site. Morbidity of up to 25% has been reported [79], and residual pain may persist for as long as 24 months after surgery [6]. The major advantage with cages filled with bone substitutes is the avoidance of any donor site morbidity. Multisegmental corpectomy and strut graft reconstructions contribute to the majority of complications regarding anterior surgery of the cervical spine. Some authors have reported perioperative complication rates up to 60% [8, 15, 53, 58, 68, 71, 78, 94, 106]. Most of these are due to inadequate soft tissue exposure and careless handling of vessels, nerves, and esophagus. Neural injuries are usually transient and involve the relatively short C5 nerve roots [77]. Complications related to bone grafting after multiple corpectomies are very common [7, 13, 24, 39]. Graft extrusion has been reported in 5–20%, even when internal fixation is used [25]. There are even reports of increased complication rate when using internal fixation [58, 68]. In instrumented multilevel corpectomies the construct failure that is observed is due to pistoning of the graft. This occurs because rigid anterior plating reverses graft-loading mechanics and excessively loads the graft in retroflexion. This load is higher then the resistive strength of the endplates, and therefore the strut graft subsides [4, 5, 28, 61, 101]. Using titanium mesh cage, Hee et al. [38] reported a high fusion rate of 95% for multilevel corpectomies but still an overall complication rate of 33%.

Outcome

Since there are no reliable data on the natural history of CSM, its treatment remains controversial. However, the anterior decompression and stabilization of the stenotic cervical spine reliably arrests myelopathy progression, and there is measurable objective improvement [7, 13, 15, 23, 25, 37, 57, 59]. Other authors report even a cure rate in excess of 50% and a regression rate of 5% [77]. A mean morbidity rate of 31% has been reported, which emphasizes the challenging nature of this kind of surgery [64, 84, 92, 106]. In an independent matched-cohort analysis comparing corpectomy vs. laminoplasty for multiple cervical myelopathy Edwards et al. [22] reported similar clinical outcome in the two cohorts, with fewer complications in the laminoplasty group. In the long term surgical benefits are maintained but functional capacity deteriorates. This is age related and may be an expression of a slow progression of cord dysfunction [104]. The surgical outcome from anterior decompression of the myelopathic spine is predictable. In monosegmental procedures the fusion rate is high, and the pseudarthrosis rate ranges from 4 to 6%. In the multilevel segmental fusion the pseudarthrosis rate increases due to the increased number of surfaces to fuse [39, 55, 83]. Preliminary experience in our clinic with anatomically shaped cages suggests a significant decrease in pseudarthrosis rate in multisegmental decompression and fusion. After solving the early complications with strut grafts in multilevel corpectomies the surgical outcome seems to be successful. In different series fusion rates above 90% have been reported without respect to plating as well [25, 23, 43, 72, 106].

In conclusion, the anterior approach to the myelopathic cervical spine is a logical answer to a specific pathological substrate. It is a challenging and rewarding surgery, which must be tailored to the individual patient.

References

1. Abraham DJ, Herkowitz HN (1998) Indications and trends in use in cervical spinal fusions. Orthop Clin North Am 29:731–744
2. An HS, Simpson JM (1994) Surgery of the cervical spine. In: An H, Simpson J (eds) Spinal instrumentation. Dunitz, London
3. An HS, Simpson JM, Glover JM, Stephany J (1995) Comparison between allograft plus demineralised bone matrix versus autograft in anterior cervical fusion: a prospective multicenter study. Spine 20:2211–221
4. Anderson PA, Budorick TE, Easton KB, Henley MB, Salciccioli GG (1991) Failure of halo vest to prevent in vivo motion in patients with injured cervical spines. Spine 16 [Suppl 10]:S501–S505
5. Askins V, Eismont FJ (1997) Efficacy of five cervical orthoses in restricting cervical motion: a comparison study. Spine 22:1193–1198
6. Banwart JC, Asher MA, Hassanein RS (1995) Iliac crest bone graft harvest donor site morbidity. A statistical evaluation. Spine 20:1055–1060
7. Bernard TN Jr, Whitecloud TS III (1987) Cervical spondylotic myelopathy and myeloradiculopathy. Anterior decompression and stabilization with autogenous fibula strut graft. Clin Orthop 221:149–160
8. Bernhardt M, Hynes R, Blume H, White A (1993) Current concepts review: cervical spondylotic myelopathy. J Bone Joint Surg Am 5:119–127
9. Bernhardt M, Hynes RA, Blume HW, White AA (1993) Cervical spondylotic myelopathy: current concepts review. J Bone Joint Surg Am 75:119–128
10. Bohlman HH (1995) Cervical spondylosis and myelopathy. Instr Course Lect 44:81–98
11. Bohlman HH, Emery SE, Goodfellow DB, Jones PK (1993) Robinson anterior cervical discectomy and arthrodesis for cervical radiculopathy. J Bone Joint Surg Am 75:1298–1307
12. Bolesta MJ, Rechtine Gr, Chrin AM (2000) Three and four-level anterior cervical discectomy and fusion with plate fixation: a prospective study. Spine 25:2040–2044
13. Boni M, Cherubino P, Denaro V, et al (1984) Multiple subtotal somatectomy. Technique and evaluation of a series of 39 cases. Spine 9:358–362
14. Brain WR, Nortfield D, Wilkinson M (1952) The neurological manifestations of cervical spondylosis. Brain 75:187–225
15. Brown AJ, Havel P, Ebraheim N, Greenblatt SH, Jackson WT (1988) Cervical stabilization by plate and bone fusion. Spine 13:236–240
16. Caspar W (1987) Anterior stabilization with trapezoid osteosynthetic technique in cervical spine injuries. In: Kehr P, Weidnner A (eds) Cervical spine. Springer, Berlin Heidelberg New York, pp 198–204
17. Clements DH, O'Leary PF (1990) Anterior cervical discectomy and fusion. Spine 15:1023–1025
18. Connolly PJ, Esses SI, Kostuik JP (1996) Anterior cervical fusion: outcome analysis of patients fused with or without anterior cervical plates. J Spinal Disord 9:202–206

19. DiAngelo DJ, Foley KT, Vossel KA, Rampersaud YR, Jansen TH (2000) Anterior cervical plating reverses load transfer through multilevel strut-grafts. Spine 25:783–795
20. Doh ES, Heller JG (1998) Multi-level anterior cervical reconstruction: comparison of surgical techniques and results. Program and abstracts of Cervical Spine Research Society 26th Annual Meeting, 3–5 December 1998, Atlanta
21. Ebraheim NA, DeTroye RJ, Rupp RE, at al (1995) Osteosynthesis of the cervical spine with an anterior plate. Orthopedics 18:141–147
22. Edwards CC II, Heller JG, Murakami, H (2002) Corpectomy versus laminoplasty for multilevel cervical myelopathy. Spine 27:1168–1175
23. Emery Se, Bohlman HH, Bolesta MJ, et al (1998) Anterior cervical decompression and arthrodesis for the treatment of cervical spondylotic myelopathy: two-to seventeen-year follow-up. J Bone Joint Surg Am 80:941–951
24. Fernyhough JC, White JI, LaRocca H (1991) Fusion rates in multi-level cervical spondylosis comparing allograft fibula with autograft fibula in 126 patients. Spine 16:561–S564
25. Fessler RG, Steck JC, Giovanini MA (1998) Anterior cervical corpectomy for cervical spondylotic myelopathy. Neurosurgery 43:257–265
26. Friedlaender GE, Huo M (1991) Bone grafts and bone graft substitutes. In: Frymoyer JW (ed) The adult spine: principles and practice. Raven, New York, pp 565–574
27. Friedlander GE, Mankin HJ (1979) Bone banking: current methods and suggested guidelines. Instr Course Lect 30:36–55
28. Garfin SR, Botte MJ, Waters RL, Nickel VL (1986) Complications in the use of the halo fixation device. J Bone Joint Surg Am 8:320–325
29. Geer CP, Papadopoulos SM (1999) Instrumentation after anterior cervical fusion: the argument for single-level anterior cervical discectomy and fusion with anterior plate fixation. Clin Neurosurg 45:25–29
30. Goldberg VM, Stevenson S (1987) Natural history of autografts and allografts. Clin Orthop 225:7–16
31. Gore DR, Sepic SB 1984) Anterior cervical fusion for degenerated or protruded discs. Spine 9:667–671
32. Grob D (1998) Surgery in the degenerative cervical spine. Spine 23:2674–2683
33. Groff MW, Sriharan S, Lee SM, Maiman DJ (2003) Partial corpectomy for cervical spondylosis. Spine 28:14–20
34. Guha SC, Poole MD (1983) Stress fracture of the iliac bone with subfascial femoral neuropathy: unusual complications at a bone graft donor site: case report. Br J Plast Surg 36: 305–306
35. Hacker RJ, Cauthen JC, Gilbert TJ, et al (2000) A prospective randomized multicenter clinical evaluation of an anterior cervical fusion cage. Spine 25:2646–2655
36. Hall DJ, Webb JK (1991) Anterior plate fixation in spine tumor surgery: indications, technique and results. Spine 16 [Suppl]:80–83
37. Hanai K, Fujiyoshi F, Kamei K (1986) Subtotal vertebrectomy and spinal fusion for cervical spondylotic myelopathy. Spine 11310–315
38. Hee HT, Majd ME, Holt RT, Whitecloud TS III, Pienkowski D (2003) Complications of multilevel cervical corpectomies and reconstruction with titanium cages and anterior plating. J Spin Disorders Techn 16:1:1–9
39. Herkowitz HN (1989) The surgical management of cervical spondylotic radiculopathy and myelopathy. Clin Orthop 239:94–108
40. Hoogendoorn HA, Renooij W, Akkermans LMA, et al (1984) Long-term study of large ceramic implants (porous hydroxyapatite) in dog femora. Clin Orthop 187:281–288
41. Hukuda S, Ogata M, Katsura A (1988) Experimental study on acute aggravating factors of cervical spondylotic myelopathy. Spine 13:15–20
42. Ito T, Oyanagi K, Takahashi H, Takahashi H, Ikuta F (1996) Cervical spondylotic myelopathy: clinicopathologic study of the progression pattern and thin myelinated fibers of the lesions of seven patients examined during complete autopsy. Spine 21: 827–833
43. Jamjoom A, Williams C, Cummins B (1991) The treatment of spondylotic cervical myelopathy by multiple subtotal vertebrectomy and fusion. Br J Neurosurg 5:249–255
44. Johnston FG, Crockard HA (1995) One-stage internal fixation and anterior fusion in complex cervical spinal disorders. J Neurosurg 82:234–238
45. Kale AA, DiCesare PE (1995) Osteoinductive agents: basic science and clinical applications. Am J Orthop 24:752–761
46. Kalfas IH (1996) The anterior cervical spine locking plate: a technique for surgical decompression and stabilization. In: Fessler RG, Haid RW (eds) Techniques in spinal stabilization. McGraw-Hill, New York, pp 25–33
47. Kang JD, Bohlman HH (1996) Cervical spondylotic myelopathy. Curr Opin Orthop 7I:13–21
48. Katsuura A, Huduka S, Imanaka T, Miyamoto K, Kanemoto M (1996) Anterior cervical plate used in degenerative disease can maintain cervical lordosis. J Spinal Disord 9:470–476
49. Kaufmann HH, Jones E (1989) The principles of bony spinal fusion. Neurosurgery 24:264–270
50. Kettler A, Wilke HJ, Claes L (2001) Effects of neck movements on stability and subsidence in cervical interbody fusion: an in vitro study. J Neurosurg 94 [Suppl 1]:97–107
51. Kostuik JP, Connolly PJ, Esses SI, et al (1993) Anterior cervical plate fixation with the titanium hollow screw plate system. Spine 18:1273–1278
52. Kreuz FP, Hyatt GW, Turner TC, Bassett AL (1951) The preservation and clinical use of freeze-dried bone. J Bone Joint Surg Am 33:863–872
53. Law MD, Bernhardt M, White AA (1994) Evaluation and management of cervical spondylotic myelopathy. J Bone Joint Surg Am 6:1420–1433
54. Law M. Bernhard M, White AA (1995) Evaluation and management of cervical spondylotic myelopathy. Instr Course Lect 44:99–110
55. Levine DN (1997) Pathogenesis of cervical spondylotic myelopathy. J Neurol Neurosurg Psychiatry 62: 334–440
56. Limbeek J van, Jacobs WCH, Anderson PG, Pavlov PW (2000) A systematic literature review to identify the best method for a single level anterior cervical interbody fusion. Eur Spine J 9:129–136
57. Lunsford LD, Bissonette DJ, Jannetta PJ, et al (1980) Anterior surgery for cervical disc disease. I. Treatment of lateral cervical disc herniation in 253 cases. J Neurosurg 53:1–11
58. MacDonald R, Fehlings M, Tator C, Fleming J, Bernstein M, Tasker R (1997) Multilevel anterior cervical corpectomy and fibular allograft fusion for cervical myelopathy. J Neurosurg 86:990–997
59. Majd ME, Vadhva M, Holt RT (1999) Anterior cervical reconstruction using titanium cages with anterior plating. Spine 24:1604–1610
60. Maurice-Williams RS, Dorward NL (1996) Extended anterior cervical discectomy without fusion: a simple and sufficient operation for most cases of cervical degenerative disease. Br J Neurosurg 10:261–266
61. Müller ME, Allgöwer M, Schneider R, Willenegger H (1991) Manual of internal fixation: techniques recommended by the AO-ASIF group, 3rd edn. Springer, Berlin Heidelberg New York

62. Muschler G, Lane JM (1992) Spinal fusion: principles of bone fusion. In: Rothmann RH, Simeone FA (eds) The spine, vol 2, 3rd edn. Saunders, Philadelphia
63. O'Brien TJ, Rapoff AJ, Ghanayem AJ, et al (1997) Anterior plate stabilization of multilevel cervical corpectomies: a biomechanical analysis of alternative plating techniques. Proceedings of the Cervical Spine Research Society 24th Annual Meeting. Orthop Trans 24:474
64. Okada K, Shirasaki N, Hayashi H, et al (1991) Treatment of cervical spondylotic myelopathy by enlargement of the spinal canal anteriorly, followed by arthrodesis. J Bone Joint Surg Am 73:352–364
65. Orr RD, Zdeblick TA (1999) Cervical spondylotic myelopathy approaches to surgical treatment. Clin Orthop 359:58–66
66. Panjabi MM, Isomi T, Wang JL (1999) Loosening at the screw-vertebra junction in multilevel anterior cervical plate constructs. Spine 24: 2383–2388
67. Papadopoulos SM, Kalfas IH, Sonntag VKH (1993) Anterior Instrumentation of the cervical spine. In Whitecloud TS III, Dunsker SB (eds) Anterior cervical spine surgery. Raven, New York, pp 89–103
68. Paramore CG, Dickman CA, Sonntag VKH (1996) Radiographic and clinical follow-up review of Caspar plates in 49 patients. J Neurosurg 84:957–961
69. Pelker RR, Friedlander GE, Markham TC (1984) Biomechanical aspects of bone autografts and allografts. Orthop Clin North Am 18:235–239
70. Rejeda BV, Peelan JG, de Groot K (1977) Tricalcium phosphate as a bone substitute. J Bioeng 1:93–97
71. Riew KD, Palumbo M, Hilibrand A, Carlson G, Bohlman H (1998) Complications of anterior cervical corpectomy in postlaminectomy patients. Federation of Spine Associations, Thirteenth Annual Meeting, New Orleans, Louisiana, March 1998
72. Riew KD, Sethi NS, Devney J, et al (1999) Complications of buttress plate stabilization of cervical corpectomy. Spine 24:2404–2410
73. Riley LH, Robinson RA, Johnson KA, Walker AE (1969) The results of anterior interbody fusion of the cervical spine. J Neurosurg 30:127–133
74. Rish BL, McFadden JT, Penix JO (1976) Anterior cervical fusion using homologous bone grafts: a comparative study. Surg Neurol 5:119–121
75. Robinson RA, Walker AE, Ferlic DC, Wiecking DK (1962) The results of anterior interbody fusion of the cervical spine. J Bone Joint Surg Am 4: 1569–1587
76. Rushton SA, Albert TJ (1998) Cervical degenerative disease. Spinal Fusion 29:755–777
77. Russegger L, Monstadt H, Wenz F (1997) First experiences with a distractible titanium implant in ventral cervical disc surgery: report on 30 consecutive cases. Eur Spine J 6: 70–73
78. Saunders RL, Bernini PH, Shirreffs TG, Reeves AD (1991) Central corpectomy for cervical spondylotic myelopathy: a consecutive series with long-term follow-up evaluation. J Neurosurg 74:163–170
79. Sawin PD, Traynelis VC, Menezes AH (1998) A comparative analysis of fusion rates and donor-site morbidity for autogenetic rib and iliac crest bone grafts in posterior cervical fusions. J Neurosurg 88:255–265
80. Schaffer JW, Field GA, Goldberg VM, Davy DT (1985) Fate of vascularized and nonvascularized autografts. Clin Orthop 197:32–43
81. Schimandle JH, Boden SD (1992) Bone grafts and bone graft substitutes for spinal fusion. In Rothman RH, Simeone FA (eds) The spine, vol 2, 3rd edn. Saunders, Philadelphia, pp 1610–1629
82. Schneider JR, Bright RW (1976) Anterior cervical fusion using preserved bone allografts. Transplant Proc 8 [Suppl]:73–6
83. Seifert V (1995) Anterior decompressive microsurgery and osteosynthesis for the treatment of multisegmental cervical spondylosis. Pathophysiological considerations, surgical indications, results and complications: a survey. Acta Neurochir (Wien) 135:105–121
84. Seifert V, Stolke D (1991) Multisegmental cervical spondylosis: treatment by spondylectomy, microsurgical decompression and osteosynthesis. Neurosurgery 29:498–503
85. Shapiro S (1996) Banked fibula and the locking anterior cervical plate in anterior cervical fusions following cervical discectomy. J Neurosurg 84:161–165
86. Smith GW, Robinson RA (1958) The treatment of certain cervical spine disorders by anterior removal of the intervertebral disc and interbody fusion. J Bone Joint Surg Am 40:607–624
87. Stahlman GC, Hanley EN, Phillips E (1992) Allograft bone in spinal surgery. In Rothman RH, Simeone FA (eds) The spine, vol 2, 3rd edn. Saunders, Philadelphia, pp 1601–1606
88. Summers BN, Eisenstein SM (1989) Donor site pain from the ilium: a complication of lumbar spine fusion. J Bone Joint Surg Br 71:677–680
89. Takeda M (1985) Experience in posterior lumbar interbody fusion: unicortical versus bicortical autogenous grafts. Clin Orthop 193:120–126
90. Tegos S, Rizos K, Papthanasiu A, Kyriakopoulos K (1994) Results of anterior discectomy without fusion for treatment of cervical radiculopathy and myelopathy. Eur Spine J 3:62–65
91. Thalgott JS, Fritts K, Giuffre JM, Timlin M (1999) Anterior interbody fusion of the cervical spine with coralline hydroxyapatite. Spine 24: 1295–1299
92. Tippets RH, Apfelbaum RI (1988) Anterior cervical fusion with the Caspar instrumentation system. Neurosurgery 22:1008–1013
93. Vaccaro AR, Balderston RA (1997) Anterior plate instrumentation for disorders of the subaxial cervical spine. Clin Orthop 335:112–121
94. Vaccaro Ar, Falatyn SP, Scuderi GJ, et al (1998) Early failure of long segment anterior cervical plate fixation. J Spinal Disord 11:410–415
95. Vanichkachorn J, Albert TJ, Silveri CP, et al (1998) The anterior junctional plate in the cervical spine. Spine 23:2462–467
96. Wang JC, McDonough PW, Endow K, Kanim LE, Delamarter RB (1999) The effect of cervical plating on single-level anterior cervical discectomy and fusion. J Spinal Disord 12:476–471
97. Wang JC, McDonough PW, Endow KK, Delamarter RB (2000) Increased fusion rates with cervical plating for two-level anterior cervical discectomy and fusion. Spine 25:41–45
98. Watters WC, Levinthal R (1994) Anterior cervical discectomy with and without fusion: results, complications, and long-term follow-up. Spine 19: 2343–2347
99. Weikel AM, Habal MB (1977) Meralgia paresthetica: a complication of iliac bone procurement. Plast Reconstr Surg 60:572–574
100. Weiland AJ, Phillips TW, Randolph MA (1984) A radiologic, histologic and biomechanical model comparing autografts, allografts and free-vascularized bone grafts. Plast Reconstr Surg 74:368–379
101. White AA, Panjabi MM (eds) (1990) Clinical biomechanics of the spine. Lippincott, Philadelphia

102. White AA, Southwick WO, DePonte RJ, Gainor JW, Hardy R (1973) Relief of pain by anterior cervical spine fusion for spondylosis: a report of sixty-five patients. Bone Joint Surg Am 5:525–534
103. Williams JL, Allen MB, Harkess JW (1968) Late results of cervical discectomy and interbody fusion: some factors influencing the results. J Bone Joint Surg Am 50:277–286
104. Yonenobu K (2000) Cervical radiculopathy and myelopathy: when and what can surgery contribute to treatment? Eur Spine J 9:1–7
105. Yonenobu K, Fuji T, Ono K, Okada K, Yamamoto T, Harada N (1985) Choice of surgical treatment for multisegmental cervical spondylotic myelopathy. Spine 10:710–716
106. Zdeblick TA, Bohlman HH (1989) Cervical kyphosis and myelopathy. Treatment by anterior corpectomy and strut-grafting. J Bone Joint Surg Am 71:170–182
107. Zdeblick TA, Ducker TB (1991) The use of freeze-dried allograft bone for anterior cervical fusions. Spine 16: 726–729
108. Zdeblick TA, Cooke ME, Wilson D, Kunz DN, McCabe R (1993) Anterior cervical discectomy, fusion and plating. A comparative animal study. Spine 14:1974–1983
109. Zoega B, Karrholm J, Lind B (1998) One-level cervical spine fusion. A randomised study, with or without plate fixation using radiostereometry in 27 patients. Acta Orthop Scand 69:363–368
110. Zoega B, Karrholm J, Lind B (1998) Plate fixation adds stability to two-level anterior fusion in the cervical spine: a randomised study using radiostereometry. Eur Spine J 7:302–307

Kazuo Yonenobu
Takenori Oda

Posterior approach to the degenerative cervical spine

K. Yonenobu (✉)
Department of Orthopaedic Surgery,
Osaka-Minami National Hospital,
2-1 Kidohigashi, Kawachinagano,
586–8521 Osaka , Japan
Tel.: +81-721-535761,
Fax: +81-721-538904,
e-mail: yonenobu-k@umin.ac.jp

T. Oda
Department of Rheumatology
and Orthopedics,
Osaka-Minami National Hospital,
Osaka, Japan

Abstract Laminoplasty has been gradually accepted as a treatment for choice for cervical compression myelopathy. The historical perspective of laminoplasty is described. The aims of laminoplasty are to expand the spinal canal, to secure spinal stability, to preserve the protective function of the spine, and to preserve spinal mobility. Laminoplasty is indicated in myelopathic patients with a developmentally narrow spinal canal or multiple-level involvement combined with a relatively narrow canal. Several laminoplasty techniques and supplementary techniques are described, together with expected outcomes and complications of surgery.

Keywords Laminectomy · Laminoplasty · Cervical myelopathy · History · Surgical technique

Laminectomy was the sole procedure by which to access the spinal canal until Robinson and Smith [24], and Cloward [2] devised the anterior procedures, and was a choice of treatment for cervical spondylotic myelopathy (CSM) or ossification of the posterior longitudinal ligament (OPLL). However, laminectomy for these conditions was not always rewarded. The following reasons for undesirable surgical results can be enumerated:

1. *Spinal cord injury during and immediately after surgery.* The insertion of surgical instruments such as a Kerrison rongeur or a curette into the spinal canal without awareness of canal narrowness, or uneven decompression of the spinal cord during resection of the laminae, can impinge or distort the spinal cord and result in worsening of neurological function. Several authors have pointed out the hazard of postoperative loss of neural function due to surgical intervention [1, 4, 18]. Hematoma in association with swelled nuchal muscles may compress spinal cord that has lost the protective shield of laminae.
2. *Instability and malalignment of the cervical spine.* Instability and malalignment are notorious as a reason for deterioration of neurological symptoms after laminectomy. The thick scar formation – so-called laminectomy membrane – occasionally seen subsequent to postlaminectomy hematoma may increase cord compression due to kyphotic deformity.
3. *Inadequate decompression caused by limited laminectomy.* Adequate posterior shift of the spinal cord cannot be expected if the laminectomy is limited [25].

Because of these shortcomings of laminectomy, many surgeons switched from posterior to anterior access to the spinal canal, and this led to the development of anterior techniques such as subtotal corpectomy and recent expansion of cervical plate systems. At the same time, several surgeons continued to try to improve the shortcomings of laminectomy. Kirita developed extensive simultaneous decompression laminectomy to avoid distorting the spinal cord by the edges of the resected laminae [20]. Hattori devised an expansive Z-shaped laminoplasty in which the posterior wall of the spinal canal was preserved by Z-plasty of the thinned laminae [23]. He attempted in this way to prevent the invasion of scar tissue, which was believed to be a cause of late neurological deterioration. He also expected that the laminae reconstructed by Z-plasty would preserve function of the cervical spine as a supportive structure. The introduction of a high-speed air-driven bar allowed the successful development of these procedures.

In 1977, Hirabayashi developed an epoch-making laminoplasty, the expansive open-door laminoplasty [7]. He described the advantages of this procedure; multiple levels of the spinal cord can be decompressed simultaneously; better postoperative support of the neck allows earlier mobilization of the patients; postoperative kyphotic deformity of the cervical spine can be prevented; and mobility of the cervical spine is reduced postoperatively, which helps to prevent late neurological deterioration as well as the progression of OPLL.

Subsequent to Hirabayashi's laminoplasty, various modifications and supplementary procedures have been devised for further improvement of the safety and efficacy of decompression, as well as the stability of the spine, especially by Japanese orthopedic surgeons. The high incidence of OPLL and CSM in Japan may have promoted the evolution of cervical spine surgery in this country. The mean developmental anteroposterior canal diameter of the cervical spine has been reported to be smaller in the Japanese than that in white Western populations.

Aims, advantages, and disadvantages of laminoplasty

Aims

The aims of laminoplasty are to expand the spinal canal, to secure spinal stability, and to preserve the protective function of the spine. Preservation of spinal mobility is also the goal of this procedure.

Nuchal muscles and spinal ligaments which were totally or partially detached to expose laminae can be reattached to preserved posterior spinal structures, and this may prevent development of the cervical instability which often happens after laminectomy, particularly in those subjects below 50 years of age. The spared laminae preserve the protective function of the spine, shielding the spinal cord from pressure from hematoma during the early postoperative period and preventing the invasion of scar tissue subsequent to hematoma in the late convalescent period. Development of kyphosis in combination with a thick peridural scar following laminectomy is a notorious cause of late neurological deterioration in laminectomy.

Advantages

1. Basically, no instrument needs to be inserted into the canal for laminotomy. Furthermore, the site of the laminotomy or hinge for laminoplasty is uniformly at the junction of the lamina and facet, whereas in laminectomy the site of the laminotomy is variable. Both these factors make laminoplasty more predictable and safer.
2. Expansion of the spinal canal is obtained without much loss of spinal stability, as mentioned above.
3. Decompression of the spinal cord is accomplished without removal of spondylotic protrusion impinging on the neural tissue. Removal of the osteocartilaginous protrusion or ossified ligament encroaching on the already compromised neural tissue is known to be the most hazardous part of the procedure when surgeons use the anterior approach to treat CSM and OPLL respectively.
4. Supplementary procedures for nerve root decompression or reinforcement of spinal stability can easily be performed. Facetectomy for nerve root decompression is optional except for the facets on the hinge side of the laminae. Bone grafting for stabilization either in single or multiple segments is easily applicable.

Disadvantages

1. Upper extremity palsy. Details are described in the complications section.
2. Neck discomfort. The incidence of neck pain after laminoplasty is reported to be high, and this is one of the most discouraging complications [11]. The pathomechanism of postoperative neck discomfort has not yet been clarified, although several hypotheses have been advocated such as prolonged neck immobilization, facet joint damage, and nuchal muscle damage.
3. Reduction of mobility of the cervical spine. Although preservation of spinal mobility is one of the aims of laminoplasty, the range of motion (ROM) usually decreases by 30–70% of the preoperative range. This becomes more marked when laminotomy or hinges are located at the facet in either expansive open-door laminoplasty or spinous process splitting laminoplasty.

Indications

Laminoplasty is indicated for myelopathy secondary to:

- Developmental spinal canal stenosis (an anteroposterior canal diameter less than 13 mm)
- Continuous or mixed type of OPLL
- Multisegmental spondylosis associated with a relatively narrow spinal canal(13–14 mm) [32, 35]
- Distal type of cervical spondylotic amyotrophy [3] with canal stenosis

For younger patients laminoplasty should be borne in mind. Laminoplasty is preferable to laminectomy because it can be lessen postoperative kyphosis and instability. Laminoplasty with stabilization (fusion) has been widely indicated for myelopathy secondary to multilevel subaxial subluxation in patients with rheumatoid arthritis.

At present, no type of laminoplasty can correct a fixed kyphotic deformity into a lordotic curve. Accordingly, a kyphotic cervical spine is an absolute contraindication for posterior decompression. Suda and his coauthors reported that patients having local kyphosis exceeding 13° showed poor surgical results and recommended anterior surgery or posterior decompression with correction of kyphosis [26]. For (radiculo)myelopathy secondary to multisegmental spondylosis associated with athetoid cerebral palsy, laminoplasty combined with a proper fusion procedure can be indicated, provided that the athetoid movements of the neck can be properly controlled with a halo vest in the postoperative period.

Laminoplasty can be indicated for myelopathy secondary to soft disc herniation when the condition is associated with a developmentally narrow canal. Spontaneous withdrawal of disc fragments after laminoplasty has been reported [14].

Techniques of laminoplasty and supplementary procedures

Although several types of laminoplasty have been reported, most of them can be classified into two types: the open-door type of Hirabayashi [7] and the French-door type of Kurokawa [10]. The basic concept of most of procedures is similar to one of these two procedures (Fig. 1). Hence these two procedures are described in more detail. For further details of other procedures, the reader is referred to the original articles [5, 10, 13, 16, 17].

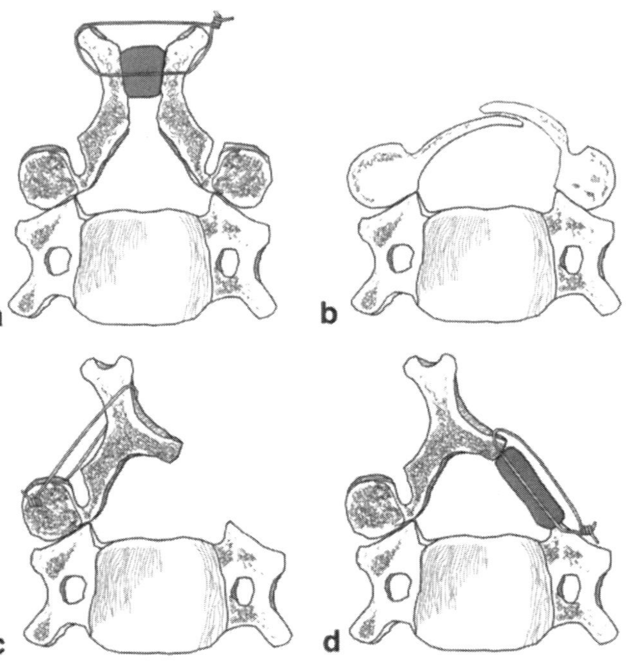

Fig. 1a–d Various types of laminoplasty. **a** Kurokawa; **b** Hattori; **c** Hirabayashi; **d** Itoh and Tsuji

The patient is placed in the prone position on a laminectomy frame to decrease the abdominal pressure. A three-point pin fixation device such as Mayfield's tongs is recommended to secure the head and maintain cervical alignment in the neutral position or slight extension. When spinal fusion is required, the cervical spine is adjusted to its proper alignment after laminoplasty.

Through a posterior midline incision, the nuchal ligament is divided at the midline. Typically, in CSM, the extent of decompression is from C3 to C7 for complete posterior migration of the spinal cord. Decompression should also be wide enough for the spinal cord to migrate posteriorly. When an ossified lesion extends up to C2, undercutting of the C2 lamina (dome-shaped laminoplasty) or a spinous process splitting type of laminoplasty is added.

Unilateral hinge laminoplasty (Hirabayashi)

For the expansive open-door laminoplasty of Hirabayashi [7, 9], the spinous processes are exposed from C2 to T1, with care being taken not to damage the supraspinous and interspinous ligaments. After exposure of the laminae from C2 to T1, a gutter is made at the junction of the articular processes and the laminae. We employ a steel burr to cut the outer cortex and cancellous bone of the laminae, and then make the inner cortex progressively thinner using a diamond burr. With adequate irrigation and suction, the color of the cortex can be seen to change from ivory to dark red as the epidural venous plexus becomes evident. The cranial part of each lamina is thicker than the caudal part and is covered by the caudal portion of the lamina above, so it needs more grinding than the caudal part to equalize the thickness of the inner cortex. Then a scalp clip holder is inserted into the gutter and opened to separate both edges of the gutter by fracturing the thinned inner cortex. With this technique, no instruments need to be inserted into the canal. After laminotomy, another gutter is made on the hinge side with a steel burr, being set more laterally than the gutter on the opening side. Opening of the laminae is secured by sutures placed on the facet joint capsules on the hinge side and the corresponding laminae.

If the lifted laminae are not fixed firmly, loss of enlargement of the spinal canal can occur. In order to avoid this loss, a prop bone graft from C7 and T1 spinous process supporting the lifted lamina was devised by Itoh and Tsuji [13], known as en-bloc laminoplasty.

Foraminotomy on the opening side can be combined with this technique. If spinal fusion is required, a block bone graft from the ilium is placed to bridge the segments to be fused and is secured with wire.

Bilateral hinge laminoplasty

In the spinous process splitting laminoplasty of Kurokawa [10], the dorsal part of each spinous process is removed and the fragments are used as bone grafts in the space made by spinous process splitting. Gutters for the hinge are produced as in the expansive open-door laminoplasty. The laminae are then cut at the midline with a diamond burr and bone grafts from the spinous processes or ilium are shaped to fit the spaces. When spinal fusion is required, a long bone block is positioned to connect the desired spinous processes. A ceramic spacer can also be substituted for an autogenous bone graft [5, 10, 22].

Procedures supplementary to laminoplasty

The nuchal muscles and ligaments are believed to be an indispensable structure helping to stabilize the cervical spine in lordosis. In fact, the nuchal muscles are displaced laterally and ventrally in patients who develop kyphotic deformity after laminectomy, indicating that these muscles and ligaments play an important role in stabilization of the cervical spine. The following procedure attempting soft tissue reconstruction for restoration of stability in lordosis has been practiced, although its clinical significance has not yet been fully clarified.

For reattachment of the nuchal muscles to the spinous process of the axis (Fig. 2), the rectus major, inferior oblique, and semispinalis cervicis muscles attached to the spinous process of the axis are detached from their origins along with small fragments of the spinous process tip, and the lamina and articular processes of C3 are exposed by retracting the semispinalis cervicis muscles laterally. After laminoplasty, the muscles are reattached to their origins by suturing the bony fragments to the tip of the spinous process. The other nuchal muscles are also repositioned and sutured to each other in order to form a suspensory nuchal ligament.

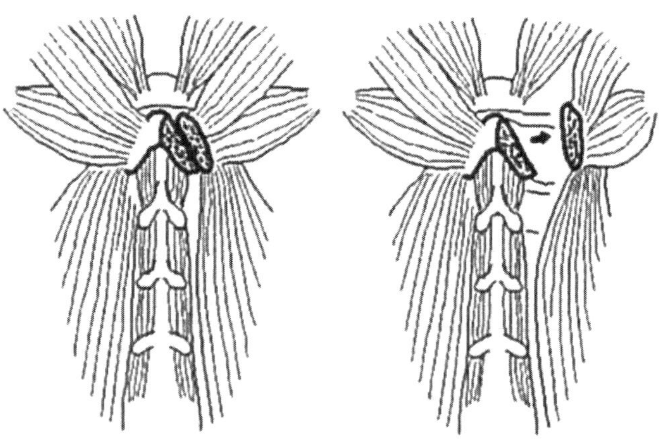

Fig. 2 Reattachment of the nuchal muscles to the spinous process of the axis

Postoperative management

A couple of days after surgery, patients are allowed to leave bed without wearing a collar. When a patient complains of neck pain, a collar is recommended until the patient can stand the pain. If a patient does not feel pain, a gentle active ROM exercise of the neck is recommended. Three weeks after surgery, isometric neck muscle exercises are started. When spinal fusion is required, immobilization of the neck with the collar should last until consolidation of the graft is confirmed roentgenographically.

Surgical results and complications

Neurological results

Since the Japanese Orthopaedic Association proposed a scoring system for cervical myelopathy in 1975, Japanese orthopaedic surgeons have used this system (the JOA system). Recently, a new scoring system has been proposed to improve assessment of shoulder and elbow function and to subdivide the assessment scale for sensory function. Inter- and intrarater reliability of the system has been verified [36]. In most of the Japanese studies, neurological results were assessed by the JOA system and evaluated from the postoperative score and the recovery rate determined by the method of Hirabayashi [7].

There are many reports on surgical results after various types of laminoplasty, and the mean recovery rate ranges from 53% to 86%, with a median of approximately 65%. The duration of symptoms is reported to be one of the most significant prognostic factors. The transverse area of the spinal cord at the maximally compressed level is another significant prognostic factor; an area less than 35 mm^2 indicates poor surgical results. The significance of a high-signal-intensity area in the cord on T2-weighted magnetic resonance imaging is still a controversial subject.

Several comparative studies of anterior surgery and posterior surgery have been conducted [12, 14, 29, 35]. However, no conclusion that has statistical significance has been drawn.

Regarding laminoplasty techniques, no procedure has been proven to be statistically superior to any others with regard to the neurological and roentgenographical results. Few studies have been done with respect to this question. Tsuzuki and coauthors employed six different procedures for CSM and reported that there was no difference in the degrees of improvement of long-tract signs of CSM [28]. We compared the results of two procedures, en-bloc laminoplasty with reconstruction of the nuchal muscle attachments and spinous process splitting laminoplasty in patients with multisegmental spondylotic myelopathy. There was no significant difference between the two groups regarding to postoperative score and recovery rate.

Concerning the difference of surgical results by disease, Miyazaki and his colleagues found that 86.8% of patients with OPLL treated by extensive simultaneous laminectomy showed useful improvement, compared with 75.5% of CSM patients after the same procedure [21]. They also reported that increased instability of the spine after laminectomy influenced the surgical results, and they therefore added posterolateral fusion to laminectomy. When posterolateral fusion was added, the results were improved, and were better than those for OPLL. Kawai and his associates analyzed the results of expansive Z-laminoplasty and reported that outcomes for spondylotic myelopathy were better than those for OPLL [16]. Therefore, better surgical results could be expected in spondylotic myelopathy if the laminoplasty is properly carried out. Of course, the severity of the myelopathy will certainly influence the surgical results.

Decompression of the nerve roots is usually impossible when the bilateral hinge type of laminoplasty is selected. With the unilateral hinge type of laminoplasty, however, foraminotomy or facetectomy can be done on the open side. Herkowitz compared the results of anterior cervical fusion, laminectomy, and laminoplasty for multiple level spondylotic radiculopathy, and concluded that although anterior cervical fusion provides the best results, laminoplasty provides an effective alternative to anterior fusion [6].

Roentgenographic outcome

Kyphotic deformity after laminectomy is a notorious problem, especially when the procedure is carried out in young patients [31, 33]. The incidence of kyphotic deformity after laminectomy for CSM, developmental cervical canal stenosis, and OPLL is probably lower than has been believed. Mikawa and his coworkers reported that no deformity developed after multilevel laminectomy for spondylosis, and that deformity developed more often in OPLL [19]. In our series, 21% of laminectomy patients showed deterioration of neurological symptoms due to cervical spine instability. Approximately half of them had a straight spine before surgery and their symptoms worsened in association with the development of kyphosis triggered by minor trauma.

All of the patients with kyphotic alignment before surgery showed worsening of their alignment after laminoplasty, while no patient with lordotic alignment before surgery showed deterioration after en-bloc laminoplasty. The degree of lordosis in the patients with lordotic alignment before surgery decreased slightly, but no patient developed kyphotic deformity of the cervical spine. After spinous process splitting laminoplasty in our series, 26.9% of the patients showed deterioration of spinal alignment. Hirabayashi and his associates did not note any postoperative malalignment of the cervical spinal lateral curvature after expansive open-door laminoplasty [8]. The difference between the procedures is not clear.

A cervical spine with OPLL tends to be kyphotic, although the reason for this is not clear. Fortunately, few patients deteriorated due to kyphotic deformity after laminoplasty. Formed laminae prevent infiltration of scar tissue into the spinal canal and maintain room for the spinal cord.

Hirabayashi and coworkers reported the progression of OPLL after laminectomy and suggested the usefulness of laminoplasty in this respect [7]. Although progression of OPLL (defined as 2 mm or more growth in thickness or length) was also observed in about 60% of laminoplasty patients, none of them complained of worsening of their neurological symptoms secondary to this progression.

Regarding listhesis, little is known because originally laminoplasty was not indicated for patients with marked spinal instability. In our series, all of the patients having instability as defined by White and Panjabi [30] revealed improvement of stability, and their results were not different from those of the patients without instability.

No procedure has been proven to completely prevent further progression of kyphotic deformity of the cervical spine and to create cervical lordosis in patients with a pre-existing kyphotic deformity. Except when supplemented with spinal fusion, no type of laminoplasty is able to guarantee lifelong spinal stability. To obtain a more consistent outcome after laminoplasty, procedures to reconstruct the supporting soft tissues and rehabilitation programs should be improved.

Postoperatively, the ROM of the neck usually decreases, with the extent of the decrease ranging from 30% to 70%. The type of laminoplasty, the extent of exposure, the position of the laminotomy, the use of bone graft, and the postoperative rehabilitation program including the period of neck immobilization may all influence the degree of loss of ROM. Many surgeons believe that the loss of ROM has a favorable effect on the neurological outcome through a partial stabilization of the spine. Few patients complain of the inconvenience of decreased ROM of the neck, which generally occurs after multisegmental anterior spinal fusion. Hence, patient complaints of ROM reduction after laminoplasty may derive from a combination of stiffness and neck discomfort.

Long-term results

Laminoplasty was developed in the late 1970s, and various modifications were reported in the early 1980s. As yet, only a few follow-up studies over 10 years have been published [15, 29]. Miyazaki and coworkers carried out a study with a mean follow-up of 12 years and 11 months, and reported that improvement after surgery was maintained [21]. Kawai and his associates followed up patients who had undergone a Z-laminoplasty for 10 years on average, and reported that spondylotic myelopathy was stable, in contrast to the results for OPLL [16]. The reasons for this difference were not described in detail. However, OPLL patients frequently have diabetes mellitus and ossification of spinal ligaments in the thoracic and lumbar spine, which also causes myelopathy. These factors might influence the long-term results of surgical treatment to varying degrees.

Complications

Generally, the complications of laminoplasty are similar to those of laminectomy. However, nonneurological complications are relatively rare compared with other procedures including laminectomy. Delayed healing or dehiscence of the surgical wound may occur slightly more frequently after laminoplasty than with laminectomy, and this may be related to the bulk of the elevated laminae. The incidence of neurological complications attributed to this operation is less in laminoplasty because of simultaneous decompression and the use of air-driven instruments. There are, however, complications characteristic to this procedure, which are nerve root palsy and axial (neck and shoulder) pain.

Neurological deterioration due to hematoma has decreased since the reconstructed or preserved laminae still have a protective function to diminish blood pooling and soft tissue swelling after surgery. We have experienced this complication in only 0.3% of laminoplasty patients in contrast to 2.4% of laminectomy patients [34].

Fracture of a hinge or loss of spinal canal enlargement due to insufficient fixation of the lifted lamina is reported to cause nerve root or spinal cord palsy when a lamina migrates into the spinal canal. Computerized tomography (CT) is useful for delineating the pathology in this case, and total or partial removal of the lifted lamina is necessary. The prognosis is usually good if salvage is carried out promptly. For prevention, the inner cortex of the lamina destined to be the hinge should be thinned step by step, while assessing its mobility, until the surgeon is very familiar with the procedure.

Nerve root palsy due to thermal damage or mechanical injury to the nerve root is known to develop occasionally following posterior decompression, and a different type of nerve root palsy is reported to occur after laminoplasty [27, 28, 34]. The initial symptom is severe pain in the shoulder and upper arm, which is followed by paresis or paralysis of the deltoid and biceps brachii muscles. There is a motor-dominant type of nerve root paralysis. The former symptom is the more frequent form of this complication. It occurs on the 1st, 2nd, or 3rd postoperative day, and not immediately after surgery. The fifth cervical nerve root is most frequently involved, followed by the sixth and seventh, in that order. The eighth nerve root is rarely affected. Out of 239 laminoplasty patients in our series, 12 patients developed fifth or sixth nerve root palsy, 3 patients had seventh nerve root involvement, and 1 patient had an eighth root complication. The long-tract signs and symptoms are usually improved, and no regression of the long-tract signs and symptoms can be detected.

The incidence of this complication varies between surgeons and procedures. Tsuzuki and his coworkers studied its incidence in relation to the surgical procedure in their own series [28]. A higher incidence of this complication was encountered in both closed types of laminoplasty with foraminectomy (C4/5, 5/6), while the closed laminoplasties without foraminectomy or facetectomy showed a lower incidence.

This complication has been rarely reported to occur after laminectomy, and the mechanism of this complication has not yet been fully clarified. Nerve root tethering due to posterior migration of the spinal cord has been suggested to be the major cause [26, 27, 33].

This entity may be differentiated from nerve root or spinal cord palsy due to mechanical compression by CT scanning with or without contrast medium. Pain can be controlled with nonsteroid anti-inflammatory drugs and/or analgesics. Neck traction in the neutral position may also reduce pain. The motor paralysis usually recovers to normal or good grade within 12 months. Severe spondylotic changes, especially at the root tunnel, and spinal cord atrophy are thought to be predisposing factors for this complication. Although the alignment of the cervical spine, the relative position of the facets to the vertebral body, and the distance from the cord to the dura–nerve root junction were all analyzed, no factor was proven to be a sole predictor of this complication.

Foraminotomy or facetectomy has not been proven to be a preventive measure. However, controlled opening of the lamina can prevent this problem – although a definitive method for control of opening has not been found.

Postoperatively, patients with laminoplasty complain of various axial symptoms such as nuchal pain and stiffness of the neck and shoulder muscles. Neck stiffness usually appeared on the hinge side in our en-bloc laminoplasty series. In our series, 59.7% of laminoplasty patients complained of some axial symptoms within 1 year after surgery, in contrast to 27.2% of laminectomy patients and 19.2% of subtotal corpectomy and fusion patients. After spinous process splitting laminoplasty, a few of the patients complained of neck and/or shoulder pain. The symptoms were usually distributed on both sides. The causes of these symptoms are not clear. However, changes in and around the facet joints caused by surgical intervention may be the cause. The symptoms resolved by about 1 year after surgery in most patients. However, axial symptoms are the chief complaint in some patients, and their cause should also be clarified. Thermal therapy and active mobilization of the neck and shoulder is recommended for treatment. Nonsteroidal anti-inflammatory agents and muscle-relaxant drugs have little effect. Recently, several surgeons have started to assess the usefulness of various postoperative muscle exercises and neck motion programs to prevent these complaints as well as to maintain or create a cervical lordosis after laminoplasty, but none of these programs has been proven to be useful so far.

References

1. Bohlman HH (1977) Cervical spondylosis with moderate to severe myelopathy. Spine 2:151–162
2. Cloward RB (1958) The anterior approach for removal of ruptured cervical discs. J Neurosurg 15:602–617
3. Ebara S, Yonenobu K, Fujiwara K, Yamashita K, Ono K (1988) Myelopathy hand characterized by muscle wasting. A different type of myelopathy hand in patients with cervical spondylosis. Spine 13:785–791
4. Graham JJ (1989) Complications of cervical spine surgery. In: Shark HH, et al (eds) The cervical spine, 2nd edn. Lippincott, Philadelphia, pp 831–837
5. Hase H, Watanabe t, Hirasawa Y et al (1991) Bilateral open laminoplasty using ceramic laminas for cervical myelopathy. Spine 16:1269–1276
6. Herkowitz HN (1988) A comparison of anterior cervical fusion, cervical laminectomy, and cervical laminoplasty for the surgical management of multiple level spondylotic radiculopathy. Spine 3:774–780
7. Hirabayashi K, Miyagawa J, Satomi K, Maruyama T, Wakano K (1981) Operative results and postoperative progression of ossification among patients with ossification of cervical posterior longitudinal ligament. Spine 6:354–364
8. Hirabayashi K, Watanabe K, Wakano K, Suzuki N, Satomi K, Ishii Y (1983) Expansive open-door laminoplasty for cervical spinal stenotic myelopathy. Spine 8:693–699
9. Hirabayashi K (1994) Expansive open door laminoplasty. In: Shark HH, et al (eds) The cervical spine. An atlas of surgical procedures. Lippincott, Philadelphia, pp 233–250
10. Hoshi K, Kurokawa T, Nakamura K, Hoshino Y, Saita K, Miyoshi K (1996) Expansive cervical laminoplasties – observations on comparative changes in spinous process lengths following longitudinal laminal divisions using autogenous bone or hydroxyapatite spacers. Spinal Cord 34:725–728
11. Hosono N, Yonenobu K, Ono K (1996) Neck and shoulder pain after laminoplasty: a noticeable complication. Spine 21:1969–1973
12. Hukuda S, Mochizuki T, Ogata M, Shichikawa K, Shimomura Y (1985) Operations for cervical spondylotic myelopathy. A comparison of the results of anterior and posterior procedures. J Bone Joint Surg 67-B:609–615
13. Itoh T, Tsuji H (1985) Technical improvements and results of laminoplasty for compressive myelopathy in the cervical spine. Spine 10:729–736
14. Iwasaki M, Ebara S, Miyamoto S, Wada E, Yonenobu K (1996) Expansive laminoplasty for cervical radiculomyelopathy due to soft disc hernia. A comparative study between laminoplasty and anterior arthrodesis. Spine 21:32–38
15. Iwasaki M, Kawaguchi Y, Kimura T, Yonenobu K (2002) Long-term results of expansive laminoplasty for ossification of the posterior longitudinal ligament of the cervical spine: more than 10 years follow-up. J Neurosurg (Spine) 96:180–189
16. Kawai S, Sunago K, Doi K, Saika m, Taguchi T (1988) Cervical laminoplasty (Hattori's method). Procedure and follow-up results. Spine 13:1245–50
17. Matsuzaki H, Hoshino M, Kiuchi T, Toriyama S (1989) Dome-like expansive laminoplasty for the second cervical vertebra. Spine 14:1198–1203
18. Mayfield FH (1976) Complications of laminectomy. Clin Neurosurg 23:435–439
19. Mikawa Y, Shikara J, Yamamuro T (1987) Spinal deformity and instability after multilevel cervical laminectomy. Spine 12:6–11
20. Miyazaki K, Kirita Y (1986) Extensive simultaneous multisegment laminectomy for myelopathy due to the ossification of the posterior longitudinal ligament in the cervical lesion. Spine 11:531–542
21. Miyazaki K, Hirohuji E, Ono S, et al (1994) Extensive simultaneous multisegmental laminectomy and posterior decompression with posterolateral fusion. J Jpn Spine Res Soc 5:167
22. Nakano K, Harata S, Suetsuna F, Araki T, Itoh J (1992) Spinous process-splitting laminoplasty using hydroxyapatite spinous process spacer. Spine 17:S41–43
23. Oyama M, Hattori S, Moriwaki N (1973) A new method of posterior decompression (in Japanese). Chubuseisaisi 16:792–794
24. Robinson RA, Smith GW (1955) Anterolateral cervical disc removal and interbody fusion of the cervical spine. Johns Hopkins Med J 96:223–224
25. Rogers L (1961) The surgical treatment of cervical spondylotic myelopathy. Mobilization of the complete cervical cord into an enlarged canal. J Bone Joint Surg 43B:3–6
26. Suda K, Abumi K, Ito M, Shono Y, Kaneda K, Fujiya M (2003) Local kyphosis reduces surgical outcomes of expansive open-door laminoplasty for cervical spondylotic myelopathy. Spine 28:1258–62
27. Tsuzuki N, Zhogshi L, Abe R, Aiki K (1993) Paralysis of the arm after posterior decompression of the cervical spinal cord. 1. Anatomical investigation of the mechanism of paralysis. Eur Spine J 2:191–196
28. Tsuzuki N, Abe R, Aiki K, Okai K (1993) Paralysis of the arm after posterior decompression of the cervical spinal cord. 2. Analysis of clinical findings. Eur Spine J 2:197–202
29. Wada E, Suzuki S, Kanazawa A, Matsuoka T, Miyamoto S, Yonenobu K (2001) Subtotal corpectomy versus laminoplasty for multilevel cervical spondylotic myelopathy: a long-term follow-up study over 10 years. Spine 26:1443–1447
30. White AA, Panjabi MM (1990) The problem of clinical instability in the human spine. Clinical biomechanics of the spine, 2nd edn. Lippincott, Philadelphia, pp 302–326
31. Yasuoka S, Peterson HA, Maccarty CS (1982) Incidence of spinal column deformity after multilevel laminectomy in children and adults. J Neurosurg 57:441
32. Yonenobu K, Fuji T, Ono K, Okada K, Yamamoto T, Harada N (1985) Choice of surgical treatment for multisegmental cervical spondylotic myelopathy. Spine 10:710–716
33. Yonenobu K, Okada K, Fuji T, Fujiwara K, Yamashita K, Ono K (1986) Causes of neurological deterioration following surgical treatment of cervical myelopathy. Spine 11:818–823
34. Yonenobu K, Hosono N, Iwasaki M, Asano M, Ono K (1991) Neurological complications of surgery for cervical compression myelopathy. Spine 16:1277–1281
35. Yonenobu K, Hosono N, Iwasaki M, Asano M, Ono K (1992) Laminoplasty versus subtotal corpectomy. A comparative study of results in multisegmental cervical spondylotic myelopathy. Spine 17:1281–1284
36. Yonenobu K, Abumi K, Nagata K, Taketomi E, Ueyama K (2001) Inter- and intra-observer reliability of the Japanese Orthopaedic Association Scoring System for evaluation of cervical compression myelopathy. Spine 26:1890–1894

Max Aebi

Spinal metastasis in the elderly

Abstract Bony metastases are a frequent problem in elderly patients affected by cancer, and those with bony metastases involve the spine in approx. 50%. The most frequent spinal metastases (60%) are from breast, lung, or prostate cancer. The chance that an elderly patient (60–79 years old) is affected by bony metastases is four times higher in men and three times higher in women than a middle-aged patient (40–59 years old). Since the medical treatment with all the adjuvant treatment options prolong the survival of this particular patient group, the spinal metastases may become a mechanical issue, thus requesting surgical treatment. Different classification systems have been proposed to rationalize surgical indications, some concentrating solely on the local spinal tumor involvement and some including the overall clinical situation. Since most of the surgical options are of palliative character, it is more important to base the decision on an overall clinical classification including the different treatment modalities – irradiation, chemotherapy, steroids, bisphosphonates, and surgery – to make a shared decision. In case surgery is indicated – neural compression, pathological fracture, instability, and progressive deformity, nursing reasons – the most straightforward procedures should be chosen, which may not need an intensive care unit stay. In the thoracolumbar spine a posterior decompression and posterolateral vertebral body resection through a posterior approach only, with a concomitant reconstruction and stabilization, has shown to work sufficiently well. In the middle and lower cervical spine the anterior approach with anterior decompression and anterior column reconstruction is most effective and has a low morbidity, whereas the occipitocervical junction can generally be treated by posterior resection and stabilization. The outcome should be determined by the survival time in an ambulatory, independent status, where pain is controlled, and the patient is not hospitalized. Surgical management shows the greatest improvement in pain reduction, but also in other domains of quality of life. Since prospective randomized studies comparing different treatment modalities for spinal metastases including surgery are not available and are ethically difficult to achieve, each case remains an interdisciplinary, shared decision making process for what is considered best for a patient or elderly patient. However, whenever surgery is an option, it should be planned before irradiation since surgery after irradiation has a significant higher complication rate.

Keywords Spinal metastases · Vertebral metastases · Elderly · Spinal tumor · Vertebral tumor

M. Aebi (✉)
Institute for Evaluative Research in Orthopedic Surgery,
University of Berne,
Murtenstrasse 35, P.O. Box 8354,
3001 Berne, Switzerland
Tel.: +41-31-6328713,
Fax: +41-31-6320928,
e-mail: maebi@orl.mcgill.ca

Introduction

Bony metastases are a frequent event in breast, prostate, lung, kidney urinary bladder, and thyroid cancer as well as in multiple myeloma and other hematological malignancies which may, however, be considered as primary tumors. About 10% of the cancer patients are attained by metastases located in the spine [23, 36] (incidence 1999, SEER and NPCR Registries, United States Cancer Statistics; SEER Cancer Statistics Review 1975–2000, National Cancer Institute). Among adults 60% of spinal metastases are either from breast, lung, or prostate cancer. Renal and gastrointestinal malignancies each account for about 5% of spinal metastases, and thyroid carcinomas and melanomas occurring with a lesser frequency [2, 24] (incidence 1999, SEER and NPCR Registries, United States Cancer Statistics; SEER Cancer Statistics Review 1975–2000, National Cancer Institute). Since these tumors are increasingly accessible to treatment by surgery, radiation therapy, and chemotherapy, thus prolonging the survival of the affected patients, there is also an increased probability of them being affected by metastases, i.e., with the improved survival, previously silent spinal metastases are becoming clinically apparent and significantly impairing quality of life. Metastatic disease involving the spine most often affects the vertebral bodies of the thoracic, lumbar, cervical, and sacral spine. Siegal et al. [46] estimated that approx. 5% of patients with cancer metastases develop cord compression. In patients with spinal metastases approx. 20% have a cord compression.

Many of the above primary tumors affect persons of advanced age (60% of cancer patients are older than 65 years; incidence 1999, SEER and NPCR Registries, United States Cancer Statistics; SEER Cancer Statistics Review 1975–2000, National Cancer Institute; World Health Organization report: "Pain in the elderly with cancer," www.whocancerpain.wisc.edu), and therefore the metastases become a major issue in the elderly. The average age of patients affected by secondary spinal tumors is 55 – 60 years [23] when considering all metastases; however, it is significantly higher when considering tumors that are more prevalent in the elderly such as prostate cancer and multiple myeloma (Table 1). Prostate cancer, for example, is at least six times more frequent in men aged 60 – 79 years than in those 40 – 59 years old. Breast cancer is almost double and lung cancer five times higher in the elderly (60 – 79 years) than in the middle-aged (40 – 59 years). Although cancer is one of the major causes of morbidity and mortality, elderly persons are often excluded not only from clinical cancer studies but also from standard treatment, and generally also from cancer screening because comorbidity and frailty alter the risk benefit of screening (World Health Organization report: "Pain in the elderly with cancer," www.whocancerpain.wisc.edu). There is clearly an underrepresentation of older persons in drug studies, as documented by the United States Food and Drug Administration (http://cbsnewyork.com, 19 July 2003).

Spinal metastases can become a major burden for elderly because it usually affects the quality of life by reducing the endurance, the capacity to ambulate, and the ability for physical activity. Due to their age these patients often have other diseases which already limit their quality of life or have metastases in other skeletal areas, therefore limiting even more the therapeutic options which may still be considered in younger patients.

Table 1 Probability of developing invasive cancer (percentages) at selected ages with spinal metastasis (from [23])

	40–59 years old	60–79 years old
Breast cancer	4.06 (1 in 25)	6.88 (1 in 15)
Prostate cancer	1.90 (1 in 53)	13.69 (1 in 7)
Lung cancer		
Male	1.29 (1 in 78)	6.35 (1 in 16)
Female	0.94 (1 in 106)	3.98 (1 in 25)
All sites		
Male	8.17 (1 in 12)	33.65 (1 in 3)
Female	9.23 (1 in 11)	22.27 (1 in 4)

Pathological anatomy and classification

Malignant metastatic cells most frequently spread to the spine hematogenously with tumor emboli following the paravertebral plexus (plexus of Batson) [3, 11, 45, 53] that is characterized by a lack of valves. It is postulated that the venous blood return is shifted into the paravertebral plexus via the intervertebral and basivertebral veins due to increased intra-abdominal and intrathoracic pressure. As a result metastases which follow this pathway result in the characteristic pattern of bony spread because tumor cells are seeded by this mechanism into the capillary network of the vertebral bodies. Due to its avascular nature the disc is usually spared from tumor involvement: however, the most frequently and severely affected part of the vertebra is the vertebral body (in about 80%) followed by the pedicles and the posterior elements. This constellation explains why most of the spinal metastasis are located in front of the spinal cord or dural sac ending up with an anterior epidural compression. More than 90% of spinal metastases are extradural and only 5% intradural and less than 1% intramedullar [45]. Less frequently cancer cells spread into the spine through aortic segmental arteries, for example, in lung cancer [45, 49]. Finally there is also the option of direct spread through direct tumor infiltration into the spine, e.g., the Pancoast's tumor of the lung.

There have been several attempts to classify and stage spinal tumors [7, 8, 9, 13, 16, 17, 27, 28, 50, 51]. DeWald et al. [13] suggested a classification system for spinal metastases that is oriented mainly towards surgical treat-

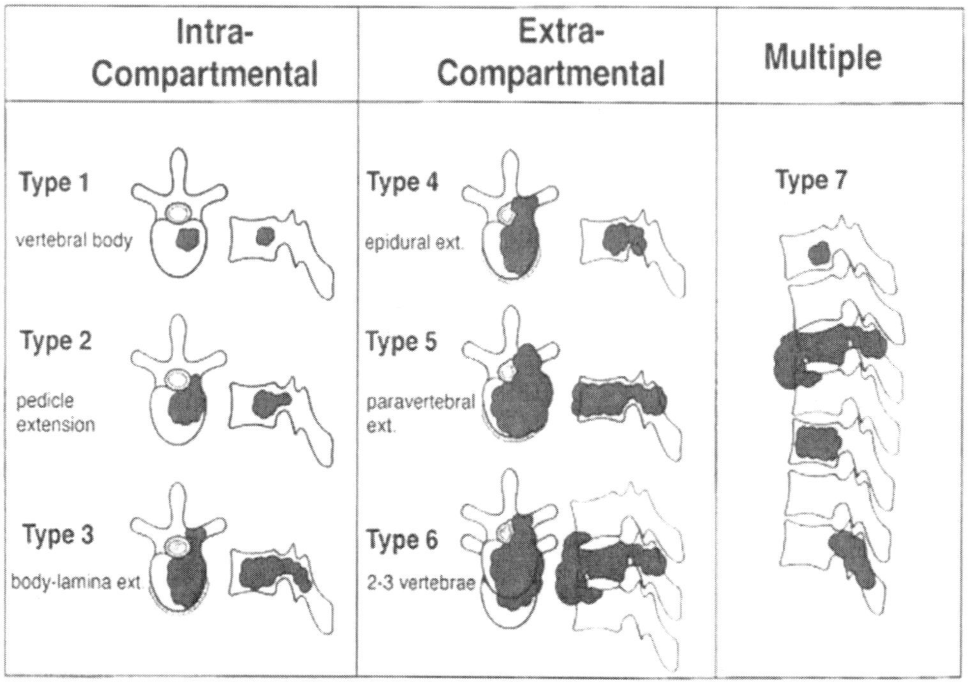

Fig. 1 Tokuhashi et al. [50] scoring system to establish preoperative prognosis of metastatic spine tumor

ment. They proposed the following five classes with subgroups covering most of the possibilities of spinal metastases appearance:

- Class I: destruction without collapse but with pain.
- Class II: the addition of moderate deformity and collapse with immune competence. This class is considered a good risk for surgery.
- Class III: patients are immunocompromised with moderate deformity and collapse. This class carries greater risk for surgery.
- Class IV: includes patients with paralysis, collapse, and deformity with immune competence. This class is considered a relative surgical emergency.
- Class V:adds immune incompetence to paralysis, collapse, and deformity. This class is not considered a good operative risk.

This classification allows consideration of the tumor, potential instability, and patient physiology, which is a sensible approach to a difficult problem. Enneking et al. [17] developed a staging scheme for malignant tumors of the spine in particular in adaptation to the staging of musculoskeletal tumors in general. The WBB Surgical Staging System was been introduced in 1997 primarily for primary bone tumors of the spine [9]. This can be applied for metastatic spine tumors; however, there are presently few reports on the system's correlation with, for example, outcome when applied for surgical indications. Tokuhashi et al. [50] introduced a scoring system for the preoperative evaluation of metastatic spine tumor prognosis that, instead, allows a correlation of the tumor extent with the prognosis [51]. The system differentiates between intracompartmental, extracompartmental, and multiple tumor involvement. The first two categories include types 1 – 3 and types 4 – 6, respectively, whereas multiple tumor involvement is categorized as type 7 (Fig. 1). This scoring system found increasing application in recent years as a baseline in publications to make the results comparable among different scientific publications. K. Tomita et al. [51] applied this system to propose their surgical strategy in spinal metastatic disease.

Clinical presentation and Imaging

The clinical presentation of metastatic spine disease is predominantly pain, neurological deficit, progressive deformity, and general weakness. Pain may be localized to a certain structure and region of the spine and may be of radicular or medullary origin. The pain is either caused by increased intraosseous pressure in the vertebral bodies due to cellular invasion of the cancellous bone, by compression of neural structures such as roots or nervous fibers, by a secondary instability due to the osteoligamentous destruction of parts of the axial skeleton, or by the infiltration of the dura or other neuroanatomical structures. Pain is usually indicated as more or less constant, dull, however with a predominance of night pain and often not to be influenced by the regulation of the physical activities. Generally speaking, slowly progressive, dull neck or back pain which occurs in a patient with a known cancer disease or which may become apparent in an elderly patient without a history of a tumor, should be considered as caused by a spinal metastases until proven otherwise [20].

The neurological deficit appears clearly with a delay of weeks to months after the initial presentation of pain. The period between initial pain and neurological deficit is for the cervical and thoracic spine weeks to months but in the lumbar spine days to weeks [1, 31]. The patients may have motor or sensory deficit or both, whereas there is the option of pure radicular and/or a medullary compression. Since most tumors start in the vertebral body, an anterior cord compression can be expected which is represented by a deficit of the corticospinal pathways with the clinical presentation of a spastic paraparesis which may finally result in an inability to ambulate [20, 46]. Spastic paraparesis appears usually before sensory disturbances. It can progress slowly but always have the potential to deteriorate within days.

Many patients who present to the spine surgeon with a paraparesis reveal a long history of preliminaries for weakness when specifically asked [2]. The loss of the ambulatory capacity may arrive quickly. Sensory disturbances may start with tingling sensation and other dysesthesias that may, again, fairly quickly convert into a loss of most the sensory modalities, even within hours. Further compression may lead to a paresis of the bladder and sphincter and sensory deficits as well as sensory dysfunction in general may become apparent and finally incapacitate the patient. Bladder and sphincter dysfunction are usually irreversible if they last more than 48 h or even shorter [12, 13, 18, 25]. Sphincter disturbances also present rather late, and in elderly persons less attention may be given to this issue, since men may have preexisting micturation difficulty with a prostate problem and women with the bladder/uterus relationship as well as a weak pelvic floor. Obviously there may be an urine retention present or difficulty to initiate the micturation as well as a bladder with an overflow or a weakness, presenting as incontinence. These clinical presentations are often irreversible and are nonfavorable prognostic factors.

The cerebrospinal fluid acts as a puffer for a compressive process, and even in case the cord is already compressed it is first a deterioration in the capillary circulation in the spinal cord which only secondary causes relevant cord damage [26]. Segmental or even multisegmental instability may be a major pain generator as well as generator for neurological functional deficit through temporary or dynamic mechanical compression of neurostructures. This instability occurs with the destruction of the dominant stabilizing elements of the spine, i.e., the posterior elements such as the facet joints, pedicles, laminae, and spinous processes including the soft tissue including ligaments and joint capsules which all contribute to the stability. Since most of the vertebral metastases affect primarily the vertebral bodies which are the major structure of the anterior column, metastases do not necessarily coincidence with instability, as long as the vertebral body contours are intact. Only when the bony structure of the vertebral body is weakened by the replacement of bone by tumor tissue (osteolytic metastases) with the result of a pathological fracture, may the anterior column be weakened sufficiently to make it collapse. Usually the posterior elements are also involved to some extent at this point and render the segment definitely unstable. Osteoblastic tumor metastases are prone to pathological fractures with fragment displacements only if there is a certain mix with osteolytic components. Osteoblastic metastases can reach a considerable hardness which makes a fracture rather improbable; however, they can initiate radicular or medullar compression due to the solidity of the tumor tissue.

In elderly patients who complain of slowly increasing pain which occurs also during sleeping in the low back region, gluteal region, groin, knee, or generally in the lower extremity, may have a hip or knee problem, however, remain suspicious for a metastatic bone cancer, specifically if they have a tumor history or clinical signs of a consuming disorder. Also newly appearing neck pain in an elderly person should be taken seriously by the first consulted physician and not just automatically considered as an expression of a degenerative cervical spine disease.

The advent of magnetic resonance imaging (MRI) has certainly added a new dimension to the tumor diagnostic of the spine, although computed tomography (CT), specifically combined with myelography may still have a relevant role to play, since CT may show more precisely the bony involvement. However, as a search methodology and for appreciation of the spinal tumor involvement MRI is the diagnostic tool of choice. It is noninvasive, in contrast to myelography, which may even be promoting a neurological deterioration combined with CT. It cannot be overlooked, however, that MRI may be overinterpreted by the examiner, and sometimes in cases in which a precise preoperative diagnostic work-up is necessary for the surgical planning CT may be more appropriate. The MRI offers a good visualization of the soft tumor involvement. In T1-weighted images metastatic tumors appear usually in a hypodense form, whereas in T2-weighted images tumors of the spine are rather hyperdense as an expression of an increased water content or replacement of the fatty marrow of the bone by tumor cells [26]. Metastases show gadolinium enhancement. In the tumor work up a bone scintigraphy may play its role as search tool for skeletal metastases. A radioisotopic study has a sensitivity of 65–70%; however, it is preferred to the other studies because the whole body can be searched. For a more specific search in an anatomical region, for example, the cervical, thoracic, or lumbosacral spine the MRI has a higher sensitivity than the bone isotope study [20].

Treatment modalities

Although there is no class I evidence (double-blind randomized placebo-controlled trial) for any of the treatment modalities indicated in the treatment of spinal metastases,

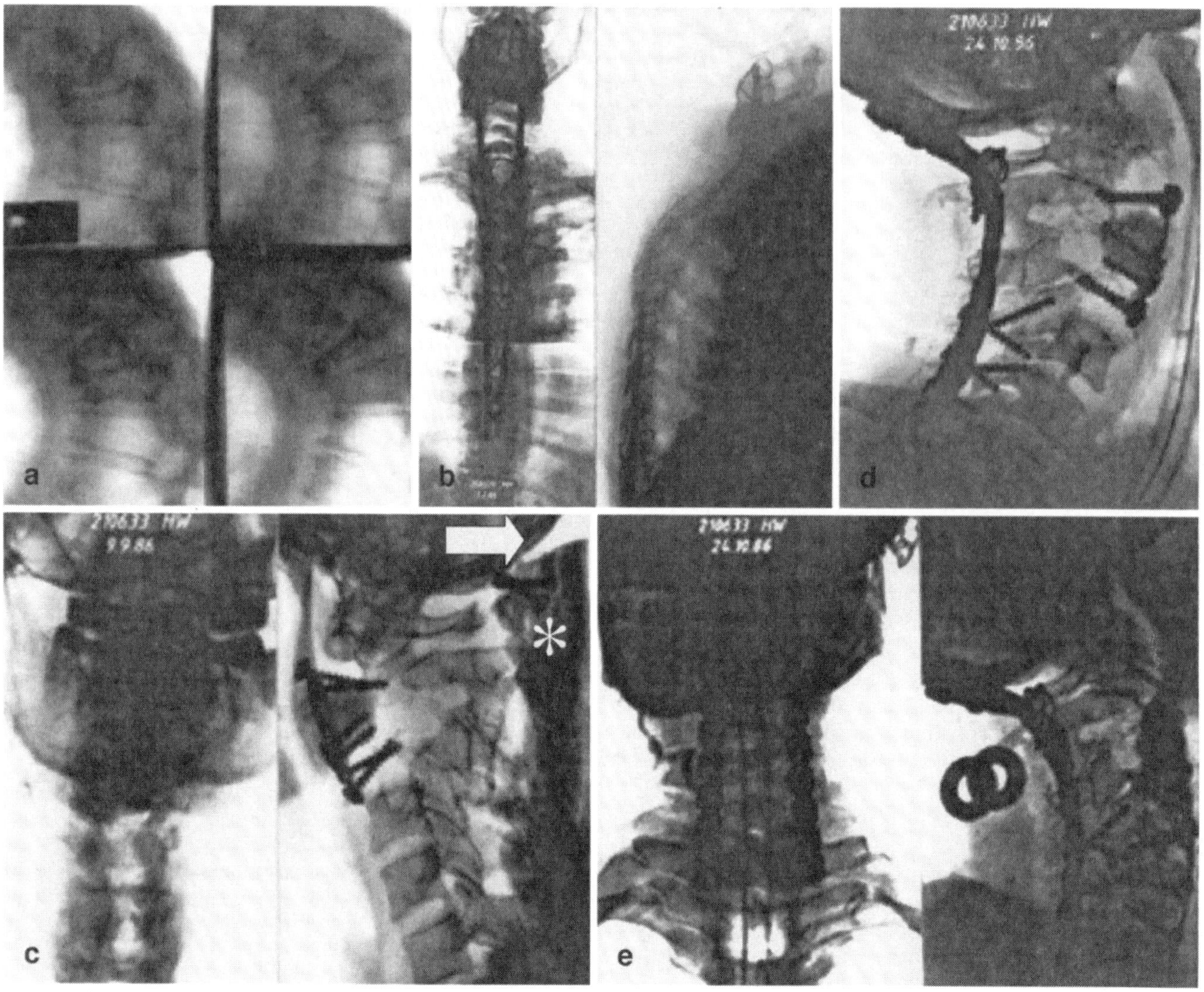

Fig. 2 Long fixation in progressing deformity and instability **a** A 62-year-old woman with multiple-level involvement of the cervical, thoracic, and lumbar spine metastases of a breast cancer with neurological deficit and pain due to progressing deformity and instability. **b** Long fixation (sublaminar wiring-metal-cement compound) and partial correction from C1 to the lower thoracic spine in combination with irradiation was most efficient in reducing pain and neurological deficit for more than 3 years. **c** A 58-year-old man with a hypernephroid carcinoma and cervical involvement had previous anterior surgery and a cement block posteriorly (*asterisk*) with consecutive progression of the tumor, loosening of the fixation and a nonunion at the cement-bone interface (*arrow*). **d** Posterior removal of the cement block and stabilization were followed by **e** anterior revision and restabilization after a previous embolization of the tumor and occlusion of one of the vertebral arteries. The patient died 2 years after this surgery from metastatic complications other than the cervical spine

there are several treatment options recommended. In the case of neurological deficit dexamethasone is the only treatment, which has proven evidence of therapeutic efficacy [29, 35, 40, 52]. The therapeutic decision in elderly frail patients is particularly difficult when they also have significant comorbity. Nevertheless there are today essentially four modalities of treatment available after the administration of steroid: (a) irradiation, (b) surgery, (c) bisphosphonates, and (d) rarely chemotherapy and hormonal therapy as an adjuvant therapy in well defined tumor types [47]. A fifth possibility is a combination of all the above. The efficacy of these diverse treatment modalities and the survival rate of patients depend on the histological tumor type, tumor stage, therapeutic control of the primary tumor, and tumor spread. Overall survival in this patient category is around 12 months [12, 15, 33, 48, 51, 54, 56].

The indications for treatment are given not merely by the neurocompression but also alsol by the major determinants of quality of life: (a) pain, be it radicular, medullar, or of dural origin caused by direct or chronic compression through instability and/or progressive deformity of the vertebral column, or be merely by intravertebral pressure elevation due to tumor invasion, (b) loss of mobility, and (c) nursing reasons. This decision-making process is difficult since a surgical option is often declined because of the possible comorbities, which, however, have never been evaluated in an appropriate controlled study.

Nevertheless it is clinical experience that patients who had surgery and were not delayed in the postsurgical recovery phase due to relevant medical problems and complications belong to the most grateful patients in spinal surgery although the surgery is purely palliative. This obviously raises the question of whether the surgery can be simplified and minimized in elderly patients to prevent as much as possible the adverse effects of surgery [37, 38]. Furthermore there is a still ongoing debate as to whether patients should be treated with radiation therapy alone or in combination with decompression, both modalities enhanced by the administration of high-dose steroids [14, 18, 58]. The general opinion has long been influenced – and still is – by a study in the 1980s which showed no significant difference between patients who had irradiation alone or decompression through laminectomy alone [58] with respect to pain relief, motor performance, and sphincter function. The combination of radiotherapy and laminectomy did not change the outcome significantly compared to radiation therapy alone. A major argument today, however, is that decompression alone in form of a laminectomy without a concomitant stabilization is in most cases insufficient to affect the pain relevantly; in fact decompression alone may even increase the instability and further contribute to pain syndrome and neurological deficit. Furthermore a laminectomy compared to a vertebrectomy or at least an anterior decompression cannot achieve the same degree of decompression since 80% of the tumor compressions arise anteriorly where it cannot be reached by laminectomy. The role of the decompression through laminectomy in spinal metastases has become increasingly debatable with the enhanced experimental biomechanical knowledge as well as in vivo studies in monkeys, where the spinal cord hemodynamics could never be restored after laminectomy alone demonstrating the insufficient effect of a laminectomy alone [14]. The clinical experience with the introduction of instrumentation shows that the realignment of a multiply involved collapsing spine has significantly improved the neurological deficit of patients with spinal metastases (Fig. 2) [5, 6, 10, 13, 32, 41, 48, 57].

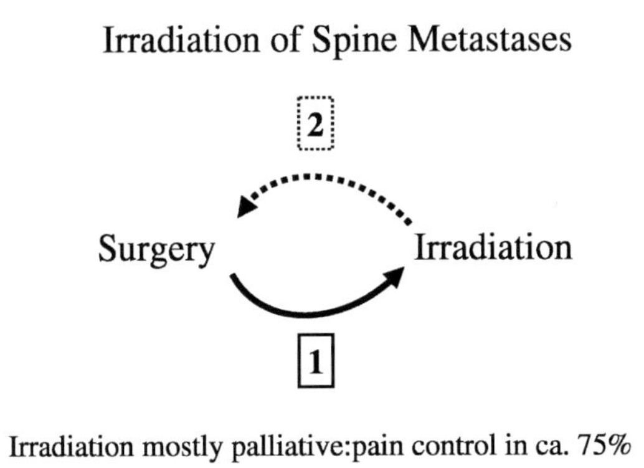

Fig. 3 Surgery ideally should be carried out before irradiation [1]. Irradiation which preceding surgery [2] has a significantly higher complication rate [21]

Today the debated question is whether irradiation alone is sufficient for most of the patients or whether it must be combined with decompression and stabilization, and, if so, whether the surgery comes first followed by the irradiation or in the opposite sequence. From the surgical stand point of view surgery should definitely be before irradiation if there is any probability that irradiation alone may not be sufficient to treat the patient (Fig. 3). Surgery into irradiated tissue has a significantly higher infection rate (30%) and is more difficult to perform than done before the irradiation [12, 15, 21, 34].

Surgical options

Indications for surgery are:

- Pain due to mechanical compression of the different pain-producing structures or clear instability
- Symptomatic mechanical compression of neurostructures (neurological deficit)
- Rapidly progressing neurological deficit due to mechanical compression
- Unknown primary tumor with clearly defined metastatic involvement of the spine
- Radioresistant tumor
- Neurological deterioration or increasing pain during or after radiotherapy (should be avoided by a careful evaluation of the tumor potential before irradiation is decided) [21]

Surgery generally is said to be indicated when the patient is still in a general condition which safely allows surgery, and if life expectancy is at least 6 months. The latter increasingly depends on the kind of surgical procedures and approaches which need to be chosen. This 6-month rule may be overruled by the possibilities of less invasive surgical procedures which allow a faster recuperation and cause less surgical trauma.

Many of the criteria are used to make a surgical indication cannot be handled rigidly and must be weighted in an interdisciplinary decision-making process. For example, there is substantial debate over what is exactly an unstable spine, and consequently there may be patients who are definitely overtreated with all the technical options available today on the base of an obscure understanding of instability. For example, applying the Denis classification for traumatic thoracolumbar fractures may not be appropriate as indication basis for surgical indications. There are more appropriate concepts developed in oncological surgery which should be applied to the metastatic spine [13, 16, 32, 50, 51].

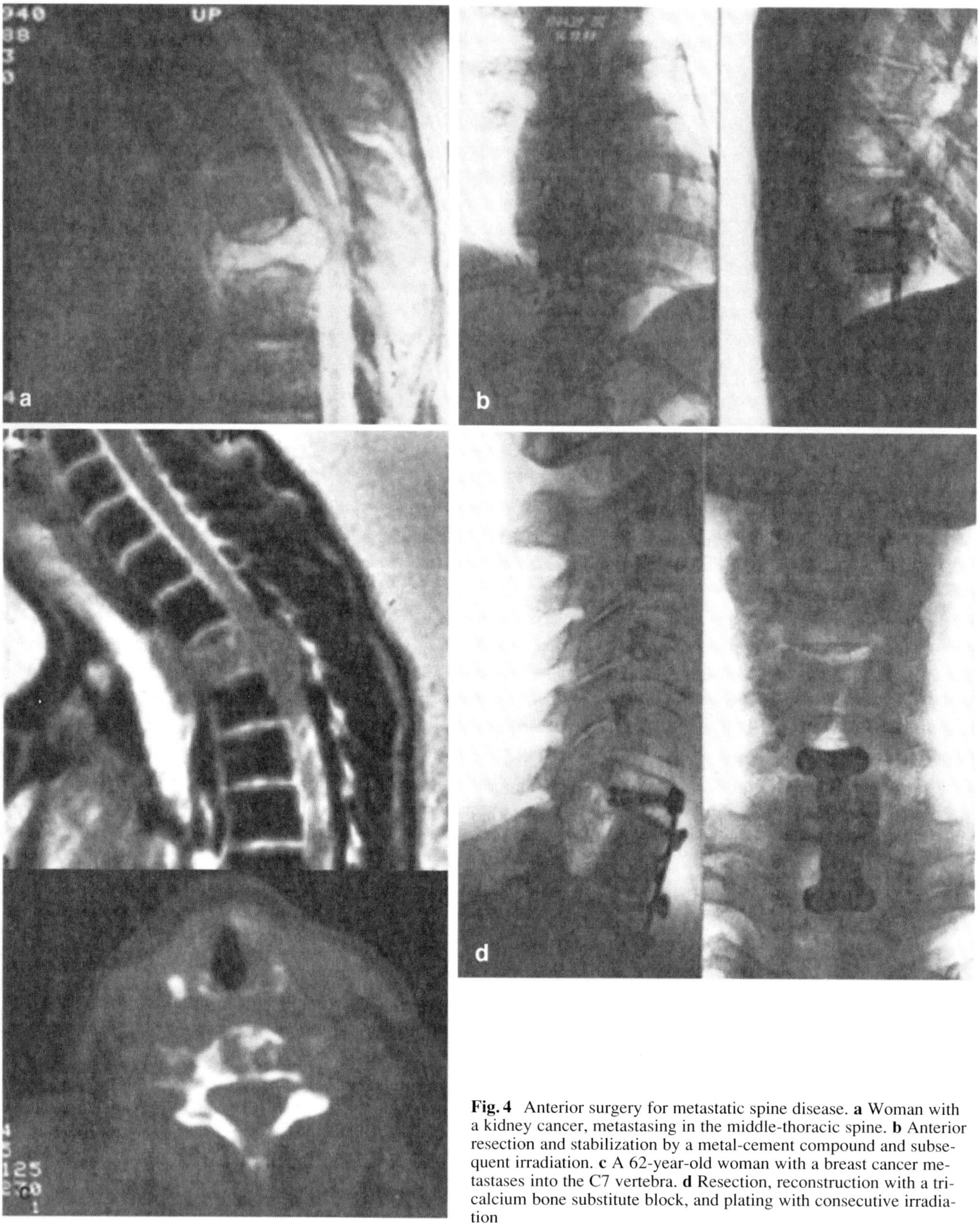

Fig. 4 Anterior surgery for metastatic spine disease. **a** Woman with a kidney cancer, metastasing in the middle-thoracic spine. **b** Anterior resection and stabilization by a metal-cement compound and subsequent irradiation. **c** A 62-year-old woman with a breast cancer metastases into the C7 vertebra. **d** Resection, reconstruction with a tricalcium bone substitute block, and plating with consecutive irradiation

In most instances the need to operate as radically as possible is usually also an overkill since radicality in most instances is not really possible, and most studies show that the local surgery of the spine does not fundamentally change the survival rate of these tumor patients, and very rarely the operated local spinal tumor is the cause of the mortality [16, 24, 25, 33, 36, 54, 55, 56]. This, again, needs to be kept in mind when deciding for surgery. The severity and extent of surgery can be influenced by adjuvant measures that may moderate the surgical intervention to an acceptable degree. One such measure is the preoperative embolization in vascularized spinal metastases or primary tumors. This can reduce blood loss and consequently morbidity and mortality drastically and facilitate the surgeon's work significantly. Kidney tumors, multiple myeloma, and thyroid tumors should definitely be considered for preoperative embolization to reduce the blood loss.

Technically a spinal tumor located predominantly in the vertebral body can be approached by anterior surgery alone (Fig. 4) or in combination with a posterior procedure (Fig. 2c–e), or it can be performed entirely through a posterior approach leaving the patient with less morbidity (Fig. 5). However, is must be recognized that endoscopic anterior surgery for vertebral tumors, specifically in the thoracic spine, where the surgeon can profit from the natural thoracic cavity in contrast to the lumbar spine, may considerably diminish the morbidity of extensive anterior surgery in the elderly. The goal is in any case to operate on the patient in such a way that stay in the intensive care unit can be avoided. Again, with modern retractor systems and less invasive technology it is possible to perfect the posterolateral approach to the anterior spine elements of the thoracolumbar spine through a midline incision which allows a laminectomy, a vertebral body resection, the anterior column reconstruction and posterior stabilization in a single approach (Fig. 5) [41, 42]. In the middle and lower cervical spine the anterior approach is most straightforward and yields little morbidity (Fig. 4c–d). In rare cases

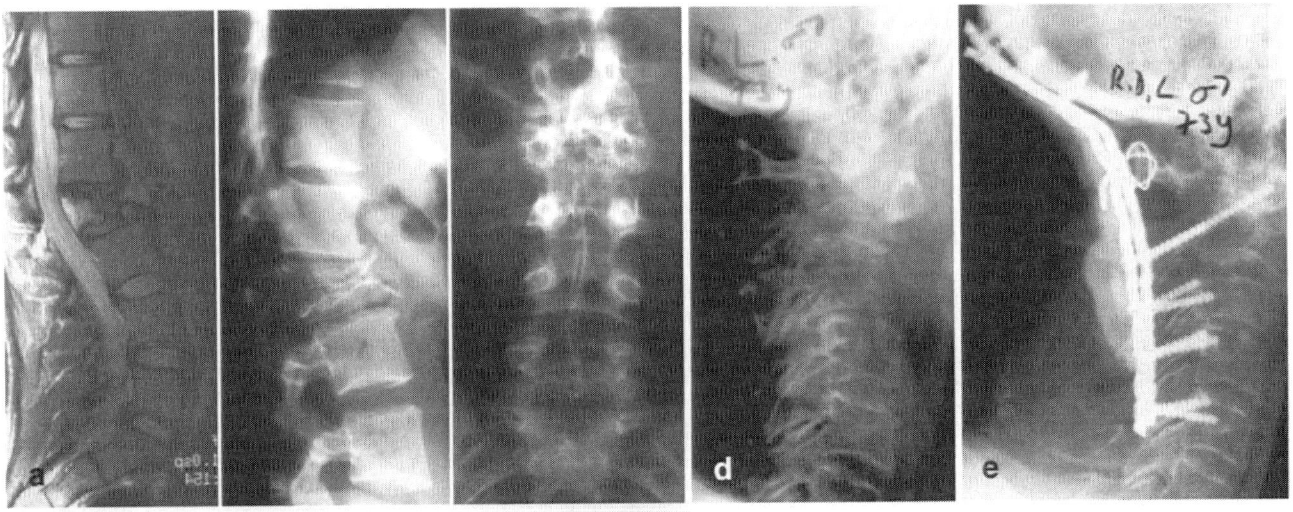

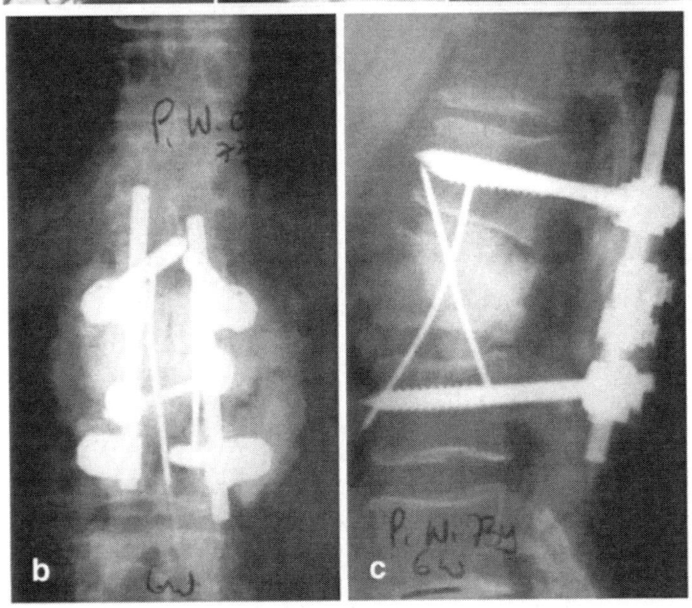

Fig. 5 Posterior surgery for metastatic spine disease. **a** A 73-year-old man with a metastases in L2 from a stomach cancer. **b**, **c** Through a single median posterior incision laminectomy, posterolateral resection of the vertebral body through both pedicles, and posterior reconstruction and stabilization with a short pedicular, angle stable system combined with an anterior column reconstruction with metal-cement compound through the posterior approach. **d**, **e** Partial resection and posterior stabilization of the upper cervical spine involved by lung metastases followed by irradiation in a 73-year-old man. Note the combination of a metal-cement compound posteriorly instead of bony fusion

a combined procedure may be indicated to control the pain mostly due to the instability (Fig. 5). At the occipitocervical junction a posterior resection and stabilization combined with irradiation is generally sufficient as palliative measure. Some authors have recently enthusiastically advocated minimally invasive technology to approach certain lesions in particular in the vertebral body involvement: Vertebroplasty or kyphoplasty as palliative technique may increasingly gain significance in patients with high morbidity index or elevated risk for open surgery [37, 38].

Reconstruction of the anterior column for stability reasons as well as realignment of the spine is rarely carried out with autologous bone because the average life expectancy does not justify it, and a possible postoperative irradiation would damage the healing potential of an autograft. Today this reconstruction is performed either with a metal-cement compound as in building construction or with the use of metal or ceramic spacers in combination with cement, which may or may not be filled with bone substitutes. Major allograft may be an alternative; however, the biological conditions for its integration are not satisfactory, specifically in the case of adjuvant irradiation and possible chemotherapy.

The stability of a diseased segment after tumor resection can certainly be enhanced by a strong posterior instrumentation in combination with the anterior reconstruction of the anterior column and is biomechanically superior to a purely anterior reconstruction, even with anterior instrumentation [32]. The surgeon needs to keep in mind that the major goal of the surgery is to put the patient in a condition to be as soon as possible independently mobile without any brace, which is an additional burden in those severely ill and often rather cachectic patients with the potential of pressure sores and unease with external fixation devices.

Option of irradiation

The general principles that govern the outcome of treatment of patients with malignant tumors of the spine are the same as those for tumors at any other site. First, for patients to be considered cured all tumor cells at the primary, regional, and distant sites must be inactivated or removed. Second, the determinants of probability of success are the anatomical site and size of the tumor and the histopathological type and grade of the tumor. Malignant lesions of the spine are often not respected with secure margins because of the constraints imposed by the proximity of the spinal cord and nerve roots, major vessels (especially along the thoracic column), and organs (e.g., esophagus). An intact spine is critical to an individual's anatomical integrity. Also, the role of radiation therapy for malignant tumors of the spine is often severely limited by the necessity to include the spinal cord in the high-dose region because tumor abuts on the dura and/or cord.

The patients in whom symptomatic spinal cord compression develops often represent a debilitated and elderly population with considerable surgical risks. Not all patients can safely undergo surgery either anteriorly or posterolaterally or even in combination – although mostly not necessary – with appropriate stabilization procedures. Nevertheless, a considerable number of these are sufficiently treated by irradiation, either because there are only minimal neurological symptoms, or because an aggressive surgical approach is deemed inappropriate at initial presentation [12]. The widespread use of MRI of the spine to detect metastatic disease in patients with cancer, results in the early diagnosis of epidural metastatic disease, which often is irradiated since not really symptomatic. For many reasons therefore more previously irradiated patients present to the hospital with symptomatic spinal cord compression. The number of major wound complications is high in this population. Recent studies showed that spinal irradiation before surgical decompression for spinal cord compression is associated with a significantly higher major wound complication rate. In addition, preoperative spinal irradiation might adversely affect the surgical outcome [4], (Fig. 3).

Irradiation is an appropriate palliative pain treatment in many patients; however, the indications need to be rationalized if we do not want to deal increasingly with cases after irradiation who need surgery because irradiation did not stop the tumor. Therefore the indications for irradiation in most of the frequent bony and spinal metastases (breast, prostate, lung, colon cancer, and multiple myeloma) are [40]:

- Radiosensitive tumor (malignant lymphoma, myeloma, small-cell lung cancer, seminoma, neuroblastoma, and Ewing's sarcoma).
- A lesion to the spine which does not compromise the stability or the neurological function of the spinal cord or its roots, but where the leading symptom is pain which is difficult to control by medication alone.
- Mild compression of neurostructures without relevant clinical neurological signs where it can be anticipated that the irradiation will stop the further progression of the tumor, or the patient's life expectancy is less than 3–6 months.
- Paraplegia more than 24 h.
- Multiple level involvement of the spine where surgery may be useless to control the metastatic disease. In this case the irradiation is a desperate attempt to palliatively influence the bony pain and to delay neurological complication depending from the biological/histological characteristics of the tumor.
- Disseminated disease with life expectancy less than 3–6 months.
- Tumor involvement for which recalcification of the irradiated vertebra can be anticipated from the biological behavior of the tumor more rapidly than a pathological fracture in a weakened vertebra.

– A general condition of the patient with a reduced resistance rendering a surgical intervention impossible.

Patients who have a relevant symptomatic neurocompression or instability or a failed pain management after irradiation should no longer undergo irradiation, but a surgical option needs to be evaluated. This shared decision-making process, once again should, be handled in a multidisciplinary team. Irradiation generally should not be performed without a histological diagnosis, with very few exceptions. In all those cases in which the primary tumor is unknown or not sure, a biopsy is recommended of the suspected vertebra either by a posterolateral percutaneous approach or by the pedicle of the patient with a Yamshidi needle of sufficient diameter (≥3 mm), usually in local anesthesia and by image guidance to obtain a proper tissue sample allowing a histological diagnosis. This can be a simple hand-guided biopsy under image intensifier or a computer-assisted one.

There is no radiotherapeutic regimen showing consistent superiority in the treatment of spinal metastases, although multiple treatment protocols have been carried out. Usually 30y in 10 fractions (over 2 weeks) are applied. Other commonly used regimens vary between 8 Gy in a single fraction and 40 Gy in 20 fractions over 4 weeks [12].

Pharmacological options

Here we may consider chemotherapy, bisphosphonates, and in some specific tumors hormonal therapy (breast, prostate, thyroid cancer) and as a general medication steroids such as dexamethasone. This is the most frequently used corticosteroid despite the fact that in the literature there is no valid comparison of dexamethasone and methylprednisolone [35, 40]. Two dosing regimen are used: the high-dose dexamethasone regimen comprises an initial bolus of 100 mg with subsequent dose of 96 mg/day. This regimen seems to have only a historical value since significant side effects have been associated with its use. It should be administered only to patients with rapidly progressing neurological deficit. The moderate-dose dexamethasone regimen starts with 10 mg intravenous bolus and continues with 16 mg/day four times daily [40, 52]. This dosage is well tolerated, and it is the regimen of choice in symptomatic patients. No steroids are proposed in nonparetic ambulatory patients.

Recently a new dimension in the treatment of bony metastases has been advocated. Since it is well established that bony metastases in general and of the spine in particular increase treatment costs and may significantly prolong hospital stay, new means of simple treatment of bony metastases are being evaluated [24]. Bisphosphonates have stood the test of time in the treatment of bony complications because they stop the vicious circle of tumor progression and pathological bone turnover. Under the effect of the tumor cells the balance between bone resorption and new bone formation is disturbed; tumor cells seed in the bone under the attraction of growth factors [43]. There they deliberate mediators which stimulate both the osteoclasts and osteoblasts, which start to turnover the bone in an unphysiological way. Again, growth factors are released which stimulate tumor cells for proliferation. The vicious circle of pathological bone remodeling and tumor progression starts. Subsequently bone quality and bone density diminish. The stability of the bone strongly decreases. Bisphosphonates show a high affinity to bone and are augmented mainly in locations with high bone turnover. They are therefore ideal medications to stop the vicious circle of bone metastasing and damaging [42]. The most successful medication is pamidronate (second-generation bisphosphonate) which is successful mostly in bony metastases of breast cancer and in osteolysis in multiple myeloma [4]. Zoledronic acid is one of the most recently developed agents and is characterized by an imidazol ring. In animal experiments the effect was 100–850 times better than that with the older pamidronate [30, 39, 44].

The objective clinical success of the bisphosphonate depends significantly on the reduction and delay of skeletal complications (SREs=pathological fracture, spinal cord compression, need for irradiation or surgery for stabilization) [19, 22]. It can be anticipated today that the bisphosphonates have an immediate antitumoral effect. Bisphosphonate treatment has the goal of diminishing the incidence of bony complications, vertebral body fractures, pain, and osteoporosis. The outcome should be determined by the survival time – once a spinal metastasis is detected – in an ambulatory, independent status, where pain is controlled, and the patient is not hospitalized. The mean survival time is 14– 18 months depending obviously on the patient's condition before entering treatment for the spinal problem. Wise et al. [56] report a mean survival time of 15.9 months after surgery for spinal metastasis, whereas Weigel [55] reports a 13.1 months mean survival time with 11.1 months mean time at home after surgery. In our own material of 67 fully documented cases between 1996 and 2001 the mean survival after surgery was 14.2 months (unpublished data). Tomita et al. [51] published recently survival times that were longer in cases in which wide or marginal excision was made (38.2 months), with only 7% local tumor recurrence, and the survival time in patients treated with intralesional excision was 21.5 months and 31% local tumor recurrence whereas only in patients with palliative surgery and stabilization the survival was 10.1 months and the local tumor recurrence 28%. They based their surgical decision making on a new prognostic scoring system. Sundaresan et al. [49] reported a mean survival time of 30 months in patients with surgery for solitary metastases of the spine and with a survival of 5 years and more in 18% of their cases. Mazel et al. [42] achieved a mean survival rate of 16.7 months in 21 of 35 patients who died and 38.2 months in 14 of 35 patients who were alive at follow-up with a so-called radical excision of tumors of thoracic and cervicothoracic metastases.

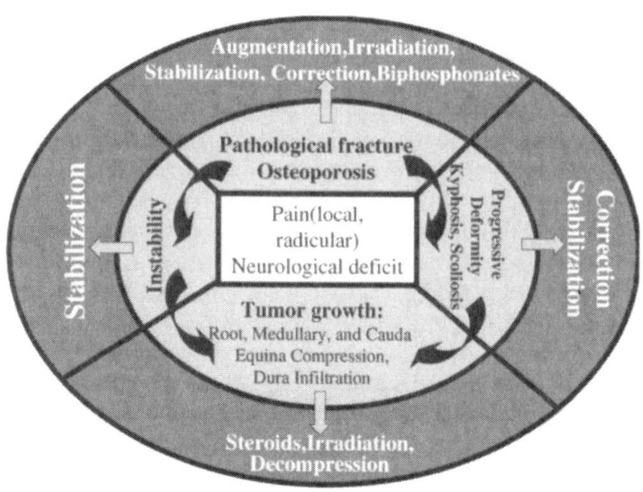

Fig. 6 Decision algorithm of the treatment tailored to the individual patient's need and therapeutic option

These results also suggest a concept of differentiated surgery with more radical options than just palliative surgery. The neurological outcome is crucial and depends on the initial neurological deficit before surgery. About one-half of the paraparetic patients at the time of diagnosis regain the ability to walk, but only fewer than 5% of patients, who are paraplegic regain ambulation [2]. Postoperative complications are frequent and are found in 15 – 30% of cases [55, 56].

Wai et al. [54] assessed prospectively the overall quality of life after surgical management of metastatic spine disease, using a validated global health status quality-of-life instrument (Edmonton Symptoms Assessment Scale). They found the greatest improvement in the domain of pain reduction, but there was also improvement in other domains of quality of life. The clinical results of nonsurgical treatment for spinal metastases has been presented in a prospective analysis of 101 patients who were treated with radiation therapy and/or chemotherapy. Of these, 66% remained neurologically stable or improved after treatment; 67% had pain relief, and 64% improved functionally, which was more related to the general debility than local tumor recurrence [33]. Unfortunately no prospective study has compared nonsurgical and surgical treatment of spinal metastases with clearly defined conditions and parameters to allow a differentiated decision about the best solution for the patient. It has also been considered that such a study may be extremely difficult to execute also for ethical reasons.

This leaves us with the necessity to assess every patient individually and to weigh the different elements in shared decision making of an interdisciplinary team together with the patient. It is a complex algorithm tailored to the patient's individual problem and therapeutic options available (Fig. 6). It cannot be emphasized enough that a decision for a conservative treatment, specifically with irradiation, should not be taken unless there is a clear understanding that a later surgical option is very improbable. There is no doubt that preoperative irradiation has a significantly negative effect on surgical outcome [21].

References

1. Abdu WA, Provencher M (1998) Primary and metastatic tumors of the cervical spine. Spine 23:2767–2776
2. Bartanusz V, Porchet F (2003) Current strategies in the management of spinal metastatic disease. Swiss Surg 9:55–62
3. Batson OV (1940) The function of the vertebral veins and their role in the spread of metastases. Am Surg 112: 138–145
4. Berenson JR, Hillner BE, Kyle RA, Anderson K, Lipton A, Yee GC, Biermann JS, American Society of Clinical Oncology Bisphosphonates Expert Panel (2002) American Society of Clinical Oncology practice guidelines: the role of bisphosphonates in multiple myeloma. J Clin Oncol 20:19–36
5. Bilsky MH, Boland P, Lis E, Raizer JJ, Healey JH (2000) Single-stage posterolateral transpedicle approach for spondylectomy, epidural decompression, and circumferential fusion of spinal metastases. Spine 25:2240–2250
6. Bilsky MH, Shannon FJ, Sheppard S, Prabhu V, Boland PJ (2002) Diagnosis and management of a metastatic tumor in the atlantoaxial spine. Spine 27: 1062–1069
7. Boriani S, Chevalley F, Weinstein JN, Biagini R, Campanacci L, De Iure F, Piccill P (1996) Chordoma of the spine above the sacrum. Treatment and outcome in 21 cases. Spine 21:1569–1577
8. Boriani S, Biagini R, De Iure F, Bertoni F, Malaguti MC, Di Fiore M, Zanoni A (1996) En bloc resections of bone tumors of the thoracolumbar spine. A preliminary report on 29 patients. Spine 21:1927–1931
9. Boriani S, Weinstein JN, Biagini R (1997) Primary bone tumors of the spine. Terminology and surgical staging. Spine 22:1036–1044
10. Bridwell KH, Jenny AB, Saul T, Rich KM, Grubb RL (1988) Posterior segmental spinal instrumentation (PSSI) with posterolateral decompression and debulking for metastatic thoracic and lumbar spine disease. Limitations of the technique. Spine 13:1383–1394
11. Coman DR, DeLong RP (1951) The role of the vertebral venous system in the metastasis of cancer into the spinal cord: experiments with tumor cell suspensions in rats and rabbits. Cancer 4: 610–618
12. DeLaney TF, Suit HD (2000) Treatment of spine tumors: radiation therapy. Curr Opin Orthop 11:502–507
13. DeWald RL, Bridwell KH, Prodromas C, Rodts MF (1985) Reconstructive spinal surgery as palliation for metastatic malignancies of the spine. Spine 10: 21–26
14. Doppman JL, Girton RT (1976) Angiographic study of the effect of laminectomy in the presence of acute anterior epidural masses. J Neurosurg 45:195–202
15. Dürr HR, Wegener B, Krödel A, Müller PE, Jansson V, Refior HJ (2002) Multiple myeloma: surgery of the spine. Spine 27:320–326

16. Enkaoua EA, Doursounian L, Chatellier G, Mabesoone F, Aimard T, Saillant G (1997) Vertebral metastases. A critical appreciation of the preoperative prognostic Tokuhashi Score in a series of 71 cases. Spine 22:2293–2298
17. Enneking WF, Spanier SS, Goodman MA (1980) A system for surgical staging of musculoskeletal sarcoma. Clin Orthop 153:106–120
18. Findlay GFG (1984) Adverse effects of the management of malignant spinal cord compression. J Neurol Neurosurg Psychiatry 47:761–768
19. Fleisch H (2000) Bisphosphonates in bone disease. From the laboratory to the patient. Academic, San Diego
20. Gerszten CP, Welch W (2000) Current surgical management of metastatic spinal disease. Oncology 14:1013–1024
21. Ghogawala Z, Mansfield FL, Borges LF (2001) Spinal radiation before surgical decompression adversely affects outcomes of surgery for symptomatic metastatic spinal cord compression. Spine 26:818–824
22. Green JR, Müller K, Jaeggi KA (1994) Preclinical pharmacology of CGP 42'446, a new, potent, heterocyclic bisphosphonate compound. J Bone Miner Res 9:745–751
23. Greenlee RT, Murray T, Bolden S, Wingo PA (2000) Cancer statistics, 2000. CA Cancer J Clin 50:7–33
24. Groot MT et al (2003) Costs of prostate cancer metastasis to the bone in The Netherlands. Eur Urol 43:226–232
25. Grosman R. Rouchal M, Chalupka R (2000) The long-term results of surgical management of spine metastatic tumours from breast cancer. Scripta Med (Brno) 73:169–172
26. Grossman RI, Yousem DM (1994) Neuroradiology. The requisites. Mosby Year Book, St. Louis, pp 491–495
27. Gunterberg B (1997) Point of view: a system for surgical staging and management of spine tumors. A clinical outcome study of giant cell tumors of the spine. Spine 22:1783
28. Hart RA, Boriani S, Biagini R, Currier B, Weinstein JN (1997) A system for surgical staging and management of spine tumors. A clinical outcome study of giant cell tumors of the spine. Spine 22:1773–1782
29. Heiss JD, Papavassiliou E, Merrill M et al (1996) Mechanism of dexamethasone suppression of brain tumor-associated vascular permeability in rats. J Clin Invest 98:1400–1408
30. Hortobagyi GN, Theriault RL, Lipton A et al (1998) Long-term prevention of skeletal complications of metastatic breast cancer with pamidronate. J Clin Oncol 16:2038–2044
31. Jenis LG, Dunn EJ, An HS (1999) Metastatic disease of the cervical spine. Clin Orthop 359:89–103
32. Kanayama M, Cunningham BW, Abumi K, Kaneda K, McAfee PC (1999) Biomechanical analysis of anterior versus circumferential spinal reconstruction for various anatomic stages of tumor lesions. Spine 24: 445–450
33. Katagiri H, Takahashi M, Inagaki J, Kobayashi H, Sugiura H, Yamamura S, Iwata H (1998) Clinical results of nonsurgical treatment for spinal metastases. Int J Radiat Oncol Biol Phys 42: 1127–1132
34. Khan DC, Malhotra S, Stevens RE, Steinfeld AD (1999) Radiotherapy for the treatment of giant cell tumor of the spine: a report of six cases and review of the literature. Cancer Invest 17:110–113
35. Koehler PJ (1995) Use of corticosteroids in neuro-oncology. Anticancer Drugs 6:19–33
36. Landis SH et al (1999) Global cancer statistics. CA Cancer J Clin 49:33–64
37. Lemke DM, Hacein-Bey L (2003) Metastatic compression fractures – vertebroplasty for pain control. J Neurosci Nurs 35:50–55
38. Lieberman IH, Dudeney S, Reinhardt MK et al (2001) The initial outcome and efficacy of 'kyphoplasty' in the treatment of painful osteoporotic vertebral compression fractures. Spine 26: 1631–1636
39. Lipton A, Theriault RL, Hortobagyi GN et al (2000) Pamidronate prevents skeletal complications and is an effective palliative treatment in women with breast carcinoma and osteolytic bone metastases. Long-term follow-up of two randomized, placebo-controlled trials. Cancer 88:1082–1090
40. Loblaw DA, Laperriere NJ (1998) Emergency treatment of malignant extradural spinal cord compression: an evidence-based guideline. J Clin Oncol 16:1613–1624
41. Marchesi D, Arlet V, Aebi M (2003) Treatment of spinal metastases by posterolateral decompression and pedicle screw fixation. Spine (in press)
42. Mazel C, Grunenwald D, Laudrin P, Marmorat JL (2003) Radical excision in the management of thoracic and cervicothoracic tumors involving the spine: results in a series of 36 cases. Spine 28:782–792
43. Mundy GR (1999) Bisphosphonates as cancer drugs. Hosp Pract (Off Ed) 34: 81–94
44. Rosen LS, Harland SJ, Oosterlinck W (2002) Broad clinical activity of zoledronic acid in osteolytic to osteoblastic bone lesions in patients with a broad range of solid tumors. Am J Clin Oncol 25:19–24
45. Schick U, Marquardt G, Lorenz R (2001) Intradural and extradural spinal metastases. Neurosurg Rev 24:1–5
46. Siegal T, Siegal T (1989) Current considerations in the management of neoplastic spinal cord compression. Spine 14:223–228
47. Smith MR et al (2003) Zometa increases bone mineral density in men receiving androgen deprivation therapy for nonmetastatic prostate cancer. J Urol 169:2008–2012
48. Sundaresan N, Galicich JH, Lane JM, Bains MS, McCormack P (1985) Treatment of neoplastic epidural cord compression by vertebral body resection and stabilization. J Neurosurg 63: 676–684
49. Sundaresan N, Rothmann A, Manhart K, Kelliher K (2002) Surgery for solitary metastases of the spine. Rationale and results of treatment. Spine 27: 1802–1806
50. Tokuhashi Y, Matsuzaki H, Toriyama S. Kawano H, Ohsaka S (1990) Scoring system for the preoperative evaluation of metastatic spine tumor prognosis. Spine 15:1110–1113
51. Tomita K, Kawahara N, Kobayashi T, Yoshida A, Murakami H, Akamaru T (2001) Surgical strategy for spinal metastases. Spine 26:298–306
52. Vecht CJ, Haaxma-Reiche H, van Putten WLJ, de Visser M, Vries EP, Twijnstra A (1989) Initial bolus of conventional versus high-dose dexamethasone in metastatic spinal cord compression. Neurology 39:1255–1257
53. Vinholes J et al (1996) Effects of bone metastases on bone metabolism: implications for diagnosis, imaging and assessment of response to cancer treatment. Cancer Treat Rev 22:289–331
54. Wai EK, Finkelstein JA, Tangente RP, Holden L, Chow E, Ford M, Yee A (2003) Quality of life in surgical treatment of metastatic spine disease. Spine 28:508–512
55. Weigel B, Maghsudi M, Neumann C, Kretschmer R, Müller FJ, Nerlich M (1999) Surgical management of symptomatic spinal metastases. Postoperative outcome and quality of life. Spine 24:2240–2246
56. Wise JJ, Fischgrund JSA, Herkowitz HN, Mongomery D, Kurz LT (1999) Complications, survival rates, and risk factors of surgery for metastatic disease of the spine. Spine 24:1943–1951
57. York JE, Berk RH, Fuller GN, Rao JS, Abi-Said D, Wildrick DM, Gokaslan ZL (1999) Chondrosarcoma of the spine: 1954 to 1997. J Neurosurg 90 [Suppl 1]:73–78
58. Young RF, Post EM, King GA (1980) Treatment of spinal epidural metastases: randomized prospective comparison of laminectomy and radiotherapy. J Neurosurg 53:741–748